When Bodies Remember

The California Series in Public Anthropology emphasizes the anthropologist's role as an engaged intellectual. It continues anthropology's commitment to being an ethnographic witness, to describing, in human terms, how life is lived beyond the borders of many readers' experiences. But it also adds a commitment, through ethnography, to reframing the terms of public debate—transforming received, accepted understandings of social issues with new insights, new framings.

Series Editor: Robert Borofsky (Hawaii Pacific University)

Contributing Editors: Philippe Bourgois (UC San Francisco), Paul Farmer (Partners in Health), Rayna Rapp (New York University), and Nancy Scheper-Hughes (UC Berkeley)

University of California Press Editor: Naomi Schneider

1. *Twice Dead: Organ Transplants and the Reinvention of Death*, by Margaret Lock
2. *Birthing the Nation: Strategies of Palestinian Women in Israel*, by Rhoda Ann Kanaaneh (with a foreword by Hanan Ashrawi)
3. *Annihilating Difference: The Anthropology of Genocide*, edited by Alexander Laban Hinton (with a foreword by Kenneth Roth)
4. *Pathologies of Power: Health, Human Rights, and the New War on the Poor*, by Paul Farmer (with a foreword by Amartya Sen)
5. *Buddha Is Hiding: Refugees, Citizenship, the New America*, by Aihwa Ong
6. *Chechnya: Life in a War-Torn Society*, by Valery Tishkov (with a foreword by Mikhail S. Gorbachev)
7. *Total Confinement: Madness and Reason in the Maximum Security Prison*, by Lorna A. Rhodes
8. *Paradise in Ashes: A Guatemalan Journey of Courage, Terror, and Hope*, by Beatriz Manz (with a foreword by Aryeh Neier)
9. *Laughter Out of Place: Race, Class, Violence, and Sexuality in a Rio Shantytown*, by Donna M. Goldstein
10. *Shadows of War: Violence, Power, and International Profiteering in the Twenty-First Century*, by Carolyn Nordstrom
11. *Why Did They Kill? Cambodia in the Shadow of Genocide*, by Alexander Laban Hinton (with a foreword by Robert Jay Lifton)
12. *Yanomani: The Fierce Controversy and What We Can Learn from It*, by Robert Borofsky
13. *Why America's Top Pundits Are Wrong: Anthropologists Talk Back*, edited by Catherine Besteman and Hugh Gusterson
14. *Prisoners of Freedom: Human Rights and the African Poor*, by Harri Englund
15. *When Bodies Remember: Experiences and Politics of AIDS in South Africa*, by Didier Fassin

When Bodies Remember

EXPERIENCES AND POLITICS OF AIDS
IN SOUTH AFRICA

Didier Fassin

Translated by
Amy Jacobs and Gabrielle Varro

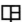

UNIVERSITY OF CALIFORNIA PRESS

BERKELEY   LOS ANGELES   LONDON

University of California Press, one of the most distinguished university presses in the United States, enriches
lives around the world by advancing scholarship in the hu-
manities, social sciences, and natural sciences. Its activities
are supported by the UC Press Foundation and by philan-
thropic contributions from individuals and institutions.
For more information, visit www.ucpress.edu.

University of California Press
Berkeley and Los Angeles, California

University of California Press, Ltd.
London, England

The illustration on the cover is a sketch of a serigraph by
Ernest Pignon-Ernest, inspired by the photograph of Hector Petersen's death, a tragic symbol of the Soweto uprising and resistance to apartheid. This work, which evokes
the ravages of AIDS, appeared in 2003 on the walls of
Soweto and Warwick. The author is deeply grateful to
artist for authorizing its reproduction without charge.

This book was published and translated with the support
of ANRS, the French Agency for Research on AIDS.

Library of Congress Cataloging-in-Publication Data

Fassin, Didier.
    [Quand les corps se souviennent. English]
    When bodies remember : experiences and politics of
AIDS in South Africa / Didier Fassin ; translated by Amy
Jacobs and Gabrielle Varro.
        p. cm. — (California series in public anthropology)
    Includes bibliographical references and index.
    ISBN-13: 978-0-520-24467-2 (cloth : alk. paper)
    ISBN-10: 0-520-24467-2 (cloth : alk. paper)
    ISBN-13: 978-0-520-25027-7 (pbk. : alk. paper)
    ISBN-10: 0-520-25027-3 (pbk. : alk. paper)
    1. AIDS (Disease)—Social aspects—South Africa.
2. AIDS (Disease)—Political aspects—South Africa.
3. AIDS (Disease)—Government policy—South Africa.
1. Title.
    RA643.86.S6F3714 2007
    362.196'979200968—dc22   2006026404

Manufactured in the United States of America

15   14   13   12   11   10   09   08   07   06
10   9   8   7   6   5   4   3   2   1

This book is printed on Natures Book, which contains
50% post-consumer waste and meets the minimum re-
quirements of ANSI/NISO Z39.48–1992 (R 1997) (Permanence of Paper).

For Thomas, Baptiste, and Camille,
and for the children of Soweto and Alexandra they have met
on the threshold of a world they will share

Past and present are Ineinander,
each shrouded-shrouding
—and this is the flesh

MAURICE MERLEAU-PONTY
Le visible et l'invisible

"*Perhaps by the end of the winter,*" *I think,* "*when hunger truly bites us, when we are cold and starving, or when the barbarian is truly at the gate, perhaps then I will abandon the locutions of a civil servant with literary ambitions and begin to tell the truth.*"

J.M. COETZEE
Waiting for the Barbarians

CONTENTS

INTRODUCTION

POLITICAL ANESTHESIA AND ANTHROPOLOGICAL CONCERN

No one will knead us again out of earth and clay,
no one will speak upon our dust.
No one.

PAUL CELAN
"Psalm"

In the mid-1990s, as project coordinator for health issues in a major program of the Centre National de la Recherche Scientifique, France's main
research institution, I proposed that we develop projects with South
Africa, which had just ended its half century of apartheid and was showing clear signs of becoming a hub of the new world politics. The director
replied that studies of South Africa could make no claim to global appli-
cability as the situation there was too singular. Actually, in those years no
African country figured among the stated priorities of the Centre. Ten
years later I was looking for a publisher for the French edition of this book,
having already received a positive response for an English edition. The series editor of a major Paris publishing house had recommended it to one
of the directors, who replied that the readership for an anthropological
study of AIDS in South Africa was so small that she could not approve

publication. These two converging assessments say much about the contemporary world.

One always has profound reasons for entering into the long and painful process of writing a book. For me, it has been the will to resist political anesthesia, as it was expressed—anecdotally but significantly—by the representatives of the research and publishing institutions whose choices assume, reflect, and, of course, reinforce "our" lack of interest in what is happening with "them," even when what is at stake is the deaths of millions of people. However, as the editors of a special issue of *Daedalus* (2001) affirm, South Africa matters.[1] It is never superfluous to demonstrate interest in the Other.

Cultural anesthesia, Allen Feldman (1994: 410) writes in his examination of the foundations of our perception of violence in the world, is a gloss of "Adorno's insight that, in a post-Holocaust and late capitalist modernity, the quantitative and qualitative dissemination of objectification increases the social capacity to inflict pain upon the Other and . . . to render the Other's pain inadmissible to public discourse and culture. It is upon this insight that a political anthropology of the senses in modernity can be elaborated." Causing suffering and ignoring suffering are for Feldman the two faces of the same contemporary reality. "Generalities of bodies—dead, wounded, starving, diseased, and homeless"—as the media allow us to apprehend the global disorder, whether through war, famine, epidemic, or disaster, depersonalize the others undergoing these events, including them physically in our world while excluding them morally. We are no more interested in the almost six million persons infected with HIV in South Africa than we are in the three million men, women, and children killed over the past decade in the African Great Lakes region. We know that they exist because the press tells us so and television shows them to us, but we feel no need to know more.

Political anesthesia in such conditions does not mean denouncing the weakness of international commitments to fight against HIV/AIDS or to actively promote peace; that is not the issue here, though it is a closely related one. It simply suggests that we do not feel we need to know any more than we already know. We have read or heard that in South Africa AIDS is a problem of sexual behaviors and peculiar beliefs, such as the often-mentioned belief that raping a young virgin will purify the contaminated perpetrator. We have read or heard that the South African government has denied scientific facts and contested medical authority as a way to justify its scandalous refusal to make life-saving drugs available. Similar commonplaces are readily encountered concerning the massacres perpetrated in the eastern part of the Democratic Republic of Congo, in Sierra Leone, or in Liberia. In these cases the commonplaces are about the protagonists' barbarity. Moreover, in these diverse situations, we speak of "genocide," thus paradoxically distancing ourselves still farther from the events because those accused of committing the atrocities seem to have excluded themselves from humanity and their victims, by the very inhumanity of the acts perpetrated against them, become inaccessible to us.

The fragmentary information we receive from an absolute elsewhere is enough for us because it confirms our sense that cultures are incommunicable and, more radically, that social worlds are incommensurable. Clearly we do not share representations or values with these others. We may therefore give up trying to understand them. They are unintelligible—except perhaps to anthropologists, whom we turn to for interpretation of exotic oddness and remote savagery. In the tension described by Zygmunt Bauman (1998: 3) between "the global elite" and "ever more localized rest," there is no inequality more disturbing than that by which we decide what is interesting and what is not, who can still interest us and who no longer does. This statement also applies to relations between north and south or, as people on the African continent see it, the West and the rest. Moreover, in South African society, the same borders are drawn internally along class and color lines.

Through this intellectual and moral retreat from otherness, we renounce politics considered as a way of "dealing with the community and reciprocity of different human beings," in Hannah Arendt's (1995: 31) terms. In a state of political anesthesia, which makes us insensitive to the fate of others foremost by making these others appear incomprehensible to us, only difference counts; neither community nor reciprocity is possible. Against this declared or assumed impossibility, my purpose and hope here is to affirm the principle of intelligibility and provide a means for a kind of understanding in which others are taken fully into account—an understanding based on a sense of shared destiny. The anthropological implications of this project are strong. As Johannes Fabian (1983: 143) wrote in a book that has greatly influenced the discipline, "anthropology emerged and established itself as an allochronic discourse: it is a science of other men in another time." The necessary reversal of this perspective involves understanding that "anthropology's Other is, ultimately, other people who are our contemporaries." This postulate has important consequences, the first of which pertains to the fact that we are different from the others, the second to the fact that we are contemporaneous with them.

Otherness must thus be taken seriously. We must strive to grasp representations, practices, social facts themselves as inscribed in local history and apprehended by local actors. AIDS in South Africa cannot be understood through the sort of ethnocentric, atemporal perspective that has often prevailed but rather on the basis of historiography-informed ethnography. As Michael Herzfeld (1991: 55) puts it, we are dealing with "multiple pasts and multiple presents" that enter in "conflict." The president of South Africa, a Treatment Action Campaign (TAC) activist, a nurse working in the rural clinic of a former homeland, and a person living with AIDS in a shack do not share the same understanding or representation of the problem, its causes and solutions. It is the whole of this "scene" that must be made comprehensible; it must be viewed and analyzed from the diverse local vantage points, encompassing the tensions and contradictions of local experiences, in the scientific arenas as much as in the townships, among political leaders as well as among village inhabitants. The point is not to fetishize ethnographic fieldwork by pretending it can offer a definitive anthropological truth but simply to consider it as irreplaceable. The epidemiological situation in South Africa has often been presented in dramatic terms, and this is readily understandable given its seriousness, the complexity of its causes, and the urgency of finding solutions. But this sense of the tragic has often led to cutting short the observation and interview time necessary to comprehension. If we step back we see that the hurried analyses and acrimonious denunciations have only made it more difficult to determine and implement effective social responses. It is not too late to get down to work.

Contemporaneousness asserts belonging to a common world experienced simultaneously in its convergences and confrontations, a world to which we all belong but experience differently. AIDS in South Africa involves policies that are defined in relation to programs and strategies deployed in international development forums and by global economic regulation authorities and multinational pharmaceutical companies but also in relation to representations and practices operative outside the health sphere, involving racism and discrimination, terrorism and sovereignty. And in the everyday and ordinary life of neighborhoods and villages, AIDS also involves men and women who suffer and die, the professional and volunteer workers who provide health care, the churches and associations that mobilize actors, the implementation of testing and treatment regimes. This has to be constructed against "anthropological culturalism," which by essentializing difference produces "subtly dehistoricizing, dehumanizing effects" (Malkki 1995: 17). What I claim is that though we share the same world, we share it unequally; that we are dealing with the same set of representations, values, and demands on which public policy are based, but the means of acceding to the resources assumed by those references are not distributed equitably; and, finally, that an AIDS patient's experiences in South Africa cannot and must not be considered foreign to us, despite the vast difference and distance between our social conditions. The politics of knowledge underlying this statement is not an abstract universalism. It represents a critical vantage point that requires thinking of our shared humanity less in terms of difference than inequality, less as a matter of culture than history.

If, as Achille Mbembe (2001: 2) writes with regard to Africa, "the theoretical and practical recognition of the body and flesh of 'the stranger' as flesh and body just like mine, the idea of a common human nature, a humanity shared with others, long posed, and still poses, a problem for Western consciousness," then this "problem of the 'I' of others and of human beings we perceive as foreign to us" presupposes a two-part imperative: we must not focus exclusively on either otherness or contemporaneousness but rather do ethnography of the local and sociology of the global. To invert Paul Ricoeur's (1990) formula, we must think of Other as self. Rather than a culture-bound, specialized, Africanist study, therefore, this is an exploration in general anthropology. What is at stake is how people can live together, not only in South African society, from which we nevertheless have more to learn than is commonly supposed, but also in a global society, whose injustices and divergences are rooted in ways of thinking that ignore or justify them. This book will have fulfilled its purpose if it manages to interest readers in the history of South Africa and bring closer to them the politics of life and death and political arrangements that are developed every day surrounding AIDS. It will have attained its goal if fieldwork conducted in the townships and former homelands helps us to grasp local and global worlds that escape us because we do not make the necessary effort to understand them.

My concern here is about bodies and memory, about the inscribing of historical time onto flesh, the social determinations of individuals' biological fate, and the remembering through which they seek to give meaning to their present. Through Pierre Nora's "lieux de mémoire" (1997: 3), French historiography provided us with the first systematic inventory of the material and symbolic spaces and objects that construct, illustrate, and make explicit a national narrative. "One only speaks so much about memory because nothing is left of it," he writes. But here I am interested in another sort of memory, that which resists its celebration, that which remains burning. I do not want to grasp a past that is being instituted as official but rather a past that is being unveiled. In South Africa the places where memory has left its mark are not those where the national epic was written. They are not the Vortreeker Monument in Pretoria signifying the glory of the Afrikaners or the Apartheid Museum in Johannesburg celebrating liberation from that oppression but rather words and gestures, silences and attitudes that expose the grim realities experienced by those who have been on the wrong side of history. Here it is less a question of places than nonplaces. What they reveal does not pertain to commemoration. It is, more profoundly, traces of an everlasting past.

My concern is the experience and politics that make up the period of uncertainty that has followed on apartheid. Experience and politics that, while coming after a spectacular break from the dark, hated past, nonetheless continue to take their very matter from it. Despite facile academic use of the prefix *post-*, this can indeed be called the postapartheid period. No other term expresses so well the dialectic of a social world that has survived its own supposed disappearance. "To articulate the past historically does not mean to recognize it the 'way it really was.' It means to seize hold of memory as it flashes up at a moment of danger," asserts Walter Benjamin (1968: 257). There is no greater peril for South Africa than the AIDS epidemic: with its almost six million infected persons, the country is the hardest hit on the planet. And there is no harsher test than AIDS for this new democracy whose actors have worked so hard to found it on the reuniting of a ravaged people: the disease precisely exposes its fracture lines and obscure areas. My thesis here is that the story of AIDS in South Africa, the spectacular spread of the epidemic in the past decade, the inextinguishable controversy over its causes and treatment, run in terrible counterpoint to the happy narrative of national reconstruction. At a moment of danger what comes to the fore is a truth very different from the reconciliation courageously undertaken by an instituted commission, a truth reopening wounds presumed to have healed, revealing memories supposed to have been buried, but not.

This book is thus about the moment when bodies remember, to use an expression close to those of Paul Connerton (1989) and Arthur Kleinman and Joan Kleinman (1994), which I discovered long after I had finished writing it. It opens with two parallel narratives: on the one hand, South Africa's President Thabo Mbeki on a crusade before international audiences against the certitudes of medicine, invoking the national past and recalling the continent's profound misfortunes to justify his heterodoxy and discredit his opponents; on the other, the story of Puleng, a young woman in the terminal phase of AIDS, reconstituting, in her dark, noisy basement the coherence of her life to account for the context of her infection and efface the stigma of her contamination before she dies (chapter 1). No two situations seem farther apart than the luxurious setting of the International AIDS Conference at Durban and a corrugated metal shack in Alexandra township. And yet the two narratives recount the same story. The president links the spread of the epidemic to the experience of apartheid; the young woman understands and presents her infection as a consequence of the structural violence of the township. Conducting a political anthropology study of AIDS means holding on to both these extremities of history in South Africa: history at work at the global level and history as lived in local space; the state policies and the politics of subjects. I begin with history at the global level and move gradually into history as lived in local space, keeping in view the ways in which the two mirror and alternately shed light on each other. The book's construction should thus be understood as a progression from macropolicies to micropolitics—or better, an exploration into the heart of darkness of everyday politics of life and death.

The AIDS controversy is considered by many commentators the most salient in South Africa's recent political life as well as the most resounding failure of Thabo Mbeki's government. It is usually situated in the first years of the twenty-first century around two heresies with respect to scientific and medical discourse. The first refers to the etiology of AIDS, for which poverty has been presented as a more decisive cause than the virus. The second pertains to antiretroviral drugs rejected as both too costly and potentially harmful. In both instances links established with a network of Western dissidents have been highlighted. If, however, we seek to apprehend the breadth and meaning of the controversy, it is necessary to analyze it as an epidemic of disputes (chapter 2). It began to develop soon after the 1994 democratic elections around what appear to be highly diverse events: a financial scandal surrounding a musical comedy designed to promote prevention of the infection; the spectacular announcement of a locally produced drug supposed to be effective in treating the disease; criticism of the pharmaceutical industry's international policies; the contesting of national mortality statistics; the refusal of prophylactic treatment for rape victims;

the interruption of prevention of mother-to-child transmission. In this constellation of controversies, a common rhetorical line was being developed that brought together the notions of race war, conspiracy theory, and national regeneration.

The South African political scene as it became structured and divided on the issue of AIDS has been represented in terms of two oppositions: political—between a government promoting heterodox theories and activists defending patient rights—and ideological—between the side of error and the side of truth. In-depth analysis disqualifies this reductionist version of reality, from both an epistemological and a sociological perspective (chapter 3). On the one hand, the terms of the debate cannot be restricted to truth versus falsehood, in which truth would be established once and for all and error definitively circumscribed. Scientific and moral boundaries are more slippery and porous than has usually been acknowledged. It is the case for knowledge about treatment, for which regularly updated data have often been replaced by brandished, imposed certitude. And it is the case for the ethics of research, which has often accepted hasty local definitions rather than universal principles. In general, the AIDS controversy in South Africa invites us to revise our ideas about the role of social conditions in the production of medical norms. On the other hand, description of the public space and its actors highlights the complex alliances and allegiances that, if correctly deciphered, allow for a different reading of South African political life than is commonly presented. For example, many of those who rallied behind President Mbeki did not do so because they believed in his dissident theses but because of their public health expertise on the difficulties of implementing equity in treatment or because their loyalty to the struggle first against apartheid and then in the democratic framework. Understood this way, the AIDS controversy appears more a discussion about the legacy of the past and the reactualization of political commitments than a battle merely between ideas and programs.

The violence of the exchanges between actors and the almost obsessive repetition of arguments in the debate must therefore be situated in the longer history of which they are a part, the history of public health and epidemics, of the health care system and its professionals. The violence characteristic of this history can be apprehended within two temporalities (chapter 4). The first one is inscribed in the long term. In South Africa health policies have been used to justify, first, racial segregation measures and, later, exploitation of the labor force. Tuberculosis and syphilis provided a foundation on which to construct theories of black inferiority and

African sexual promiscuity. The way people's bodies were treated thus cannot be historically dissociated from the ideological and practical domination that culminated in apartheid. The second one is embedded in the short term, the time of AIDS. But there is the time before 1994, before the epidemic. By not taking it into account, many features of today's situation, the codes of which have been designed previously, remain incomprehensible. The stigmatizing representations that the disease has given rise to are drawn from a stock of images accumulated over more than a century. Even more troubling, in the shadow of the regime that was about to be dislodged, genocidal discourses and programs were being developed. Considering this past experience, which combines the ordinariness of colonial occupation with the exceptionality of the apartheid regime whose details are only now being revealed in the public space, enables us to account for the government's statements and policies much more effectively than does the vague notion of "denialism" commonly used to describe it. In fact, two logics are at work: an economy of resentment, whereby the past constitutes an inexhaustible reservoir of painful memory, and an economy of suspicion, whereby the present is interpreted through the lens of an intense mistrust of anyone making any claims to authority.

But history is not merely a narrative or the sum of competing narratives. It is also what is inscribed within our bodies and makes us think and act as we do. South Africans' prereflexive view of the social world as run through by a color line, the interactions between men and women in matters of love or sex, the attitudes of employers to employees on the farms or in the mines, the norms of conduct people impose on themselves and their children, in sum what is called racial, gender, class, and generational relations—precisely all those relations through which HIV risk and prevention pass—are caught up in and shaped by particular experiences of time. Against the behavioral and culturalist interpretations that have been used to explain the dramatic spread of the disease, interpretations that are as ineffective as they are unjust, it is essential to give meaning to the embodiment of history (chapter 5). Inequality, violence, and mobility are the most salient elements of that history. And here what best enables us to read the complex inscription of the past in the present are life stories, the biographies of people who in most cases lived through the different periods of apartheid, from its establishment through its decline, and the successive phases of the return of democracy, from transition to disillusionment, each experiencing concrete and specific configurations of these realities.

The tragic singularity and the profound sense of contradiction that South

African society is experiencing today have to do with the fact that it has become a society living with death. Death is the individual reality of people with AIDS, their families and their friends, as much as the collective reality of the nation and those who govern it (chapter 6). With one-fifth of the adult population being HIV-positive, there are virtually no households that have not been either "infected or affected," as the expression often goes. In this context biopolitics, that is, the governmental technologies of the sovereign to protect the well-being, health, and ultimately the life of its subjects, has become necropolitics, in which the most urgent question, for families, is organizing funerals and, for the authorities, managing cemeteries. And yet life is being reinvested in two distinct ways. The first way is represented best by the notion of rebirth. Collectively, this involves a project expressed most fully by the term "African Renaissance," which has become a leitmotiv for the country's intellectual and political elites. Individually, it refers to "moral regeneration," understood in both religious and political terms. The second way, less apparent but perhaps even more fundamental, refers to survival. People often talk of "normal life." For patients, it means remaining alive, feeding oneself and one's family, fulfilling one's obligations with dignity, surviving—in the deepest sense of the word. For the government, this concern with material life has given rise to a major allocation program for the sick and the children they will leave behind, the aim being to maintain decent living conditions for them. At the frontiers of death, South African society is thus redefining what it means to live.

Historians of South Africa continue to debate whether the specificity of apartheid and postapartheid means that the country's history is unique (the exceptionality thesis) or whether it should instead be considered no more than an exacerbated version of the colonial and postcolonial situation (the exemplarity thesis). Rather than decide between the two, I want to consider what meaning South African history has for the contemporary world (conclusion). Though South African history is particular in many ways, it nonetheless sheds light on many realities beyond South Africa. The world is not only organized into an economic and political hierarchy; it is also morally and ideologically divided. September 11, 2001, and its aftermath are one expression of this division, though certainly not the only one. Relations of authority, wealth, and signification are imprinted on the bodies and minds of the rulers and the ruled. We may observe without being deterministic that these relations take the form of structural violence whose consequences may be measured in terms of mortality rates and seen in the distribution of suffering. We may observe without being functionalist that these relations are also expressed in denunciations of the Western world, in subaltern and nationalist discourses, and in the moral discourses of prophetic churches and fundamentalist ideologies. The politics of inequality as it may be read in the lives of the South African adults who are dying so young and the politics of defiance against power and science that has manifested itself in South Africa have become global issues. Attempting to understand the situation there can help us to move from our current age of anxiety to an age of *inquiétude,* worried concern open to the promise of humanity.

Classic ethnography developed through monographic studies that appeared to be characterized by spatial and social unity, the assumption being that it was possible to provide an exhaustive description of an ethnic group on its territory. In parallel, anthropology in its halcyon days was constructed on theoretical propositions that articulated analytic principles assumed to have universal value in the framework of a unifying culturalist, functionalist, structuralist, or Marxist paradigm. I would like to situate this book at the intersection of these two approaches, to see it as a type of monograph whose unit of intelligibility is theoretical. I have sought to study a problem with a concern to account both for the diversity of its components and the general nature of the issues involved. At the end of his life, Michel Foucault (1994: 545, 611) attributed primary importance to the concept of "problematization": societal productions such as madness and disease, life, language, and work were "problematized," and the practice of research itself was "perpetual reproblematizing" rather than a search for solutions. It seems to me that the problem of AIDS in South Africa, both in its most ethnographic reality and in its most anthropological meaning, can only be grasped as a problematization of the contemporary world involving relations between history and memory, power and knowledge, truth and suspicion, inequality and violence. What may on first analysis seem an overly dense, heterogeneous tissue of events, statistics, narratives, and anecdotes is very simply the compact, composite matter of which social content is made. The work of the anthropologist in these conditions is to shape problematizations through monographs.

Restitutions of this sort are usually based on narrative. But here we must be vigilant. "A reader's perception that a story 'tells itself' is a powerful illusion created by the author who extracts a story from the words of its narrator and the setting in which the story emerges," notes Charles Briggs (2003: 11) at the beginning of a chronicle of cholera in Venezuela in the 1990s cowritten with his wife, Clara Mantini-Briggs. His remark is epistemologically and ethically salutary. On the one hand, the history of AIDS recounted in these pages is the product of both intellectual choices and the practical conditions in which the interviews and study were realized. This means that someone else would have written it differently. In reading and analyzing the mounds of documents and archival material assembled over four years, the hundreds of pages of transcribed interviews and observations, I have worked to produce a certain truth, and I hope not to have failed in the labor of objectification that is part of any and all social science research. Still, it would be less than straightforward not to accept, for a subject that arouses such strong feelings and passions in citizens and researchers alike both in South Africa and in the rest of the world, that any restitution presupposes an interpretation. Rather than pretend to be objective, I have been as careful as possible not to remove myself from the circumstances in which this narrative was produced, to specify my place in the episodes here related. Moreover, it was often in the details of daily life and the interstices of informal exchanges that things appeared to me most clearly. However, as my work progressed, through the ties I established, the presentations I made, and the texts I published, I also became a local and international actor in the history of AIDS in South Africa. It would be disingenuous not to acknowledge that on what is a fairly crowded stage, where many were and are courageously engaged in trying to change national policies, I have tried to produce a kind of truth aimed, among other things, at transforming the public sphere of AIDS both in South African society and in the perceptions that the outside world has of it. By speaking repeatedly to the Western medical community, French association activists, and international cooperation circles, I often overstepped the borders defined by the rules of professional anthropology, though there is of course nothing extraordinary in that.

One last confession. Despite all my efforts, I remain an impenitent positivist. I believe my work as an anthropologist helps to produce a bit more truth (certainly not *the* truth) about South African society; that the combination of empirical study and epistemological distancing makes it reasonable to believe I have succeeded in presenting with some objectivity (while of course acknowledging my own subjective position) a situation made especially delicate by intense passions and interests; last, that there is something of science (though not the Popperian variety) in what I and researchers in my discipline do. But there is more—and worse. I must acknowledge too that my political view of anthropology is also a moral one. I believe the work presented here can be socially useful, that anthropology is not a matter of art for art's sake, that making the things of this world a bit more intelligible, especially when they appear opaque, incomprehensible, and irrational, can make them less unjust, ineluctable, or unacceptable. To put it bluntly (of course, in a Durkheimian tradition), I am convinced that social science would not be worth a moment's attention or labor if it had no political role.

The research this book is based on was supported institutionally and financially by the Agence Nationale de Recherche sur le Sida (ANRS), whose executive director, Michel Kazatchkine, and successive social science project directors, Yves Souteyrand and Véronique Doré, devotedly and unswervingly defended the program. Together with the Mission Recherche Expérimentation (MiRe) of the French Ministry of Solidarity, the ANRS funded the translation of the book into English. The Institut National de la Santé et de la Recherche Médicale (Inserm) graciously granted me a two-year leave to finish my fieldwork and write about it.

My institutional collaboration in South Africa began with the School of Public Health and its director at the time, William Pick. It continued with the Center for Health Policy at the University of Witwatersrand and its director, Helen Schneider, as well as Duane Blaauw and Loveday Penn-Kekana; our collaboration has been uninterrupted during the past six years. It was further enriched by exchanges with the Wiser Wits Institute for Social and Economic Research, in particular its director, Deborah Posel.

Nearly all the studies in the Johannesburg townships of Alexandra and Soweto and in villages of the former Lebowa and Gazankulu homelands in the north of the country, today part of Limpopo province, were conducted with the knowledgeable and friendly assistance of Frédéric Le Marcis, then research fellow, and Todd Lethata, research assistant, both at that time members of the anthropology department of the University of Witwatersrand; the "we" used in the fieldwork accounts refers most often to them. I owe grateful thanks to Regina Makwale, who was my guide several times in urban contexts, and to Dios Moaji and his wife, who were generous hosts in rural ones. Discussions with Nono Simelela, director of the National AIDS Programme; Mark Heywood, spokesman for the Treatment Action Campaign; Lulama Sulupha, coordinator of the Friends for Life association; Sokie van der Westhuysen, then in charge of the health subdistrict of Tzaneen; and many others shed valuable light on the various South African "scenes" that have developed around the issue of AIDS.

Exchanges with colleagues and students at the École de Hautes Études en Sciences Sociales have been greatly enriching, as have discussions with members of the Centre de Recherche sur la Santé, le Social et le Politique (Cresp), whose secretary, Véronique Anohan, provided valuable assistance. Though writing is fundamentally a solitary activity, it was done in this case in a stimulating and encouraging community of colleagues and friends. I am certain this book bears its trace. At times it takes no more than hearing or reading an idea in the margins of a text or in the moment of a discussion for a new line of thought to spring up. In this sense I am particularly grateful to Joao Biehl, Arachu Castro, David Coplan, Jean-Pierre Dozon, Paul Farmer, Achille Mbembe, Mariella Pandolfi, Stefania Pandolfo, Paul Rabinow, Richard Rechtman, Nancy Scheper-Hughes, Mara Viveros, and Sophie Wahnich. My translators, Amy Jacobs (introduction, chapter 1, conclusion) and Gabrielle Varro (chapters 2–6), have worked hard to get their best out of the French original: they will forgive my numerous revisions of the English version of the manuscript, which also benefited from Kate Warne's reading. The confidence shown by Naomi Schneider, sponsoring editor at the University of California Press, and François Gèze, director of La Découverte, has made it reassuringly clear that the men and women of South Africa can still be of "interest" to the world of books. And there are debts and gratitude too great to be expressed, among them mine to Anne-Claire Defossez.

Nothing has been more humanly and intellectually decisive for me in the past six years than the time spent with the men and women who told me their stories and shared with me their anxiety and anger, expectations and hopes. Some of them have died. Many more will have when these pages appear in print. While the words of the book are mine, their lives, their bodies, and their memories are its matter.

D. F.
Osny, August 2005

ONE

As If Nothing Ever Happened

The past will always be a powerful presence in the present. . . . For those of us who are survivors of the past, it is important that we do not forget.

ZAKES MDA

Preface to John Kani, *Nothing but the Truth*

"WE CANNOT AFFORD TO ALLOW the AIDS epidemic to ruin the realization of our dreams. Existing statistics indicate that we are still at the beginning of this epidemic in our country. Unattended, however, this will result in untold damage and suffering by the end of the century." At the Maputo AIDS Conference in 1990, Chris Hani, the exiled charismatic leader of Umkhonto weSizwe, the armed wing of the African National Congress (ANC), thus shared his vision of a menaced future.[1] At the time AIDS data for South Africa seemed reassuring. Whereas between 10 and 20 percent of the adult population of central Africa were HIV-positive, annual surveys of major South African cities gave figures below 1 percent. Some specialists wondered how to explain this relative immunity: did the country have an epidemiological profile similar to Western nations, where specific groups, mainly homosexuals and heroin addicts, were the most exposed to infection, rather than to African nations, where heterosexual transmission was threatening the population at large? That year, after four decades of apartheid rule, the thirty-year ban against opposition political parties was lifted and, after ten thousand days in prison, Nelson Mandela left Robben Island. The transition to democracy was under way. It would be completed in 1994 with the first free democratic elections the country had ever known. The "new South Africa" could begin. A few months before, however, Hani, who had been secretary-general of the South African Communist Party (SACP) since 1991, was assassinated by a "white extremist." He had continually called for peace and reconciliation, in a period when the issues facing postapartheid South Africa were negotiated in a climate of tension and violence.

Ten years after the Maputo call to mobilize against the scourge of AIDS, as I started my research in South Africa, the country had become the world's epicenter of the pandemic. According to the international agency UN-AIDS, in 2000 there were an estimated 36 million HIV-infected persons throughout the world; 25 million of them were on the African continent, the vast majority in sub-Saharan Africa. In the Republic of South Africa alone there were 4.5 million cases, for a total of 43 million persons. In other words, more than one infected person in ten worldwide was a South African, and more than one South African in ten was infected. A Department of Health survey conducted the same year found a nationwide rate of seroprevalence among pregnant women of 24.5 percent. The figure was as high as 36.2 percent for the province of KwaZulu Natal, whose capital is Durban, and 29.4 percent for the province of Gauteng, which encompasses Johannesburg. Ten years earlier the figure had been 0.7 percent. The effects were already showing in mortality rates. A Medical Research Council study found as many deaths from natural causes among persons ages 30 to 40 as in the 60 to 70 age group: instead of the usual regular increase of mortality from childhood on, the graphs were showing unprecedented plateaus. The proportion of deaths due to AIDS was estimated at 20 percent for all adults and 40 percent for persons ages 15 to 49. Projections from the data gave even greater cause for alarm: between 1990 and 2010 life expectancy at birth could decline from sixty to forty years.[2] Most of this dramatic evolution affected the so-called African populations. Five years later the situation has worsened: almost 6 million persons are estimated to be HIV-positive, the rate of infected women in the annual antenatal survey reaching 27.9 percent. But let us go back to the year 2000.

At Baragwanath Hospital in Soweto, the largest hospital on the African continent, which was recently renamed after Chris Hani, HIV infection had for so long been part of the daily work and life of all medical and paramedical staff that it was no longer categorized as a specific pathology, which would justify placing patients in the infectious disease ward. In gastroenterology and pneumology, in obstetrics and pediatrics, a majority of patients were HIV-positive. The infection had become one ordinary feature of the pathological profile, regardless of what service patients were in.

Moreover, barring complications, persons living with AIDS were rarely hospitalized, because other than through clinical trials no antiretroviral drugs were available for them. Very few persons with AIDS were admitted to the few charity hospices in the township to live out their last days. Most would die at home, with at best a few visits from a volunteer from a neighborhood humanitarian association. Medicine could do nothing for these people. When their families brought them to the emergency room in the terminal stage of the disease, they were usually sent back home. Ambulance companies were increasingly unwilling to transport these undesirable patients.

In one decade the prediction announced in Maputo had thus been realized. The dream of a democratic renaissance had become the nightmare of a catastrophe foretold. Delivered from the violence of apartheid, South African society had fallen prey to the disaster of AIDS. Commentators have noted the simultaneity of these facts, and it has become commonplace to say that the fight against the disease is the new battle that must be waged now that apartheid has been vanquished. Many people assert that one tragedy has been overcome only for another to take its place. On the heels of political terror has come biological horror. The same collective strength and resources must thus be mobilized in this new struggle. And, indeed, some of the actors of yesterday's struggle against apartheid are today fighting on the new front. But are the two realities as separate from each other as is often suggested, or are they irremediably entangled? Do they tell two different stories or the same one? To ask a symmetrical question, is it necessary to think of apartheid and AIDS as comparable phenomena with similar dynamics? Looked at somewhat differently, do they pertain to two sets of politics or to one?

Among the many posters designed by the Treatment Action Campaign in its mobilization for access to antiretroviral drugs, one, consigned by the Congress of South African Trade Unions (COSATU), has been especially successful. On it two photos are juxtaposed. The first is titled "15 June 1976. Hector Petersen. Age 13." A teenager in tears with a little girl at his side bears the body of a boy gunned down by the police. It is the most famous and dramatic scene from the Soweto uprising. The second photo, titled "1 June 2001. Nkosi Johnson. Age 12," shows a familiar face. Everyone in South Africa recognizes the sick boy who spoke at the opening of the Thirteenth International AIDS Conference in Durban to ask the South African president to make antiretroviral drugs available to all. Nkosi Johnson died a few months later. Yesterday's martyr with today's victim. Both images represent symbols of the past and present struggles. Apartheid not long ago and AIDS from now on. It was undeniably effective to bring the two together just after commemorating the twenty-fifth anniversary of the Soweto uprising, which itself marked the renewal of the fight against the old regime. But what truth was the poster affirming? That the life of a child is as valuable as any other life and that all political causes that attempt to save one child are of equal worth? Compassion, especially when it is directed toward children, has undeniable efficacy in swaying public opinion. Most campaigns for drug availability have been based on this "moral sentiment," as Adam Smith (1976) would have said.

However, there are other truths, as emotional as this one but less consensual. In South Africa AIDS is not just an epidemic that people fight. It is also an epidemic about which people fight each other. It is not only a matter of policy in the way we speak of health policies targeting prevention, treatment, and patient assistance. In the sense that it often sets actors and theories virulently at odds, and may well partake of the very definition of politics, it is also a political issue. As many observers have noted,[3] only a few years after the advent of democracy in South Africa, AIDS has become the main political question, not so much because of its incredibly rapid spread or even its incalculable human and economic costs, as for the violent way it confronts the frailty of political power and rends people's lives and relations.

Michael Walzer (1983), searching for the foundation of a just society, proposed as a criterion "the shared understanding of social goods," in other words, agreement on what is good for all and each. History and memory are such social goods, as they represent the relationship with time through which identities and differences are built. In South Africa such shared understanding—what may be called, more simply, history and memory—can hardly be said to exist. This is clear from the work of the Truth and Reconciliation Commission (TRC), which had difficulty getting its hearings published in full, and the tensions surrounding the procedures for compensating victims. Playing on the national reconstruction slogan, "the rainbow nation," Deborah Posel (2002) calls the contradictory versions of events that emerged in the TRC hearings, which interfered with both the reconstitution of particular stories and the production of a collective history, a "rainbow of truths." Even the remarkable charisma and consensus-reaching skill of the commission's president, Archbishop Desmond Tutu, have not been enough. Frustrations have grown in proportion to hopes placed in the process and dashed by the results, deceived expectations of reparations and too easily obtained amnesties. But more important, perhaps, the hearings have demonstrated publicly the impossibility of restoring one common historical truth, and—however honest and sincere the work of the TRC has been—the very notion of shared memory has had to be abandoned.

The most acclaimed theatrical event of the postapartheid era, *Nothing but the Truth,* tells how a father, his daughter who works as an interpreter for the TRC, and his niece who has just arrived from London are confronted with a series of revelations about the past, especially about the old man's brother who has recently died.[4] The whole family has lived the myth of the exiled hero, victim of the apartheid regime, but they discover that the father was more of a womanizer than a fighter and that he had to leave the country simply because of a love affair. Beyond the intimate wounds of these lies suddenly unveiled, however, the father suffers from not knowing the truth about his son who was killed by the police years before; no inquiry has been conducted, and the perpetrator remains free. This might be the deepest truth the TRC brought to light: on the one hand, where the present is constructed in pain and discord, there can be no unique truth about the past; on the other hand, if justice is not done, no reconciliation will be possible. Truth and justice, however relative and fragile they might be, are deeply linked.

This is attested by the social history of AIDS, whether we consider the intense controversy sparked by the South African president's declarations on the etiology of the disease and the effects of antiretroviral drugs or the deep inequalities in the distribution of the disease and access to drug treatment. On one side, opinions on Mbeki's declarations are divided along the wounds that remain in memory. Prejudices resurface; mistrust is reborn. On the other side, regarding the objective facts about who gets AIDS, the disparity reflects the violence of the past. Social differentiations are perpetuated; racial tensions sharpen. In opening this book with an analysis of the controversy surrounding the president's declarations on the virus and the autobiography of a woman dying of the disease, in working to hold together simultaneously the macro- and micro-political histories of AIDS— an approach resisted strongly in South Africa, where the first elicits condemnation and the second compassion—I hope to shed light on what I believe is in fact one reality—that through which bodies remember.

many rains later
media reports have confined the leader
to the oblivion of a secluded farm—however
now & then an outburst splutters on the front page
a croaking yell from an obstinate past
the old vulture will not be forgotten
already
fresh broods of misanthropes are on the rise
as everywhere the blood testifies.

SEITHLAMO MOTSAPI
"The Leader Reclines"

I first learned of what would become the largest political and scientific controversy in the history of AIDS in early April 2000. In an interview I was conducting on AIDS policies, an international official from a West African country whom I had known for some time opened his desk drawer and took out a fax, indicating its contents should not to be divulged publicly.[5] He told me it was a copy of a confidential letter President Mbeki had sent to several "world leaders," among them U.S. President Bill Clinton, British Prime Minister Tony Blair, and UN Secretary-General Kofi Annan, to explain his recently stated policy on AIDS. It referred to the meeting of South African and international experts that Mbeki had convened to assess knowledge on the epidemic and the means to fight against it. The Presidential Panel, as it was called, included famous scientists involved in the discovery of the virus and clinical trials on the infection but also researchers known for their dissenting view of its causes (they consider the virus an "innocent passenger" of the disease) and treatments (they claimed antiretroviral drugs were responsible for the death of most patients). In his letter Mbeki expressed his indignation at the negative reactions his initiative had provoked in the world scientific community. His intention, he wrote, was simply to understand the specificities of the African epidemic and choose solutions adapted to that context rather than merely reproduce interpretations and remedies used in Western countries, where propagation characteristics were clearly different. Obviously, the missive I had in my hands was a potentially dangerous document that I decided to safeguard. I could not have imagined that it would cause the first global controversy over AIDS.

A Contemporary Apostasy

President Mbeki's "letter to world leaders" did not remain a secret for long. On April 19, just days after I received a copy, the *Washington Post* published long excerpts of the letter, along with a lengthy commentary on its contents and the "emotional controversy" it had sparked. The South African president, the article explained, was challenging the orthodox view of the etiology of the infection and the efficacy of its treatment. Although the letter neither explicitly proposed an alternative interpretation nor openly questioned the link between HIV and AIDS, it gave credit to heterodox scientists and thus put his country in a crisis of confidence. Surprisingly, in referring to the "scientists who dispute the prevailing views in the West on the causes and treatment of the disease," the editorial writer, Barton Gellman, seemed to suggest the relevance of Thabo Mbeki's analysis, as if the theories generally accepted by researchers referred to a specifically Western position—as if scientific truth was less dependent on universal criteria than on geopolitical considerations.

The controversy grew over the next few weeks. Indignant reactions multiplied, leading an editorial writer for the celebrated British medical journal the *Lancet* to question whether it made sense for specialists the world over to attend the Thirteenth International AIDS Conference in Durban—the first time since the epidemic had begun that the conference was to be held in an African city. A large number of researchers, physicians, and activists feared that their presence would lend legitimacy to the dissidents' theses. But the scientific gathering ultimately took place. As Mbeki began his opening remarks, half the audience stood up and walked out in a spectacular expression of collective disapproval. In the weeks leading up to the conference the president had clearly manifested his skill at provocation.

In Pretoria on May 6 and 7 and later in Johannesburg on July 3 and 4, less than a week before the Durban conference, Mbeki had called meetings of his Presidential Panel. Sixty-three experts had been invited to evaluate knowledge on AIDS. Fifty-two actually participated in the working sessions, including some of the most important experts in the world. Of the two presumed discoverers of the virus, Luc Montagnier attended and Robert Gallo did not. There were institutional officials, such as Awa Marie Coll-Seck, a director of the UNAIDS program; Helen Gayle, director of the Centers for Disease Control in Atlanta; and Clifford Lane, director of the National Institutes of Health in Washington, D.C. There were South African specialists in various disciplines, including the immunologist Malegapuru William Magkoba, president of the Medical Research Council; the pediatrician Jerry Coovadia, president of the Durban conference Scientific Committee; the gynecologist James McIntyre; the infectious disease specialist Salim Abdool-Karim; and the economist Allen Whiteside. And there were the dissidents, more or less well known, to whom the panel gave an unhoped-for forum for disseminating their views and, perhaps more important, an opportunity to strengthen their network. Among this group were the Americans Peter Duesberg, David Rasnick, and Charles Geschekter; the Canadian Etienne de Harven; the Colombian Roberto Giraldo; the Austrian Christian Fiala; the Australian Elena Papadopoulos-Eleopoulos; and the South African Sam Mhlongo. The jurist Stephen Owen served as "facilitator." It had been understandably hard for representatives of legitimate science to decide if it was preferable to be on the panel or to abstain, to participate so as to defend their ideas at the risk of paradoxically seeming to support their opponents or not to take part and thereby avoid being compromised but leave the door open to heresy. Ultimately, the orthodox were more numerous than the heterodox on the panel, but on each of the select themes, there was supposed to be an equilibrium of viewpoints. President Mbeki opened the first working session with these words:

I am going to read a few lines from a poem by an Irish poet, Patrick Pearce. It will indicate some of what has been going through my mind over the last few months. The poem is titled "The Fool," and it says:

"Since the wise men have not spoken, I speak but I'm only a fool;
A fool that hath loved his folly,
Yea, more than the wise men their books or their counting houses or
    their quiet homes,
Or their fame in men's mouths;
A fool that in all his days hath never done a prudent thing . . .
I have squandered the splendid years that the Lord God gave to my
    youth
In attempting impossible things, deeming them alone worth the toil.
Was it folly or grace?"

I have asked myself that question many times over the last few months: whether the matters that were raised were as a result of folly or grace.

You will remember the letter we sent inviting you to this meeting. It included a quotation from a report by WHO on the global situation of the HIV/AIDS pandemic. It said that of the 5.6 million people infected with HIV in 1999, 3.8 million lived in sub-Saharan Africa, the hardest hit region. There were an estimated 2.2 million HIV/AIDS deaths in the region during 1999, being 85% of the global total, even though only one-tenth of the world population lives in sub-Saharan Africa. . . . It was because it seemed that the problem was so big, if these reports were correct, that I personally wanted to understand this matter better. Now, as I've said, I'm only a fool and I faced this difficult problem of reading all of these complicated things that you scientists write about, in this language I don't understand. So I ploughed through lots and lots of documentation, with dictionaries all around me in case there were words that seemed difficult to understand. I would phone the Minister of Health and say, "Minister, what does this word mean?" And she would explain. I am somewhat embarrassed to say that I discovered that there had been a controversy around these matters for quite some time. I honestly didn't know. . . .

According to these reports, clearly something changed here. In a period of maybe five, six, seven years after 1985, when it was said that such transmission in this region was not endemic in Southern Africa, there were high rates of heterosexual transmission. Now, as I was saying, being a fool, I couldn't answer this question about what happened between 1985 and the early 1990s. The situation has not changed in the United States up to today, nor in Western Europe with regard to homosexual transmission. But here it changed radically in a short period of time and increased radically in a short period of time. Why? This is not an idle question for us because it bears very directly on this question: How should we respond? . . . And so you see why I've been thinking over this matter over the last few months that perhaps I should have allowed the wise men to speak. Indeed when eminent scientists say: "You have spoken out of time," it was difficult not to think that one was indeed a fool. But I'm no longer so sure about that, given that so many eminent people responded to the invitation of a fool to come to this important meeting. Welcome and best wishes. Thank you very much.

As Thabo Mbeki's biographers, Adrian Hadland and Jovial Rantao (1999: xvi), have noted, "While many senior politicians both in South Africa and abroad charge staffers to write their speeches, Mbeki generally does them himself." He writes with particular care over long hours, perhaps as much from a literary taste for rhetoric of which he plays with virtuosity as a concern for the trace of himself he will leave to posterity. Identifying oneself as and with a fool when one is chief of state is a move not devoid of irony, and this fool was clearly there to speak the truth to all "wise men."[6] At the height of the controversy journalists and politicians did indeed call Mbeki's mental health into question, first expressing their astonishment at his "nonsense" and "irrationality," then more openly wondering about his "para-noia," finding him "depressed" or even "off the rocket," to the extent that Sonti Maseko, editorial writer for the *City Press* newspaper, felt compelled to title her piece of October 8, 2000, "President Mbeki Is Not Mad." It is characteristic of political life in South Africa for debate to become person-alized, and obviously the South African president helped the process along by taking a controversial personal stance on this sensitive issue and persist-ently using the first person. This psychopathological approach sheds little light on the polemics surrounding AIDS, and it is another line of inter-pretation that I have tried to explore.

The Fool's Truth

I long abstained from speaking out on the Mbeki issue in South African academic circles, though the politics of AIDS was the focus of my research. The controversy was too delicate a matter, I thought, and everyone was al-ready quite familiar with its substance. A Western anthropologist might say nothing relevant or innovative. It seemed preferable to leave the speaking to my South African colleagues, who had direct knowledge of and experi-ence with the situation. Moreover, if one did not immediately denounce Thabo Mbeki's ideas in a scandalized or ironic tone, one was in danger of being cast as a dissident. But I changed my mind about keeping silent in April 2001 during the AIDS in Context conference, organized as part of the History Workshop at the University of Witwatersrand in Johannesburg.[7] There I was struck by the fact that whereas the conflict of opinions was get-ting the majority of political and media attention, it was mentioned in only two of the conference's eighty-seven papers, neither of which was presented by a social scientist. However, as soon as participants left the sessions for a break or a meal, all they spoke about was what the president had said or not said, either expressing how appalled they were at his erring ways or scoff-ing at his incompetence. What was a taboo subject in the scientific inner sanctum was thus a commonplace of informal conversation and discussion among those same scientists.

There were, it seemed to me, two reasons that the researchers were silent on the controversy in their talks. First, faced with such a grave issue, they could only take sides, as many of them had previously done under apar-theid. The issue was a matter for urgent activist "involvement," not analytic "detachment," to use Norbert Elias's (1956) words. In a sense action was a necessity and science was somewhat out of place. Second, they surely per-ceived the intellectual and political risks involved in interpreting disputes that exacerbated unhealed wounds from the recent past. On this point, and though they had been rejected by all involved, the old racial oppositions resurfaced, and every time the polemic was evoked, in groups of specialists or gatherings of friends, affiliations were revealed that followed the vehemently condemned and yet very present and relevant "color line" (Du Bois [1903] 1994). In most situations the white researchers were extremely critical of Mbeki—or showed contemptuous irony—whereas their black colleagues defended him—or expressed irritation at the attacks against him. For my part, these two observations convinced me that the "affair"[8] deserved to be taken seriously and that it would no doubt provide keys to a better understanding of contemporary South African society.

Let me use a metaphorical circumlocution. In a preamble to a discussion of "historical consciousness," John Comaroff and Jean Comaroff (1992: 41) make this surprising revelation: "Paradoxically, it is a fool who taught us the most on consciousness in rural South Africa." The story they relate takes place in a psychiatric hospital in Tswana country. The protagonist is a mental patient. His eccentric outfit, in which references to the mine (boots and leggings) are mixed with references to religion (cape and miter), includes a shining sash across his chest with the letters "SAR" embroidered on it. What the white doctors saw as just another extravagant touch the black nurses and patients recognized as having meaning and power. Comaroff and Comaroff continue, "SAR was his church and he was its only incarnation. The letters corresponded to South African Railways. In fact, just as we were meeting him, the night train for Johannesburg passed by noisily taking its everyday load of migrant workers." The message on his clothes was understandable to all. The railroad stood as "a tangible link between rural and urban life" and the figure of the proletarian migrants who boarded it evoked the essential distinction between "work for oneself" and "labor for the white man," the freedom of the first and the exploitation of the second. Therein lie the seeds of historical consciousness, the authors affirm. I would venture a similar parallel. It was a man who some say is "mad" and who occasionally presents himself as the poet's "fool" who taught me most about the unconscious issues of postapartheid South Africa.

The lesson may have been missed by many of those who criticized and often caricatured the stance of Thabo Mbeki and his supporters, some because they were engaged in the battle against AIDS and saw only too clearly the human cost of the government and public administration's blatant inaction, others because they were cynically rejoicing in the first faux pas of a government they had never wanted or had quickly distanced themselves from. But thinking that the president's argument deserves attention does not mean that one wants to discredit the activists' cause or has compromised oneself by conceding to the dissidents. It is not my purpose to determine whether Thabo Mbeki did or did not say that "the virus is not the cause of AIDS," to which the South African press devoted considerable energy for over a year, but rather to try to grasp what was behind "Mbeki's crusade," as a writer for the *Weekly Mail and Guardian* titled his piece in the March 31, 2000, issue. The writer concludes that he sees no "apparent reason" for the stir raised by the president's views. But there were many reasons. The question is thus, how can the anthropologist account for them with the necessary detachment required of the disipline and without renouncing the inevitable involvement that arises from an event in which people suffer and die?

Writing on the aftermath of the September 11, 2001, attacks and their consequences for the social sciences, Hugh Gusterson (2003: 25) comments: "In such a situation where the world is polarized, what is the responsibility of the international fraternity of anthropologists? Surely the humane tradition of our discipline at its best is one not of plunging into conflicts but of seeking to recast and mediate them, to humanize and understand the other rather than taking for granted the terms in which it is vilified." He cites Faye Ginsburg interpreting the positions of the two sides in the violent abortion debate in the United States and Renato Rosaldo deciphering the meaning of headhunter practices in the Philippines. This is what Lila Abu-Lughod (2002: 789), referring to a similar international polarization on the status of women in Muslim countries, calls "respect for difference," which, she explains, has nothing to do with "cultural relativism." She rejects the idea of making male domination tolerable and even acceptable on the grounds of incommensurable values and calls instead for a scientific position that includes the acknowledgment that "we do not stand outside the world, looking out over this sea of poor benighted people." Whether we like

it or not, we are part of this world, including when we deal with a radically different Other whose positions we do not support but whose history is nonetheless inextricably linked to our own. The public sphere of AIDS in South Africa, a different historical context but related to the international tensions these authors speak of, proves similarly polarized. Tensions are so sharp between adherents of scientific orthodoxy and supporters of the government theses that over the past few years there has been no room for doing the work usually expected from social scientists: presenting and analyzing discourses, positions, and facts. It is along this uncomfortable dividing line that I propose to proceed.

The only justification I can invoke for doing so is anthropological. <u>First</u>, contrary to what is suggested by the way the debate has been personalized around the figures of South Africa's President Thabo Mbeki and, to a lesser degree, former Vice President Jacob Zuma and two successive health ministers, Nkosazana Zuma and Manto Tshabalala-Msimang, politicians have not been the only ones to contest the authority of biomedical discourse, nor are they the only ones to express thereby their distrust of Western hegemony. That the government's statements on this matter have had great resonance in South African society is not, contrary to what has often been said, because they turned highly malleable public opinion away from the truth but because there were favorable conditions for accepting their assertions. These conditions, which are historical, deserve closer attention. <u>Second,</u> the very way in which the debate developed, that is, outside the usual rules for public discussion, with invective and censure, reciprocal disqualification and anathema, reveals that what is at stake exceeds technical questions and scientific facts, though this is what was emphasized throughout the debate. Very quickly the arguments exchanged and accusations made came to involve some of the most sensitive issues in the contemporary world: race and racism, genocide and denialism. The South African experience of these issues is singularly painful. Here again these realities, shaped by history and reconstructed through memory, cry out for analysis. I believe that taking seriously the entire set of actors and arguments in the AIDS crisis and trying to understand and make intelligible all positions constitute the only anthropologically sound approach, and the only one by means of which the researcher may be useful to the citizen.

The President's Theses

Going back to the controversy itself, what did Thabo Mbeki say? The two texts mentioned—his "letter to world leaders" of April 3, 2000, and his opening speech at the Durban conference on July 9, 2000—present his argument quite clearly.[9] In the first he justifies his position to his peers <u>without clearly stating it;</u> in the second he expresses his conviction more <u>directly to the world at large.</u>

The letter begins by recalling the actions undertaken by his government in the preceding six years to fight AIDS, attesting to a real commitment to combating the disease. However, Mbeki writes, the African epidemic does not at all resemble the one in Western countries: the disease is transmitted above all through heterosexual relations and spreads much more quickly; and whereas the situation seems to have stabilized elsewhere, in Africa it continues to worsen dramatically. Does not this indicate that "specific and targeted responses" should be devised for Africa rather than "a simple superimposition of Western experience on African reality"? This, he explains, is what he had in mind when he invited international experts to assess existing knowledge of AIDS. He wants to adapt AIDS policy to African realities rather than accept "the comfort of the recitation of a catechism." And it is why he felt so indignant at hearing his initiative characterized as "a criminal abandonment of the fight against HIV/AIDS" by his opponents: "Not so long ago, in our country, people were killed, tortured, imprisoned and prohibited from being quoted in private and in public because the established authority believed that their views were dangerous and discredited. We are now being asked to do precisely the same thing that the racist apartheid tyranny we opposed did, because, it is said, there exists a scientific view that is supported by the majority, against which dissent is prohibited." And he concludes: "It may be that these comments are extravagant. If they are, it is because in the very recent past, we had to fix our own eyes on the very face of tyranny." A French diplomat remarked to me ironically, in reference to the letter, that Mbeki had known nothing of apartheid personally because he had spent a good part of his life in Britain, sheltered from the violence of the regime. Thus disqualifying his exile as golden is as historically unjust as it is uselessly disparaging.[10] That there are diverse experiences of apartheid is obvious—even more for people who have lived directly under this regime, as recent historical studies and also the hearings of the Truth and Reconciliation Commission have started to reveal, sometimes painfully. But in referring to apartheid in his letter, President Mbeki was not merely being rhetorical about memory; he was referring to a history that speaks to many citizens.

The July 9 speech reveals in greater detail the theory on AIDS that the president had been developing gradually. This time he begins by referring to the apartheid past, calling conference participants to witness: "I am certain that there are many among you who joined in the international struggle for the destruction of the antihuman apartheid system. You are therefore the midwives of the new, democratic, nonracial, nonsexist South Africa as are the millions of our people who fought for the emancipation of all humanity from the racist yoke of the apartheid crime against humanity." He then presents his thesis in a narrative form legitimized by drawing on official international sources: "Let me tell you a story that the World Health Organization told the world in 1995." The account is tragically prosaic: "This is the story. The world's biggest killer and greatest cause of ill health and suffering across the globe is listed almost at the end of the International Classification of Diseases. It is given the code Z59.5—extreme poverty." Citing numerous epidemiological statistics, he recalls the differences in life expectancy worldwide and the proliferation of infectious diseases caused by malnutrition in poor countries: "As I listened to this tale of human woe, I heard the name recur with frightening frequency: Africa, Africa, Africa!" AIDS is thus the latest avatar of the scourge that lashes the continent, its ultimate product: "One of the consequences of this crisis is the deeply disturbing phenomenon of the collapse of immune systems among millions of our people, such that their bodies have no natural defense against attack by many viruses and bacteria." Then comes the conclusion, which would cause the scandal: "As I listened and heard the whole story told about our country, it seemed to me that we could not blame everything on a single virus." Once again justifying the convening of the Presidential Panel by the "desperate and pressing need to wage a war on all fronts," he ends by enumerating his government's actions for simultane-ously combating the disease and poverty. Few heard his final words, as by then the auditorium was half empty, many attendees having left in disapproval. Nelson Mandela's closing remarks, three days later, in which he distanced himself from all dissidence, had greater success.

There is no need to engage in a subtle exegesis of Mbeki's texts or to dissect his utterances on AIDS, as the South African press did: his stance is clearly influenced by dissident theses, in particular those that reject the virus's role and invoke instead chronic malnutrition and multiple infections. Under these circumstances the analyst that I propose to be has two possibilities: Either he can dismiss the president's thinking as irrational querying of the viral etiology of AIDS, in which case the terms of the debate become radicalized but simple, or he can try to grasp the particular rationality of Mbeki's thinking, suggesting a sociological interpretation of the epidemic, in which case one seeks a kind of third way, a means of making biological and social theories compatible, as was done more than a century ago for tuberculosis.[11] The first option seems to have been chosen by most actors in South Africa, as demonstrated by the entrenched warfare between Mbeki sympathizers and opponents in the media and in political and scientific circles. The second way is possible, however, and would not involve pleading moral relativism or renouncing scientific truth but would rather imply a different reading of history and a different conception of politics.

The social sciences have certainly lost out by keeping their distance from these arenas, in South Africa and elsewhere.[12] If, as Marilyn Strathern (2000) affirms, the time has come for "new accountabilities" in public action, this should apply first to those who claim to pronounce truths about societies. Ethics, she remarks, is "a social actor frequently enrolled to justify auditing practices, yet as frequently seen as betrayed by or in resistance to them" (1). In the context of South Africa, as in many others, ethics has readily been invoked to simplify the terms of the debate and, ultimately, to preclude thinking. The president's questioning of scientifically established facts, along with his repeated refusal to make antiretroviral drugs available, has been rightly criticized. But little concern has been shown by South African actors about the fact that biomedical theories do not take into account the structural components of the development of the epidemic or the realities of the majority of the population's daily lives, which are of crucial importance for grasping the gravity of the disease and its spread.

As Shula Marks (2002: 17), whose work on the history of public health and the medical profession in South Africa sheds light on present health issues, suggests, "The speed of its expansion is because, in many ways, HIV/AIDS was a pandemic waiting to happen." She recalls that the social context at the end of apartheid created particularly propitious conditions for widespread infection, in that it multiplied "high risk situations" (Zwi and Cabral 1991), namely, poverty, urbanization, work-related migration, forced population displacements, intensifying civil war, and dislocation of social structures. As Paul Farmer (1999: 9) observes, "It is unfortunate that these topics have been neglected in the social science and clinical literature on AIDS." The role of the political economy in South Africa's epidemic remains to be analyzed. If there had been more active opposition to the resolutely behaviorist and strictly medical approaches to the disease so dominant in international public health circles during the first two decades of AIDS, this might have opened a space for critical thinking of the sort Mbeki expressed without engaging him in a dialogue in which his only interlocutors were dissidents. Of course, this is only an optimistic hypothesis, but it should certainly be considered. In any case, it engages researchers' responsibility.

That the controversy sparked by the president's letter and speech reveals an insufficiently acknowledged kernel of truth is only one reason for the present study, however. The other is what their reception reveals. Just as in their study of scientific disputes sociologists of scientific knowledge realized they had to take into account both the content of conflicting theories and the agents' social positions, as Andrew Pickering (1992) recalls, so anthropologists of political crises have to grasp both the substance of arguments used and the configuration of social space thus created. In other words, they must produce an external and internal analysis. The public conflict that so profoundly divided not just elites but the whole of South African society is crucial for what it shows not only of the past that made possible the present realities of the epidemic but also of the present, in which it is proving so difficult to give the past its rightful place. In this respect AIDS in South Africa at the beginning of the twenty-first century is similar to cholera in the nineteenth-century British Empire as studied by David Arnold (1993). It reveals often invisible or obscured realities of the social world, prejudices, tensions, and power relations that already existed but were not perceived at the time. And these realities, to which I have dedicated most of this research, is <u>unquestionably political.</u>

What is a just society? A society that remembers, replies Thabo Mbeki. That answer contains a deep truth that many of his supporters are grateful to him for uttering and that the anthropologist is called on to understand. But it also eludes two other truths. <u>The first</u> is that democracy presupposes confrontation among truths; memory has to be fought for, and indeed, there can be no official version of memory in a democracy. <u>The second</u> is that governing implies having effects on people's lives; the consequence of errors can be devastating. It is these truths, even more violent, that make up the substance of Puleng's story.

A LIFE

They want me to open my heart and tell the story of a life lived in cages. They want to hear about all the cages I have lived in, as if I were a budgie or a white mouse or a monkey. And if I had learned story-telling instead of potato-peeling and sums, if they had made me practice the story of my life everyday, standing over me with a cane till I could perform without stumbling, I might have known how to please them.

J. M. COETZEE

Life and Times of Michael K.

I first met Puleng in April 2002. She was living in the township of Alexandra, in the heart of Johannesburg. The township is the oldest trace of racial

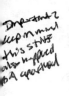

segregation in the city, dating back to long before the practice was legally instituted. Puleng lived in a cellar dug out beneath a shack made of wood and sheet metal, reached through narrow, winding alleys lined with houses and crisscrossed with laundry lines. At the bottom of a few stairs you entered a three-square-meter room that served as a kitchen and opened onto a bedroom. In the bedroom, devoid of natural light, stood only one real piece of furniture, the big bed she shared with her daughter and to which she was now nearly confined. That day, however, she had insisted on getting up for a few minutes to boil water and prepare tea. She had learned from the young volunteer worker who visited her several times a week that foreign researchers were studying AIDS in the neighborhood, and she had expressed the desire to speak to them about her illness and her life.

A Story So Simple

Puleng was twenty-nine. She must have weighed about thirty-five kilos. The angles of her emaciated body could be discerned under her nightgown; the exposed parts of her skin were covered with the disease's characteristic sores, visible in so many African patients. Her face, whose features appeared once to have been delicate and regular, was swollen with edema, especially around the eyelids, as in children suffering from kwashiorkor; she could barely open her eyes. She lay on the bed holding her face in her hands as she spoke to us.[13] She did not wait for our questions. No sooner had we sat down facing her than in a weak voice, barely audible because of the music the owners above us were listening to, Puleng began to speak.

> My name is Puleng. I was born in Baragwanath Hospital in 1973. I grew up in Soweto until the age of seven. Then I came to Alex in this same house where we are now. And this is where I always lived. When I was a child my father went away and my mother raised us alone. She tried so hard. But she drank too much. When she had taken alcohol, we used to sleep in the streets. I have a sister, she was born in 1976. I had a brother also, he was born in 1978, he was my best friend. He died when he was twenty, he was shot by the police, because he was accused of a car theft.
>
> Then came this disease. They told me about it in 1998. I never drank. I never smoked. I never had time to go to casinos. I only had four boyfriends in my whole life. The first one, when I was still in high school, he left me. The second one, I separated from him. The third one, he was married, I could not stay with him. And then the father of my child, I lived ten years with him. He was good to me. But he cheated me. I discovered he had another girlfriend. And his girlfriend died. I said to him:

"How could you do that to me? You're killing me now with this disease." When I told him about the disease, he didn't want to believe me. And he lied to me. He said to me he had done the test and when I asked the doctor, because we had the same one, he told me it wasn't true. . . . I'm not willing to have another boyfriend, now. We are living here happy with my child. She's twelve. She goes to school. I want her to be somebody.

So, you see, this is my life. A life of misery. We've been suffering so much. But I was talented. I used to write stories when I was a child. The first one, it was after reading a book on Florence Nightingale. And I liked to write poems. I even got a scholarship to study abroad. But there was a fire in my house and all my documents were burnt. I liked to study. I wanted to be a doctor, because it's nice to heal people. I was so talented. . . . Now, my life is sinking. But I'm very strong, very very strong. And I'll live until God decides I should pass away. I'd like to do many things. I told my family: "On my funeral day, I don't want you to prepare a meal." Because people act like at a party. It costs a lot of money. But what's the use, if I'm dead. It's only to put them in debt. No, I just want them to bury me. . . . But I don't think of that all the time. I thank God to have brought me in this world.

Puleng fell silent. In shadow hardly dispelled by the lightbulb, she laid her head on the pillow. She had recounted her story in one breath. We had not spoken. Later we would ask her a few questions, requesting details on certain aspects of her biography, trying to grasp what it was to live with an incurable disease that incurs social exclusion. She would relate the circumstances in which her brother was killed, she would tell us about her neighbors' rejection of her, she would criticize the government's health policy. And she would assure us too, with a sad smile, that at one time she had been "very pretty." For now, there is just the silence of the room, interrupted by the sounds coming from outside.

I have long wondered about the urgent need Puleng seemed to feel to narrate the story of her existence to us, why she confided in researchers she did not know, merely on the basis of what the volunteer worker had told her, why she gave such tight, definitive shape to her life, as if she were bearing the story inside her waiting to deliver herself of it. I have wondered too what I should do with this testimony collected on the threshold of death. What the terms of this exchange were in which I received her last, tragic gift of self. And what the trace of the life she transmitted to me, a life she knew was ending, meant.

Puleng died three months after we met. She had never received antiretroviral drugs, available then only through private pharmaceutical channels at prices utterly beyond reach of the vast majority of sick persons. She had just received approval for a disability grant, but the weeks spent going through the administrative procedures to obtain it meant that the first payment arrived just in time to pay her burial expenses. She left us the small school notebook I had brought her after she had expressed her desire to start writing again. She had only had time to write two pages, in which she basically retold the story she had related orally, concluding thus: "This is all I can share with you about my life. Thank you, all of you who make time to come and see me."

The Gift of the Self

Reflecting on the difficulty of representing violence in anthropology, Valentine Daniel ([1996] 2000: 334–335) recalls the circumstances that led him to focus on a question that he had not initially chosen to work on: "More than ten years have gone by since the responsibility of writing an anthropology of violence pierced, like a shriek in the dark, my world of other preoccupations." He was working then on Tamil culture in Sri Lanka: "I distinctly remember the moment of my commission. A daughter who had witnessed her father's murdered body being dragged away by the army Jeep to which it was tied said at one point in her interview with me: 'You're a man who has seen the world, please take this story and tell the world of what they did to my father, how they treated him.'" What the anthropologist should do seemed very clear: his mediation would make known what had been unknown until then. Through him, a truth might be told that would otherwise disappear forever. He was to carry the message to "a world where the difference between good and evil still holds, but also a world that needs to be told and must not be allowed to forget." The anthropologist's testimony thus answers for both a debt to the distant others and a moral obligation with regard to his own community.

But suddenly this obvious imperative is shaken: "At another point, in the same interview, she pleaded: 'Please don't tell anyone else this story. My father is such a dignified man. He never comes to dinner without bathing and without wearing a clean white shirt. I don't want anyone to remember him the way I see him, with his clothes torn off his body.'" To follow the new injunction, the anthropologist must then remain silent, preserve the person of the speaker and her anonymity, choose the right to confidentiality over the advent of truth. He becomes a silent witness of suffering that is ethically, if not practically, unspeakable. Or rather, the duty that falls to him is to choose "not only what story to tell and what not to tell, but how to and how not to tell a story." Clearly, this task cannot be articulated in simple prescriptive terms but, finally, seems more a matter of the researcher's inner conviction.

The position is itself potentially dangerous because like the doctor and the judge, who are "moral entrepreneurs" (Becker 1963), the anthropologist assumes the extraordinary right of deciding for the Other, and the only source of rules is, clearly enough in this example, what his "conscience" tells him. This is most likely to be the only tenable norm for the critical moment when confidences are offered,[14] when, troubling the serene confidence of scientific objectification and laying the foundation of necessarily problematic intersubjectivity, the respondent makes the interviewer the gift of her life, at least that part of it over which she still has control, what can and should be said of it. A critical moment, in that it reveals a truth about ethnography, its combined fragility and strength, the rationality on which it is based and the feelings that are mobilized, the insurmountable ambivalence that Michel Naepels (1998) calls the "ethnographic situation." Sympathy for or antipathy to one's interlocutor, adherence to or rejection of his or her ideas, implicit or explicit biases for or against persons or causes—all contribute to the social science discourse developed. A critical moment also because the researcher can no longer lay claim to "ethnographic authority," which James Clifford (1988) has shown means closing out knowledge of the Other, but must now rethink his scientific activity in terms of what could be called anthropological accountability. The statements one produces commit oneself not only with regard to one's peers but also with regard to those who agree to confide, and beyond them to the society one claims to interpret. The moment of my encounter with Puleng crystallized these questions, which for me are political as well as ethical.

In reproducing Puleng's narrative under her name and signature, thus breaking with the professional practice of anonymity that I followed in my earlier works and to which I return below, I hope not to have betrayed her intentions. It seems to me, given her choice of listeners, her willingness to be recorded, her transmission of a written text reiterating the oral version, her insistence on sharing her life story with others, that Puleng wanted to testify in the first person, to address her words directly to a world she did not know (and would have loved to travel to and discover, she told us). There is perhaps something remarkable, even suspicious, in the unlikely convergence of an anthropologist's interests, always on the lookout for stories, and the informant's interests, her longing to tell of herself—neither of them much concerned with the "biographical illusion" that Pierre Bourdieu (1986) criticized for diverting attention from the social processes underlying individual itineraries; both of them participating in the construction of contemporary societies' "culture of biographical revelation," wherein Paul Atkinson and David Silverman (1997) rightly discern the influence of the social sciences themselves.[15] No doubt anthropologists should keep in mind that "iconic figures" of misfortune have emotional rather than demonstrative value, that they illustrate their theses rather than prove them, as Leslie Butt (2002) points out for a series of recent studies in which vignettes of "the suffering other" are given as self-sufficient. Conversely, on the informants' side, they should analyze more in depth the meaning and implications of what Achille Mbembe (2002) affirms to be one of the dominant traits of African identity, a propensity to describe the self as victim.

Indeed, Puleng's act of narrating her life takes its source in a long history,[16] that of a subject speaking of self to others, or, in Foucault's terms, subjectification through "care of the self" as a specific way of being in the world. With AIDS, however, what Aloïs Hahn (1986) describes as "self-thematization," actualized in "confession rituals" and inscribed within a "process of civilization," has become a politics in the construction of which North American and European AIDS activists have played a decisive role, first in their own national spaces, then beyond their borders, in particular in Africa to which they have actively exported their models. The aim of this politics is threefold: to combat denial of the disease through sick persons' narratives and accounts; to fight against stigmatization by making it clear for all to see that large numbers of people are having similar experiences; and to hold the finality of death a bit at bay by reconstituting life stories. The South African health department created a traveling exhibition of thirty-two biographies pasted on boards, each accompanied by the person's photograph, a humanist and didactic illustration of the diverse origins and trajectories of people living with AIDS.[17] Meanwhile, at the instigation of charity and religious organizations, a practice has developed in the townships of making "memory boxes", either by the sick persons themselves or by families and friends after their deaths, assembling personal effects and autobiographical recordings, accounts destined primarily for the children that the dying leave behind.[18] Puleng's confidences were thus part of this South African social context, in which biographical or autobiographical narrative has become a political weapon for fighting AIDS. Hers was not a singular or unique initiative but rather part of an organized collective activity that has already produced many such testimonies and traces.

But the fact that her life narrative is part of a practice that may be qualified as "cultural," in the sense that it is deeply embedded in a space of conventions historically situated, does not exonerate the person who receives it from reflecting on its meaning. The narrative form, in the tight sketch version she used of it, is itself a language. It belongs to what Claude Polliak (2002) calls "ordinary ways of speaking of self." However, it reveals the presence of a code but not its meaning. The understanding of the group culture does not suspend all inquiry into the social agent's intention. Remarking that Puleng was probably unconsciously following autobiographical practices that the media, international organizations, and social science researchers have helped to spread does not mean there is no need to analyze what she meant in telling of herself. To make one's life into a story is not only to participate in the "tyranny of intimacy" denounced by Richard Sennett (1974) but perhaps above all to testify about what that life is.

Attesting to One's Existence

In defining the "human condition," Hannah Arendt ([1959: 85) described what distinguishes human and nonhuman life as follows: "The chief characteristic of this specifically human life, whose appearance and disappearance constitute worldly events, is that it is itself always full of events which ultimately can be told as a story, establish a biography; it is of this life, *bios,* as distinguished from mere *zoē*, that Aristotle said that it 'somehow is a kind of praxis.' For action and speech, which belonged close together in the Greek understanding of politics, are indeed the two activities whose end result will always be a story with enough coherence to be told, no matter how accidental or haphazard the single events and their causation may appear to be." Assembling the scattered fragments of one's life in order to give them communicable meaning is very simply what it means to live that life. Through this decision to give a biographical account of it, Puleng manifests a sense of life beyond its physiological definition, or *zoē*. And no matter how deeply determined her existence may be by the historical experience of being born and growing up in a township under apartheid, it has a unique meaning for herself and for others, which can be designated by the term *bios*. The difference between the two meanings is what makes humans human. That Puleng desired to narrate her life—"you see, this is my life"—

and to transmit that narrative—"this is all I can share with you about my life"—is enough to make that meaning a political reality, regardless of the cultural schemata her action may fit into. It is this political meaning that I propose to decipher.

Though the tone of her account is not indignant, I think that in recounting her life Puleng wanted to express a sense of the injustice of her condition. She does not speak self-pityingly. She does not look for compassion, even if she arouses it. "We've been suffering so much," she says, but immediately adds, "but I was so talented." And later: "Now my life is sinking," she laments, yet quickly insists, "but I am very strong." If we use Luc Boltanski's (1993: 16) distinction between two types of response to the pain and misfortune of the world, "politics of justice" and "politics of pity," this narrative should be understood as expressing an expectation of the former rather than the latter. The first goal of telling the story of her life is not to complain but to denounce its iniquity. It is not intended to produce tears for her suffering that she knows will end soon. It demands truth of the anthropologist and those to whom he will repeat it later. It is not only the fact of dying at twenty-nine from a disease reputed to be incurable that is an affront to the young woman; it is also and above all the accumulation of social violence that has made her existence what it is. AIDS is taking her life, but what life has it been? Her protest is not against a biological fate but against a political fact.

The violence she details is that of an ordinary existence during what was a state of emergency in the township: extreme poverty, physical insecurity, absent father, alcoholic mother, brother killed by the police, life lived in a cellar, school success never rewarded, hopes of a better future repeatedly shattered. With AIDS in the new democracy, she discovers new forms of violence: neighbors shun her when they learn what ails her; the government refuses to make effective therapeutic drugs available; she is to die in near-total destitution because the disability grant she applied for has not come; there is no hope of palliative care to soothe her last days, only the kind words of the charity volunteer. Hardly negligible is the violence of being a woman infected by an unfaithful partner, stigmatized for the moral fault that the disease is understood to carry; the violence of being abandoned by her partner, though he seems to have continued to help her for a time, of having nothing to hope for but a better existence for her daughter. Her life, she says at the end of her narrative, is that. In collecting the moments of her history precisely when they are in danger of disappearing forever, in producing this short narrative, she is seeking to show more than the disease.

Just as she insists that the deteriorating body others see was once desirable and that the drastic physical decline that drains her of all energy should not make us forget that she was a talented teenager, so she indicates that her life is not just a stretch of biological time that death is on the verge of ending but that it is also a social process inscribed in a particular collective history made of political violence, a history of which AIDS is not just the culmination but also one more episode.

Political violence extends beyond the apartheid regime's exercise of direct repression, of which Puleng's personal and family trajectory bear the indelible trace. It is also inherent in and produced by the imposition of a system based on the notion of racial inequality, with, at its core, a policy of segregation in which vast numbers of human beings are confined to narrow physical and legal space. There is political violence in separating family members as part of the overarching logic of exploiting the labor force and in devaluing people's existences through daily processes of disqualification. In describing living conditions in Brazilian favelas, Nancy Scheper-Hughes (1992) speaks of "the violence of everyday life." Paul Farmer (1997), presenting biographies of AIDS victims in Haiti, refers to "structural violence."[19] By using the term *political violence,* I mean simply to recall that politics in the broadest sense concerns the ways in which citizens are enabled to live together. Beyond the experience of the disease as suffering, it is Puleng's experience of politics as violence—historical, social, gendered, ordinary—that I believe she was seeking to transmit to us. In this sense her account is profoundly political.

Social scientists need to take a lesson from it. In fact, the anthropology of AIDS long limited itself to analyzing risk behaviors, especially in Africa.[20] As Randall Packard and Paul Epstein (1992: 354) have written, "The medical research community expected the social scientist to adhere to the dominant behavioral model. Constructed in this way, the question immediately narrowed the range of sociological data relevant for the discussion. It became not: 'What is the social context within which HIV transmission occurs in Africa'? but rather: 'What are the patterns of behavior which are placing the Africans at risk of infection?' While the first construction would have allowed for open-ended discussion of a wide range of social, political and economic conditions that might be affecting health levels in Africa, the latter formulation quickly narrowed discussion to an inquiry into the 'customs of the natives.'" Not only is this approach to the problem ineffective, as many studies conducted since have shown, it is also unjust, because it leads to laying responsibility for their affliction on people with AIDS themselves, a classic reversal of the order of things that consists in "blaming the victim." This reasoning has not been applied to Africans alone; in Europe, for instance, there has been a constructed representation of hemophiliacs as "innocent victims," implicitly suggesting that any others are not. When Puleng hurries to deny having engaged in socially deviant practices and indicates her modest number of lovers, she is rebelling against this understanding of her contamination. How can it be that she has AIDS, she who has never drunk or smoked and has known only four men? To tell her story is to denounce an injustice that consists not only in dying so young but also in not even being able to denounce this as unjust.

In passing on Puleng's words, I am not trying to illustrate an argument on AIDS, suffering, or inequality. However factually exact it may be, her narrative is of less interest to me as restitution of her biography—for which I would need more details and verifications, a larger context and a more precise chronology—than as a process of subjectification—in producing it she constituted herself as a subject. But this operation does not proceed out of Cartesian interiority (the subject of self-consciousness) to which anthropologists have no access since they know only how to listen to words and observe actions. As Veena Das (1997) says of the suffering of the Indian women whose narratives of kidnapping and rape she collected, I am tempted to say that Puleng's suffering "eludes me." I think I can apprehend it, yet it is necessarily inaccessible to me, since I can only see her body and listen to her sentences, and as Wittgenstein explained, it is illusory to think we can know the meaning that her body and sentences have for her: such a belief is what Jacques Bouveresse (1976) calls "the myth of interiority." What I do know, however, which presupposes no particular psychological hypothesis, is that Puleng wanted to meet with us, tell us her story, tell us of her life in the township, tell us that she objected to the injustice of her illness, its social causes, and others' moral judgment of her. In Puleng's case, as for so many other persons I met after her, the speaking subject speaks up and out. She affirms herself as a subject with rights. She claims her rights to a physical as well as to a social existence, to *zoē* and *bios*. The only type of subjectification process I can report on and account for is thus political.

What is a human life? To this question Puleng gives her answer, not only in recounting her own, but also in uttering through her narrative the universal truth that a life is a story within a history. It is a political experience of living with others, and, for her, of the inequality one is subjected to and of the injustice one denounces.

April 2001. In black letters on a wall in Johannesburg may be read the following words: "As if nothing ever happened." No other phrase seems to me to sum up so succinctly the complex and ambivalent relationship of South African society to its memory.

For decades South African democrats both in the country and in exile lived their history in the future tense. To use Rheinhardt Koselleck's (1990) categories for conceiving human relation to time, we could say that the struggle against apartheid was their "field of experience" and apartheid's end their "horizon of expectation." Doctor Burger, whose memory haunts the characters in Nadine Gordimer's *Burger's Daughter*, published in 1979, can stand as a fictional image of these violent years. A courageous man, devoted entirely to the antiapartheid struggle, he sacrifices the present, his family, his freedom, and ultimately his life for a better future in which blacks and whites will participate in the same democratic project. Significantly, the epigraph of the work is from an anthropologist, Claude Lévi-Strauss: "I am the place where something happened." It was a time of certitudes, the present turned toward a radiant future that could not fail to come. In 1994, with the fall of the dehumanizing regime, the longed-for future became the lived present.

For many observers, the "New South Africa" was to triumph over the detested era, the experience of which nearly everyone had an interest in repressing: those who had been victims, because it was associated for them with memories of destitution and humiliation; those who had promoted apartheid, because history had turned against them; those who had combated it, because they wanted to turn the page. The extraordinary feat of averting civil war on the eve of the first democratic elections and the improbable pacification achieved despite predictions of violent division reassured those who wanted simply to move on, especially since everything had happened so quickly. A friend of mine, a professor of medicine, who had been previously categorized as "Coloured," told me how persons who the day before had brushed past him in the hospital corridor with indifference or contempt had suddenly smiled and become friendly. Remarkable tabula rasa. In fact, this situation confirmed Renan's profound intuition: "Oblivion and I would even say factual historical error are essential factors in the creation of a nation." In order for the "rainbow" to hold, the bad memories had to be erased, or rather, contained in specific institutions, such as the Truth and Reconciliation Commission, or the Museum of Apartheid, where the history presented, however authentic and poignant, is also by definition official history or restricted to the confined spaces of historians' books and seminars, where scholarly critiques reach a small, well-educated audience.

But this is not how time flows in real life. In South Africa's new temporal configuration, the horizon of expectation has been superimposed on the field of experience, the one contradicting the other. The past has been rejected and the future has disappeared. What remains is a dense present, where the experience of today is inextricably mixed with a yesterday that dogs it, unacknowledged, and a tomorrow so long hoped-for and already disappointing. The segregation laws no longer exist, but racist practices continue. Civil liberties have been acquired, but social inequalities grow sharper. Political violence has ceased, but ordinary crime is mounting. And those who fought side by side for a better tomorrow clash at times from where they stand on the different sides of yesterday's color line. What is relevant here is the sense of despairing disenchantment in Coetzee's *Disgrace,* published in 1999. While the moral touchstones of the South Africa portrayed here are being lost, its social and race relations endure and lead to grim violence inherited from the recent past. At the end the resignation of the hero thus echoes the renouncement of the author himself who chose to leave his country for Australia.

Other responses are possible, however. I read in the newspaper one day that a friend of mine, a professor at the university, long active in the Mass Democratic Movement, had been told by the minister of health in response to a comment she had made about AIDS that, as a white person, she could not understand what black people felt about it. When I mentioned this anecdote to her, she said she did not remember and preferred in any case not to talk about it. Perhaps in choosing to be silent she was following an intuition not to deepen divisions, and she was respecting the practical wisdom of giving things time. As a citizen of the world, I can only approve of her attitude. As a social analyst, however, and from a position admittedly less difficult and delicate than that of my friend at that moment, I would rather cite Marc Bloch (1993: 61): "Ignoring the past not only harms understanding of the present but compromises present action." Exploration of the strata of time in South African lives reminds us of the obvious fact that the mark of apartheid is still deeply inscribed in bodies.

Memory, buried deep, does not disappear. History relentlessly resurfaces. In a knowing smile or a racist crime. In words blurted out and a gesture one regrets. This is what AIDS in South Africa reveals, through the experience of the sick and the violence of the controversies. Paul Ricoeur (2000: 554) understood memory as inscribed in three ways: documentary, through the "archive"; biological, in the "brain"; and last, "the most problematic but also the most meaningful" way, "consisting in the persistence of passively registered first impressions," or, to put it differently, what happens when "an event strikes, touches, affects us" and "its mark remains in our mind." I am interested here in this third type of inscription. But I believe Ricoeur's analysis is insufficient in two ways. First, it is not only a passive impression left on the mind; it is also the result of a permanent work of mobilization, reappropriation, reinterpretation. Second, it is not limited to the immateriality of the mind; it is present in the materiality of the body, in its conduct, feelings, deterioration. This embodiment of memory has two dimensions. One corresponds to the way in which past facts are inscribed in objective realities of the present; it accounts for the fact that Puleng became ill and did not have access to treatment because of her life in the township under apartheid and the immediate postapartheid years, and likewise for what Mbeki was referring to in speaking so explosively of the social causes of AIDS. The other consists in the way past facts are inscribed in the subjective experience of the present; it is what is reflected in Mbeki's references to apartheid and the accusations of racism he makes, and it is what Puleng tells us of her sense of injustice. Through this twofold inscribing, memory becomes actualized. In order for the future to continue to be what Arendt calls a "promise," it is necessary to recognize that the past is indeed present.

"As if nothing ever happened." But something did happen, of which I seek here the lasting trace.

TWO

An Epidemic of Disputes

His people wondered. They heard him softly humming,
humming a chant such as no one had ever heard.

GUY BUTLER
"Ntsikana's Bell"

"A GREAT DEAL OF ATTENTION has been devoted, locally and internationally, to issues raised by South Africa over HIV and AIDS. To put the issues
beyond doubt in the public mind, particularly so that the battle against this
scourge may proceed with full vigour, the following statement is issued by
the government. Neither the President nor his Cabinet colleagues have ever
denied a link between HIV and AIDS." On September 17, 2000, the Government Communications Service issued this astonishing statement in the
form of an advertisement in the *Sunday Independent* headlined "Response
to Enquiries and Comments on HIV/AIDS," which all the newspapers in
the country picked up over the following days. The statement was made necessary by the strong reactions to an interview with Thabo Mbeki published
in *Time* magazine on September 11. After an exchange of generalities about
economic and political life in South Africa, the reporter had posed the question she thought everyone was expecting: "Are you prepared to acknowledge
that there is a link between HIV and AIDS?" To which Mbeki had retorted
a very definite "No." At a time when all the media were urging South Africa's
president to speak up—the *Weekly Mail and Guardian* had pleaded on its
front page on September 15, "Just Say Yes, Mr. President"—his answer
seemed final indeed. The government's statement thus tried to clarify the
matter by providing evidence from "the full transcript of the President's interview," which it said could be accessed on the government homepage and

on *Time* magazine's website. It thus entered into a complicated textual analysis: "The published version, on which many critics depend, conflated his remarks in a way which could give rise to a misunderstanding over his generic or nonspecific use of the word 'no' after being asked if he was prepared to acknowledge that there is a link between HIV and AIDS. In fact the President went on to say that 'you cannot attribute immune deficiency solely and exclusively to a virus.' The context of the full transcript makes it expressly clear that he was prepared to accept that HIV might 'very well' be a causal factor." Mbeki presented his technical argument in the same interview: "If you go through the literature, ordinary standard literature available in medical schools, there will be a whole variety of things that can cause the immune system to collapse. Endemic poverty, the impact of nutrition, contaminated water, all those things will result in immune deficiency. If you take the African context, you add things like repetitive infections of malaria, syphilis, gonorrhea, etc. All of these will result in immune deficiency. Now, it is perfectly possible that among those things is a particular virus." The unusual fact that the South African administration felt it necessary to justify itself in the country's major newspapers and that it should have done so by going into muddled explanations of what was meant, publicly returning to a medical discussion that everyone thought had been settled once and for all, is evidence enough of the exceptional nature of AIDS in South Africa. Science challenged by the authorities. Politicians playing scientists. A negative adverb stirring up endless and surreal discussions to avoid being accused of denial. More than anywhere else, public health is a passionate subject in South Africa. But what is at stake is precisely what such passions reveal— and what the anthropologist must try to account for.

Studies on health policies are often tedious. When they do more than just superficially report on the policies they either criticize them for what they claim to be doing or blame them for what they have not done. But whether they accuse them of doing too much (in words) or of not doing enough (in acts), they generally reveal more of what researchers suppose is or should be good policy rather than explain the meaning of actual government action. More often than not, they teach us less about the way societies handle health care issues than about the degree to which researchers adhere or reject the rhetoric and actions of those working in the field of public health.[1] In this respect, sociologists and anthropologists might benefit from the work of historians, who, through their surveys of illnesses and the medical profession, often manage to bring the human social dimension to situations that medical language tends to disembody. The history of epidemics in the West and in the colonial empires, in particular, considerably enriched and even renewed our knowledge about those societies.[2] AIDS is thus an integral part of those long-lasting biological events that have become political facts. Of this, contemporary South Africa is a striking example.

Epidemics are moments of truth when both knowledge and power are put to the test. Doctors test their theories, and citizens expect concrete results from the authorities. This well-known and often-recorded fact, along with the transformations it brings about in the field of science and the destabilizing effect it has on the current government, has led to interpreting epidemics as factors of social change. It would be closer to reality, however, to regard them as factors that reveal states of the world that are already there but could just as well never materialize. They are revealing in the sense of unveiling. In the same vein, in her discussion of AIDS in Great Britain, Virginia Berridge (1992) has shown that though it appears to raise some new questions the epidemic is in fact part of a "preexisting agenda": the anxieties, interpretations, and answers that follow in its wake correspond to moral, cultural, and political configurations that were already hinted at in the social world. Referring to surveys conducted in France, Michaël Pollak (1992) similarly observes that discriminatory attitudes against people affected by the illness rest on "preexisting stigmas," aggravated by the negative associations connected to the infection: by defining them as risk groups, epidemiology reinforces the already existing negative images of homosexuals, prostitutes, or immigrants. The epidemic thus invents nothing; it uncovers. It is a biological phenomenon that shakes or strengthens the existing social structures and representations but does not create them ex nihilo. Seen in this way, the crises provoked by AIDS deserve our attention for what they contribute to a general history of society as much as for what they contribute to the history of illness or medicine. "We have learned very little that is new about the disease, but much that is old about ourselves," a doctor wrote during the polio epidemic in New York in 1916.[3] Much the same may be said about AIDS in Johannesburg in 2000.

The South African epidemic is thus a powerful lens on postapartheid society. But a study of the epidemic becomes obscured by the passions it unleashed and the cleavages it created. What makes understanding it especially necessary is therefore paradoxically what at the same time makes it impossible to understand. To quote Paula Treichler (1999: 2), "of all the metaphors generated by the AIDS epidemic, AIDS as a war—a long, devastating, savage, costly, expensive, and continuing war—best helps us consider this question." From this perspective, the war waged around the various meanings is certainly not less violent. It has torn apart South African society virtually since the day after the 1994 democratic elections. This semantic war is far more than a confrontation between different explanatory models. It is a confrontation between worldviews, ways of relating to history and memory, definitions of morals and politics. In the end, the choices made for prevention and treatment are about the lives of individuals and the future of populations. It is far more than a problem of good governance, of policy making and political leadership, as Sean Jacobs and Richard Calland (2002) would have us think when assessing the meaning of the controversy.

But as it is a war of meanings, it is also a test for the social sciences, since they participate in the semantics through which the meaning of the epidemic is construed. How then can we account for AIDS? How far should we distance ourselves from it? What involvement should we claim? Let us return to the historians. Charles Rosenberg (1988: 18) writes, "The most frightening and novel of nineteenth-century European and American epidemics, cholera is the closest modern analogy to AIDS." Clearly, the remark is debatable. I would, however, like to consider it here not as a theoretical hypothesis but as a methodological postulate. As such it is less a matter of carrying out a comparison between the two epidemics than of asserting that the facts about AIDS in Africa today can be studied with the same instruments and following the same procedures as those produced when Europe was overtaken by cholera. In other words, it should be possible to make a history of AIDS at the beginning of the twenty-first century in a way similar to the history of cholera at the beginning of the nineteenth. Such a proposition to introduce a study of the controversy that is presently dividing South African society, and the international scientific community as well, means claiming the right (or at least suggesting the possibility) to treat it as an object for sociological inquiry through which a better understanding of society might be gained—in other words, to consider a history of the contemporary as a legitimate discourse. In South Africa such an approach goes against the mainstream, which, on the contrary, continues to demand that everyone take sides. The desire to extract oneself from this false dilemma makes one suspect. Refusing to condemn President Mbeki and his allies means a fortiori being open to heretical theories.

To counter these prejudices, I want to defend the "principle of symmetry" that Bruno Latour (1988: 41) claimed was the basis of the anthropology of science, though this claim of course applies to all anthropology. But he adds that one should not to limit oneself to this principle alone as this would just amount to ordinary relativism: "It is useless to pretend that all systems of thought and all programs of truth are equivalent, since precisely they do their utmost not to be, to gain the upper hand in relation to the others and, in certain cases, to prevail." It is therefore necessary to "reinject a certain asymmetrical quality into the analysis," for it must be acknowledged that "nuclear physics has won over witchcraft and that this victory too must be explained." On that matter, I want to comment on a fact that I find quite troubling. Several years ago, while working on witchcraft and more generally on those acts called magic in West Africa, I was able to preserve the points of view of the actors (in that case the healers and diviners) by transmitting their own words in my written and oral presentations but never answering the question that was put to me so many times: "What do *you* think of these stories?"[4] I had thought, as far as the South African polemic on AIDS was concerned, that I might avoid expressing my convictions on the viral etiology of the illness and deal with the subject according to what seemed to me the customary ethical behavior in my field. But my optimism was short-lived, for having been challenged several times in South Africa and elsewhere, I came to realize that it was best to declare my orthodox position on biomedical affairs outright so as not to interfere with the points that were important to me—which have to do with politics more than science, domination more than dissidence.

That is where my analysis departs from the sociology of science. The issues about the role of the virus, the effectiveness of the antiretroviral drugs, or the reliability of epidemiological statistics are only pertinent from my perspective here as long as they contribute to answering, not the question, what is science? very legitimately put by Alan Chalmers (1987), but the question posed by Hannah Arendt (1995), what is politics? Dissidence is part of my research program not as a contribution to or a critique of a theory of knowledge but essentially because it echoes the preoccupations and the realities of South Africa, its leaders and its citizens. I am not interested in Peter Duesberg but in Thabo Mbeki. Or rather—as making the controversy personal blurs its understanding—it is not the cultural symptom that Duesberg and his disciples in the scientific domain represent that is important to me but the political fact that his ideas have been taken up by Mbeki and his allies. Saying this will not prevent me from exploring those ideas and discussing them, but I try to do it as a contribution to a better understanding of power relations in South Africa and the world.

I have already mentioned the apparent boredom intrinsic in many studies on health policies. There are at least two reasons for this. First, they are not fleshy enough, imprisoning their analyses in systems of norms and institutional problems. They do not allow us to see the men and women in charge, their beliefs and interests, what they disagree about and fight over. The history of South Africa reminds us, often tragically, that opposite rationales may clash, that emotions may explode, and finally that health care policies are not only about health. But, second, these studies tend to take at face value things that in my opinion do not at all go without saying; for example, that health is humankind's most precious possession and that everybody thinks so, or that sick people and doctors share the same interests, or that prevention is better than cure. There again, the South African controversy shows us that all this is not necessarily so, that the debate goes on not only about health care policies but also about health as a political issue. As can sometimes be heard in South Africa, among all the problems facing the government and society as a whole, AIDS has become high politics.

BEGINNINGS

There are so many lies in this world.

THAMI VILAKAZI

"Maskanda's Song of the City"

"Politics has inappropriately taken center stage in the South African response to the AIDS epidemic with the publication of the open letter from President Mbeki stating that 'whatever lessons we have to and may draw from the West about the grave issue of HIV/AIDS, a simple superimposition of the Western experience on African reality is absurd and illogical.'" In the eyes of the international scientific community the affair had to be quite serious since the prestigious journal *Science* dedicated its editorial to the subject on May 19, 2000, and since it was written by an African researcher—an exceptional occurrence indeed. But it also called for a great deal of courage on the part of Malegapuru William Makgoba, at that time president of the Medical Research Council, South Africa's highest scientific authority in medicine, to thus oppose in the eyes of the world the chief of state, with whom he had shared exile in Great Britain, by denouncing in no uncertain terms "the dangers of pseudo-science" (this proved the end of his special friendship with his former "comrade"). The editorial concluded: "The current political and scientific furor in South Africa, fuelled largely by dissidents' theories on HIV/AIDS and the seeming support of Mr. Mbeki, has much broader implications for South Africa and South Africans than some are prepared to admit. We cannot afford to make any more mistakes lest history judges us to have collaborated in one of the greatest crimes of our time." On July 6 the equally prestigious rival journal *Nature* published a disclaimer in the form of a petition known as the "Durban declaration," signed by more than five thousand physicians and researchers among whom, once again, was Makgoba.[5] The title of the piece, "African Scientists Join Colleagues in Affirming HIV's Role in AIDS," suggests that, for the author, the appearance of the signatures of African scientists (explicitly listed) along with those of Western ones (implicitly qualified) at the bottom of the declaration was in itself remarkable. Whatever the case may be, the publication of these two articles was a turning point in the history of the controversy. The affair was no longer simply national; it had spread worldwide. But although the global scientific community was to discover its most recent episode at the Thirteenth International AIDS Conference, the story of the epidemic had long been agitating the South African scene.[6] In fact, the story had begun in 1996.

A Scandalous Play

"At Long Last, *Sarafina III!*" The title of Robert Kirby's article on the Durban conference in the *Weekly Mail and Guardian* on July 14, 2000, was as mysterious to the foreign visitor unfamiliar with the political situation of South Africa as it was transparent for its citizens. Kirby's title refers to the musical *Sarafina,* which had received popular acclaim and to its supposedly didactic remake, *Sarafina II,* whose misadventures had occupied the government gossip column for several years. Like a political satirist, he was dishing out the old joke about the health minister looking for a new episode to continue the saga, which once unanimously popular had become a bone of contention. He was suggesting that through its bad taste and eclecticism, mixing art and politics, the inaugural ceremony of the Durban conference was just such a continuation.

The opening of the remake had taken place on World AIDS Day, December 1, 1995, in the KwaZulu-Natal province, which already was the hardest hit by the epidemic.[7] To demonstrate its will to implement preventive action among large segments of the population, the National Health Department had chosen the famous play *Sarafina* and asked its author and producer, Mbongeni Ngema, to adapt it to the educational needs of the mobilization against AIDS. Many experiments in Africa and elsewhere had already used theater as a legitimate cultural medium for prevention propaganda. Though not really original, the idea therefore showed a real desire to take the problem seriously and to look for solutions suitably adapted to local situations. A year earlier, the new health minister, Nkosazana Zuma, had also launched an ambitious program to fight AIDS, combining information programs, distribution of condoms, treatment of venereal diseases, and campaigns to stop discrimination against patients. Though the budget then allocated to AIDS amounted to only 20 million rands, Zuma announced that it would soon be multiplied by five thanks to international aid from the European Union and USAID. She stressed that, to guarantee the success of her plan, she was counting on the volunteer associations and professional groups that she knew well as former president of the strategic committee of the National Aids Co-ordinating Committee of South Africa (NACOSA).[8] Conscious, however, of the difficulty of her job, she ended her inaugural speech with a lucid and even prescient appraisal of the situation: "This gives us a fighting chance. The last government did try, but it had a history of controlling people's lives, so people saw AIDS prevention as another form of control. I don't think it's going to be easy for us, but we stand a better chance." Even this moderate show of optimism was to prove excessive.

Only a few weeks after the opening of the play, at the beginning of February 1996, the scandal exploded when the amount of money put into the show by the health minister became known. The contract signed with the successful author and producer amounted to 14 million rands (about U.S. $3 million at the time), approximately one-fifth of the budget devoted to combating AIDS. Moreover, the decision had not gone through normal channels but had circumvented the usual mechanisms for the allocation of public funds. Also, in spite of her promise to do so, Zuma had not brought the associations into the picture. In her defense, she claimed that all the provincial administrations had given their approval but that one could not expect every nongovernmental organization (NGO) to be contacted: "AIDS doesn't consult, it infects people," she declared, adding: "Perhaps people are jealous because the money was given to a black person." The director general of the Health Department, Olive Shisana, similarly justified the choice of her services and the cost of the production, explaining that it was not the South African taxpayer who was financing the project but the European Union, which had subsidized it. "Who is to say life is not worth 14 million rands?" she asked, and concluded, "We are not apologetic about what we have done. The previous government paid no attention to the AIDS crisis. The new government has allocated 70 million rands to AIDS, while the apartheid one gave only 20 million." But this was not the end of the story. The health minister was summoned in front of Parliament, where she faced virulent attacks from the opposition, especially from the Democratic Party spokesman, Mike Ellis, who demanded an audit. It was later said that the session at which she was to be confronted by the Parliamentary Health Commission, presided over by Manto Tshabalala, was postponed because of direct pressure from President Nelson Mandela himself, who was thereby hoping to contain the affair. A vain hope.

The recently appointed Public Protector, occupying the traditional function of ombudsman, was given the delicate task of evaluating the scandal and assigning responsibility for it. It was his first important assignment and was considered a test of his independence vis-à-vis the executive branch. His report, released at the beginning of June, pointed to the financial director, Hugo Badenhorst, and his deputy, Johnny Angelo, who had been responsible for allocating the funds. The health minister and the director general were spared. The conclusion was that, given the irregularities that had taken place, the play had to be closed. A few days later, Nkosazana Zuma was again in Parliament and once again violently attacked by the opposition, especially the National Party and the Democratic Party,[9] whose representatives asked for her resignation. She acknowledged her mistake in not following normal procedure but repeated she was convinced the play had pedagogical value; nevertheless, she announced it would be closed. She added that the public funds allocated to honor the contract would be canceled and that a private donation would cover the Ministry's debt. Deputy President Thabo Mbeki sent a message reiterating Nelson Mandela's continued support of his minister. The affair could have stopped there. But the press and the politicians continued their harassment.

In July, at the Eleventh International Conference on AIDS in Vancouver, Canada, the health minister was interrupted in the middle of a speech on her country's policy by Gary Lamont, an activist who, amid questions shouted by members of his Cape Town organization, Wola Nani, demanded she explain the *Sarafina II* affair. Later, in an interview by a South African paper, Lamont criticized the minister, saying that "just about every AIDS agency had lost confidence in her" and that "social upliftment is the best route to slowing the spread of AIDS." Once back in Johannesburg, Nkosazana Zuma again had to cope with the inquisitive press and members of Parliament, who were this time trying to pin down the name of the mysterious and generous donor to the production of *Sarafina II*. A couple of leaks allowed Mike Ellis to announce that this was none other than the wealthy businessman Vivian Reddy, who reacted by accusing the Democratic Party's health spokesman of launching this campaign because of his connections with the pharmaceutical lobby, which feared criticism from the health minister, and by declaring that pharmaceutical companies had paid for several of the spokesman's trips abroad. Ellis then had to admit publicly that he had indeed benefited from Smithkline Beecham and Hoechst's generosity for various trips he and his wife had made but said this was usual practice for such companies and that they had not told him how to act. Finally, President Nelson Mandela intervened to defend Health Minister Nkosazana Zuma, adding that the "*Sarafina* saga was only a smoke screen to mask the multinational firms' attempts to throw her off balance." From incident to incident and from one declaration to another, the scandal was thus periodically revived, monopolizing public mention of the epidemic, gradually weakening government action by letting the public think that at the highest level AIDS was a subject of lies and swindles.

The *Sarafina II* affair is generally considered not only the first episode in a long series of controversies that have poisoned politics in the mobilization against AIDS but also the beginning of the end of the exceptional state of grace that had blessed the new government. In hindsight, there is nonetheless a tremendous difference between the supposed seriousness of the facts and the attention they received. The criticisms are mainly of two kinds. The first is that public funds had been depleted, the allocated sums appearing excessive compared to what was being delivered; also, the messages that were supposed to be transmitted, compared to the complex realities of transmission, seemed simplistic to say the least. However, though certain people said that two million rands should have been enough to stage the musical, the amount provided for in the contract hardly seemed excessive in the light of the Department of Health's budget; and even if the didactic project about condom use only promised slim results, it was merely one aspect of the program. The second complaint was that the normal channels for allocating public funds had not been respected and that organizations active in the fight against AIDS had been left out of the decision; these mistakes were aggravated by the arrogance of the health minister and her director general in the first weeks of the crisis. Nevertheless, in contrast to the administrative dysfunction of the health authorities, other practices were in greater conformity with the rules of government action, as can be seen from the government's strict implementation of the conclusions of the Public Protector's audit.

It is thus significant that not a single voice was raised to say the new

Health Department was entitled to a few mistakes, to remind the public that no government could be expected to master in only two years all the intricacies of a democracy that the country had not previously known. Instead, the most definitive verdicts were pronounced, the most serious accusations thrown, the severest sanctions demanded. Given the country's history, this style of tongue-lashing—inherited from the activism of Western countries—seemed quite out of place for the health officials. That the criticisms appear to ignore or underestimate the accomplishments of the new regime—and that they emanate for the most part from young white men—was deeply unacceptable to the government. As Mark Heywood, then a member of the AIDS Law Project, which was to become the main pillar of the Treatment Action Campaign set up to ensure access to antiretroviral therapy several years later, was to observe: "There was an assumption that there would be immediate recognition that AIDS would be a national priority—but it wasn't. We talked about a broad response but we also talked about AIDS as if it's the only thing government had to deal with and this contributed to our failure to find an entry point."[10] Generally speaking, all those who had fought for a just society seemed to imagine that after living through the long years of apartheid in exile or in prison, government members would emerge fully armed to take on the many challenges that awaited them: such passionate reactions give the measure of their disappointment. As to the others, who had accepted the changes passively or who had tried actively to stop the democratic process, they multiplied the pitfalls and rejoiced at every false step: their fierce attacks on the politicians in charge were fueled by bitterness. The former were erasing the traces of the past; the latter were looking back with regret. Lack of realism on one side, excessive cynicism on the other: in the crisis provoked by the *Sarafina II* affair, it is likely that the government was harmed more deeply by its so-called friends than by its actual enemies.

From that point of view, the most serious consequence is that yesterday's allies lost faith in each other. On the side of the activist organizations and professional groups striving to combat AIDS, it was now a foregone conclusion that the government intended to implement its policy without them, even against them, for the health minister made no secret about it: that is how the cut in public funds allotted to the NGOs, down from 19 million to 2 million rands in 1998, was interpreted. For Gary Adler, executive director of the AIDS Foundation, the scandal "threw the national AIDS directorate into disarray and with it came the demise of a shared vision for AIDS in this country." On the governmental side and mainly from the point of view of the Health Department, the besieged fortress syndrome was uppermost; the department felt misunderstood, if not betrayed, since only the drawbacks and never the successes of their actions, however spectacular, were pointed out. In a rare moment, Nkosazana Zuma confided, "I've never received good press, everything I touch is attacked." In strong contrast to the spiteful tone of most commentators, Jim Day, in one of the only positive articles covering the government's achievements in public health, wrote, "Despite scandals, unauthorized spending and a history of putting her foot in it, Dr. Nkosazana Zuma's Health Department is systematically revolutionizing South Africa's health care system. She is blamed by many for the fourteen-million-rand Sarafina II disaster, but many health workers acknowledge the radical changes she has set in motion during the past three years. Her ministry has developed a policy of free public health care for all, has built hundreds of new clinics and has begun reallocating funds from tertiary hospitals to primary health care facilities." Day went on to list the significant advances achieved in just a few years.[11] But this balanced assessment, aside from remaining an isolated instance, came too late. The harm was done.

Aside from the strictly political ins and outs of this first crisis, one must be attentive to what it reveals about the sociology of the "New South Africa." If we look closely at the debates that have accompanied it, what most stand out are the themes that will be woven into the narrative and argumentative fabric of future controversies: apartheid as a countermodel; priority on the value of human life; the intrinsically legitimate nature of government action; insinuations that attacks by opposition members have racist overtones; the suggestion that there is a conspiracy within the international pharmaceutical industry. A second polemic, more violent still, will reinforce this pattern.

An Embarrassing Discovery

"In a special presentation to the full Cabinet today, the team of scientists said results of preliminary trials conducted in Pretoria on about a dozen patients, using a formula patented as Viroden P058, suggested a breakthrough in the fight against AIDS. The entire Cabinet stood up and applauded on completion of the presentation, at which two of the trial patients were present." The story reported by the daily *Cape Argus* on January 22, 1997, and repeated by all the South African newspapers the day after, is probably unheard of in the annals of health policy.[12] It was a bizarre venture, indeed: a laboratory technician named Olga Visser, said to have invented the miracle drug, together with a pharmacologist, Eugen Olivier, and two cardiothoracic surgeons, Dirk du Plessis and Kallie Landauer, both from Pretoria University, to substantiate their results in front of an audience of ministers, had brought along two patients in treatment and a few statistics. A no less unusual procedure consisted in having the government hear a report of scientific results even before the results had been validated by the official clinical experimentation authorities and published by traditional medical journals, with the sole justification the supposed urgency of needing 3.7 million rands to pursue their promising investigations.[13] The measures decided by the health minister when organizing this little event were, however, as exceptional as what was being promised by those scholars, whose work she had been following for some time. The newspaper editorial summed it up: "Millions of AIDS sufferers in even the world's poorest countries may benefit from a medicine developed by South African researchers, who claim it has produced far better results and is much cheaper than any other drug or combination of drugs on the market." Given the importance of the issue, this secret well kept was tantamount to a state secret.

The very next day, emotions in the country ran high. Patients rushed to get information and to offer to serve as test subjects. An article evokes the dramatic atmosphere in South Africa: "Prisoners at Pollsmoor Prison yesterday morning were among thousands of people living with HIV/AIDS who openly rejoiced at the news of a drug breakthrough only to have their hopes dashed later in the day when the claim was denied. The prisoners were so excited that they demanded to be included in trials for the new 'wonder drug,' Virodene. They are excluded from trials for expensive AZT and 3TC drug cocktails, which retail at 4,000 rands a month and have to be taken over three years." When questioned by the press, South African AIDS specialists expressed surprise but declined to say anything definite since they had never heard of the researchers or their work. As the science editor of the *Weekly Mail and Guardian* wrote, "Pretoria University was unable to provide curriculum vitae for the scientists, or information on their research achievements and funding. However, the researchers have had some international success in their field of cryogenics—the preserving of live organs." Already, the Medicines Control Council, which authorizes clinical testing and evaluates drugs before they can be put on the market, let it be known through its director, Peter Folb, that it was opposed to the continuation of the experiments, considering that ethical and methodological standards for the clinical trial were not being observed.

In the hours that followed, more information was disclosed. Olga Visser was at the origin of the discovery: while freezing rat hearts, she realized that the substance she was using had accidentally killed a virus; she then contacted her thoracic surgeon colleagues to discuss possible experiments on humans; but the composition of the product remained a mystery. It was her husband, Zigi Visser, who organized the tests and became the group's spokesman. With his wife, he created a company, Cryo-Preservation Technologies, that was already marketing the product; when asked why he had not approached the pharmaceutical industry (which would certainly be interested in such a therapeutic breakthrough) for financing the trial, he answered that they had begun working with several companies but each time results began to look promising their partners had given up. As to Professor du Plessis, he corrected the first announcement by indicating that Virodene was not a cure for AIDS but a substance that reduced the viral impact and enhanced the immune system. The government confirmed its interest in the product and considered the possibility of providing financial support for the research program but remained careful, as President Mandela's spokesman, Parks Mankahlana, commented: "The government is awaiting the outcome of the investigation into procedural and ethical questions, and in the event of these being cleared up, would wish to give the necessary encouragement to deserving efforts at combating HIV and AIDS." Officially no decision had been taken, but actually financial support had been given.

Now, after the enthusiasm of the first days and while stock in the product continued to grow, anger also grew among doctors and among AIDS associations. Head physician of the AIDS program in Cape Town, Ashraf Grimswood, said he had felt "an overwhelming joy" upon hearing the news but a few days later "utter dejection" as it became clear that things were going wrong: "The way it was handled was completely insensitive, almost as if no one, from the cabinet down, really took the time to reflect on the effects the cure hype would have. It is as if they did not care that they were dealing with people who are hanging on to life by a thread waiting for a miracle cure." The National Association of People Living with AIDS (NAPWA), the main organization of its kind, worried about the way the government was managing the affair: "The unconventional presentation of these preliminary findings together with the cabinet's support and the media reports have unfairly raised the hopes and expectations of millions." And the more details one learned, the more worrisome it was.

During the February meeting of the AIDS Consortium, consisting of about one hundred organizations, du Plessis answered questions in front of a full house: often evasive, he acknowledged nevertheless that the experiment had involved eleven patients of whom only six had been biologically tested, that the variations in the lymphocyte count on which the drug's assessment depended were in fact not statistically significant, and that, consequently, the experiment did not allow one to conclude that Virodene worked. In the course of the discussion, it also came out that the documents signed by the patients included the requirement that the experiment be kept secret, which was contrary to the principle of informed consent. It seemed there was nothing more to be said, especially since the experts' suspicions about the miracle drug's chemical formula had just been confirmed: Virodene did in fact contain dimethylformaldehyde, an industrial solvent that can be used to denaturate DNA but that does not distinguish between viral and a human DNA; the molecule was therefore toxic, especially to the liver, where it causes irreversible, potentially cancerous or deadly lesions.[14] The Medicines Control Council once again made the final decision; it refused to permit any further experimentation with Virodene.

Parallel to the scientific investigations, the political debate got under way once more. Using the fact that the government had bungled the affair so badly to their advantage the opposition representatives went into action, comparing it with the *Sarafina II* scandal. Jack Bloom, on behalf of the Democratic Party, denounced the minister's "new fiasco"; Willem Odendaal, on behalf of the National Party, accused the government of making "human guinea pigs" out of patients. At the Health Department, the officers in charge, beginning with Rose Smart, the new director of the National Programme on AIDS, had learned about Virodene in the press, but resistance to pressures from either side, scientific or political, started organizing. Trusting in the new drug despite growing evidence of its ineffectiveness and even danger and faced by four refusals to allow clinical trials, Nkosazana Zuma studied ways to circumvent established procedure and announced that she was considering setting up a new commission to evaluate the drug.[15] On World AIDS Day, December 1, 1997, speaking at Odi stadium in Mabopane, she declared, "Dying patients willing to take responsibility for their actions should not be prevented from using the still-unapproved Virodene drug." She added, with tears in her eyes, "This breaks my heart. I have a lot of compassion for AIDS sufferers, but my hands are tied. I feel no one should play God. But one day, just one day, I can't say when, I will take a firm decision about the matter. The new health law soon to be put before Parliament will enable me to take that decision." More and more, the government sought to control public health policy, in particular drug policy, both economically, by supporting local companies and not leaving control entirely in the hands of the international pharmaceutical industry, and technically, by having a say in the evaluation of the services rendered to the population and not keeping it exclusively under the medical authority. A new conception of the role of the state was emerging.

At the beginning of 1998, the debate waxed more dramatic and radical. On February 3, the Medicines Control Council rejected the application for the right to carry out experiments filed by the Pretoria University researchers for the fourth time, a decision justified by Peter Folb: "Virodene may not be used for treatment of any patient before the outstanding ethical, scientific and technical problems have been dealt with." A few days later Deputy President Mbeki made his personal public entrance on the scene:[16] "More than twelve months ago, emanating from a request the Minister of Health presented through me, the Cabinet listened to a presentation of the Virodene researchers. The Cabinet had also the privilege to hear the moving testimonies of AIDS sufferers who had been treated with Virodene, with seemingly very encouraging results. The Cabinet took the decision that it would support the Virodene research, up to the completion of the Medicines Control Council processes. So far, this has not necessitated any financial or other material support." He then mentioned the letters from academics he had received in support of the clinical trial: "Alas, this local review board still refuses to accept the application, despite its knowledge of the unanimous opinion of these 'learned and highly qualified professionals.' To confirm its determined stance against Virodene, and contrary to previous practice, it has, with powers to decide who shall live or die, also denied dying AIDS sufferers the possibility of 'mercy treatment' to which they are morally entitled. I and many others will not rest until the efficacy or otherwise of Virodene is established scientifically. If nothing else, all those infected by HIV/AIDS need to know as a matter of urgency." Folb merely responded that the most recent research carried out in the United States demonstrated that Virodene was not only toxic to humans but also liable to stimulate the development of the virus, especially in the large amounts prescribed by the protocol. What is more, his list of the points in the clinical trial that were contrary to scientific rules and ethical principles was overwhelming both for the researchers and for those who defended them.

Mbeki's accusation that the Medicines Control Council had the power to decide who shall live or die shows that two new phenomena were becoming crucial to the polemic. First, it reveals the personal involvement of the state's second most important person, and through him of the entire government, in a question that, aside from a few isolated statements by the president's spokesman, had until then remained mainly with the Health Department—though we were soon to learn that he had been holding secret meetings with the Pretoria University researchers for a long time. Second, it points to a suspected secret agenda behind the rejection of Virodene, which Mbeki made even clearer in an interview with an Afrikaaner newspaper, in which he insinuated that it was exactly because the epidemic hit mainly the African population that the evaluation of the drug was being blocked; in other words, he suspected the doctors had racist motives. During the same week in March, even more openly and this time aimed at active members of the opposition, Nkosazana Zuma declared, "The Democratic Party hates ANC supporters. If they had their way, we would all die of AIDS." By that time the controversy had taken a more directly political turn with the discovery of documents apparently pointing to a connection between the firm producing Virodene and certain members of the ANC who were supposed to have bought shares in it. Once again, Democratic Party spokesman Mike Ellis draped himself in righteousness, not hesitating to accuse the deputy president and the health minister of having a personal, vested interest in Virodene and filing a complaint with the Public Protector for what looked like a new case of corruption. Some weeks later, after the inquiry led by that institution, the two were proven innocent, but the rumor had produced its deleterious effects on the government's integrity.

However, as she had announced several months before, Nkosazana Zuma launched the reform of the Medicines Control Council while claiming that it had absolutely nothing to do with the Virodene crisis: it was only a question of adapting a tool left over from the previous regime to the new objectives of public health policy, thus also avoiding possible conflicts of interest with the pharmaceutical industry. This argument was emphasized even more as the government was now coming under pressure from the international pharmaceutical firms, which threatened to take it to court if it continued to import generic medicines at the same time as the brand names. On April 23 Peter Folb was replaced by Helen Rees, heretofore manager of the Baragwanath Hospital Reproductive Unit, who, as soon as she was in office, set up a working committee to help the Pretoria University researchers conceive and present their clinical experiment more convincingly. Where her predecessor had been inflexible about evaluation, she tried rather to develop a negotiated partnership with the team that had discovered Virodene. But the professional circles and the activist organizations did not fall for this attempt at normalization. In a letter sent to the newspapers a physician declared indignantly, "The only real victors are the skeptics who now have further potent fuel for the argument that in Africa yesterday's self-sacrificing, highly principled liberators are tomorrow's objectionable self-serving despots." Nevertheless changing the people in charge and reforming the institution was not enough to put an end to the Virodene problem. A year after this coup, the scientific and ethical conditions were not yet put together to start the clinical trials. However, it was discovered that human experimentation was being carried out secretly in South Africa and elsewhere in the world. Thus the affair was far from over.[17] But by then other battles were beginning to rage, this time over a drug completely accepted in the biomedical field, AZT.

In an editorial published on December 22, 1998, under the title "A Lesson from the Virodene Saga," the daily that had first announced the Pretoria University researchers' presentation to the government recapitulated the history of Virodene:

> With very little funding available for treatment or counter-measures, the temptation in government to grasp at Virodene as a heaven-sent panacea was powerful indeed. When its inventors requested public funding and support to develop and test the drug they presented the Cabinet with a formidable test of rational judgment and political leadership. To many, Deputy President Thabo Mbeki and Health Minister Nkosazana Zuma, the chief protagonists of Virodene, failed that test. They appeared to succumb to the desperate pressures of the moment and ignored the pleas for caution from the scientific establishment. . . . South Africa has learned a hard lesson: there is no quick fix for AIDS and in the battle ahead what we need is unity of purpose between the government and the country's scientists.

The moral of the story seemed comforting. But reality is different. In this second controversy, the government, already estranged from AIDS organizations, definitively alienated the medical and scientific community. The loss of trust, once again, was mutual. The great majority of physicians and researchers did not understand what the administration was doing in their domain of institutional competence and professional autonomy. Hesitating at first to oppose the discovery, they became more and more critical. The health minister, soon joined by the deputy president, threw themselves into the battle, both in public and behind the scenes. And the more the evidence against the miracle molecule piled up, the more each of them withdrew into an argument based on pity and compassion but also racism and hostility.

The Virodene saga is certainly not the first affair in the world in which a locally produced drug has been said to be effective against AIDS and promoted by the governments as being the national response to the plague. Three "discoveries" in Africa alone—for similar incidents have happened in other regions, particularly in Latin America and Europe—became known internationally. First came the MMI in 1987 tested by two scientists, one from former Zaire and the other from Egypt, who sealed their alliance by baptizing their drug with the initials of the names of their heads of state, Mobutu and Mubarak.[18] After making the headlines of the regional papers, the product rapidly fell into oblivion. Next was Kemron, developed in Kenya in 1990, an alpha-interferon that had first been brought into the country by a Texas veterinarian and tested on about forty patients at the Nairobi Medical Research Institute before being officially ushered in by President Arap Moi.[19] After inconclusive controls, the drug had a second life in 1992 when the National Institutes of Health in the United States was compelled by pressure groups of African American patients and medical associations to repeat the clinical trials, which once again proved fruitless. Finally, in 2001, there was a flurry of excitement among scientists and journalists in Ivory Coast when the Pharmacy Faculty of the University of Cocody announced promising results on ten patients who had received Therastim, a product of the so-called traditional pharmacopoeia.[20] Happily riding on the simultaneous introduction of antiretroviral multitherapy, with which it seemed to be in local competition, the timely drug made but a brief foray into the ongoing international debate, mainly through the warnings issued by researchers of the French Research Institute for Development.

Limiting this list to the African continent might suggest that a specific tropism exists for such "affairs" to occur there. Suffice it to remember the French episode in the mid-1980s, in which Philippe Even, head of the Pneumology Department at Laënnec Hospital, and Georgina Dufoix, minister of health and social affairs, had jointly and publicly announced the discovery of a medicine to fight AIDS, the well-known cyclosporine, on the basis of preliminary and unpublished results obtained on a few patients— a lead that was to be abandoned soon after. In all these stories the same ingredients can be found: doctors only marginally involved in research, even when they occupy academic positions; politicians in charge hoping for economic and symbolic benefits for their country, often holding forth in typically nationalistic terms; and, finally, attempts to circumvent the usual procedures of scientific validation, presented as obstacles on the road to innovation.

There is, however, something specific in the drugs developed and promoted in Africa: each announced discovery appears to serve as revenge for the colonial and postcolonial past; and, at the same time, any reservations expressed by representatives of official science are attributed to ulterior motives with racist overtones. The day MMı was announced, A. S. Mianzoukouta, an editorial writer for the major newspaper in Brazzaville, wrote, "It would be fair that such an evil, of which Africa is suspected to be the source, be vanquished by Africans. If we, who are supposed to be resistant to science, were to relieve the suffering of the world, what a wonderful lesson it would be for the champions of Aryan theories." When Kemron was tested, the National Medical Association, made up mainly of African American physicians, accused "the white medical establishment" of "prohibiting African-Americans from accessing a promising therapy from Africa," and Janet Mitchell of Harlem Hospital accused the official researchers who had shown the Kenyan product to be ineffective of being "racists who want the black populations to continue dying of AIDS." So runs the haunting thread of memory through South Africa.

The wounds that the Virodene affair both revealed and revived are the signs of a social division deeply engraved in history. The seriousness of the insinuations or the violence of critiques points to social divisions that go far beyond the partisan oppositions concealing them. Like the *Sarafina II* scandal, questions naturally arose about the need to break with the recent past, about the need to protect the country from the pharmaceutical empire, of the importance of developing a national drug policy. But what especially emerged was the theme of racial hostility, this time compounded by the accusation of being indifferent to others' suffering or even of wanting them annihilated. It went a step further in unveiling history's unresolved conflicts. To those who reproached them for having, through their incompetence, toyed with people's hopes, the health minister and the deputy president responded that they, the accusers, had toyed with their very lives and out of far less honorable motives. This argument was to become the focal point of the controversy that arose shortly after.

What a Child's Life Is Worth

"Babies Too Poor to Live," "The High Cost of Living Babies," "Save Our Babies, Dr. Zuma," "Programme Could Save 18,000 Lives." From 1998 on, the newspaper headlines alluding to government decisions concerning the administering of AZT to pregnant women dramatically threw into the balance the price of a baby's life against the cost of treatment.[21] On January 30, 1999, an editorial in the *Saturday Star* (titled "Suffer the Little Children") set the tone: "The cost of saving the life of the most pathetic, vulnerable human being, a baby, from a grim AIDS death is surprisingly small: just 400 rands. Yet Health Minister Nkosazana Zuma doesn't seem prepared to pay it." For months, economic arguments and moral pronouncements waged battle in the press and in Parliament, mingling with scientific demonstrations and political considerations. The *Sarafina II* scandal and the Virodene affair had mainly concerned questions of governance, the good management of public funds and respect for decision-making or evaluation procedures. If at all, patients were involved only indirectly, through the assumed misuse of funds supposed to go to prevention in the first case, the dashed hopes due to the premature announcement of a major therapeutic breakthrough in the second. The AZT controversy took this a step further, since it meant deciding whether a presumed efficient drug could and should be administered to patients, or to be more precise, to HIV-positive pregnant women, not for their own sake but in order to reduce the risk of transmission to their children. What was at stake was the number of human lives that might be saved. At least that is how the debate was being presented. In fact, as we saw above, during the polemic surrounding the Pretoria University researchers' miracle drug, the Medicines Control Council had already been charged with going beyond its mission and deciding who was to live or die. However, this had taken place while Virodene was still in a trial phase and not, as was now the case, when treatment had been validated; moreover, Virodene had been offered as a compassionate gesture in the last stages of the illness and not in order to prevent new infections, as it was said AZT could do. In the controversy surrounding the prevention of mother-to-child transmission, the government's accusation of the medical authorities boomeranged with far more serious consequences.

To understand the terms of the debate beyond invectives, it may be useful to remember the unstable state of knowledge on the subject at the end of the 1990s.[22] The infection of the child by the HIV-positive mother-to-be is not systematic. In the absence of all medical treatment it fluctuates between 15 and 25 percent in the West and between 25 and 40 percent in Africa, the difference apparently linked to more frequent and longer breast-feeding in the latter. Among measures that might reduce the rate of transmission to newborns, aside from obviously recommending the use of artificial milk and prophylactic cesareans, the administration of an antiretroviral drug during pregnancy and at the time of delivery was progressively developed as of 1994, when the pioneering experiments carried out jointly by North American and European teams were first publicized. They were using AZT, the first molecule whose effectiveness in the treatment of AIDS had been confirmed in 1987. The results obtained in preventing mother-to-child transmission were spectacular, since the proportion of infected infants was 25.5 percent in the control group and only 8.3 percent in the experimental group. Several further trials confirmed these results, and in some protocols applying the treatment brought the rate down to 3 percent. But all these studies concerned only rich countries. Early in 1998 an experiment carried out in Thailand with the same product but a different protocol, both less complicated and less costly and therefore supposedly better adapted to Third World countries, revealed a decrease in the rate of infection from 18.9 to 9.4 percent. The result was confirmed by another trial, in Africa this time, and the drug, associated with another molecule, 3TC, similarly reduced the number of infected babies from 17 to 9 percent.

Such spectacular data must nonetheless be put into perspective because of existing doubts as to the long-term consequences of the treatments used on children born under such conditions—a risk of cancer has been observed in rats—and because of the problems of the acceptability of such measures—surveys had shown that some women refused to take the serological tests or the antiretroviral drugs for fear their relatives would find out they were sick. In addition, little was known about the actual effectiveness of these protocols when mothers continue to breast-feed, a frequent occurrence in Africa about which preventive messages are unclear because the risk of viral transmission must be weighed against the equal risk of infections and malnutrition among bottle-fed children. A question also arose as to the possibility that these medicines may be selecting resistant viral colonies among the infected children, in a proportion estimated at about one in ten, which would mean serious difficulty for further treatment. Last, problems of cost were crucial; a British study estimated that a cost of about £28,000 per each infection might be avoided by appropriate treatment. The conclusion of Diane Gibb and Beatriz Tess's 1999 review of literature illustrates the cautious attitude of the international specialists: "In resource-poor settings, results of trials on the use of antiretroviral therapy to prevent mother-to-child transmission in breast-feeding populations are eagerly awaited but the risks and benefits of providing alternatives to breast-feeding, as well as integration of intervention into prenatal care and other HIV prevention strategies, are major obstacles which, both in African and

Asian countries, require concerted worldwide political will to overcome" (1999: S101). What should be recommended was much clearer for rich countries than for poor ones.

Thus the new political crisis concerning AIDS broke out when much was being learned about the disease but much also remained uncertain. As early as the end of 1997, the researchers involved in the international Prevention of Perinatal HIV Transmission (PETRA) clinical trial at Baragwanath Hospital leaked to the press their optimism about the positive results they were expecting, stirring up "hope to formulate a strategy to reduce the number of babies who contract HIV from their mothers." A few months later the conclusions of the Thai experiment were made public in the United States and widely discussed in South Africa. The South African government came increasingly under pressure from the medical profession and patients' organizations, which demanded that programs be rapidly implemented. In June 1998 Dr. Glenda Grey, one of the coordinators of the trial at Baragwanath Hospital, declared indignantly: "The government is sleeping while Rome burns. Every day three babies in Soweto are born HIV-positive. While we wait, babies die." And the activist Gary Lamont of the AIDS agency Wola Nani exclaimed, "Every month that the government withholds these drugs is a cumulative act of genocide for thousands." Yet Rose Smart, director of the National Program on AIDS, reported that the problem was not only a matter of cost but also, more broadly, given the way the South African medical system worked, a matter of counseling, testing, and medical follow-ups for women.

In July, at the annual International AIDS Conference in Geneva, the media reported that similar results were obtained in trials carried out in Asia and Africa. Tensions grew. Glaxo-Wellcome laboratory, which owned the patents for AZT until 2005, was also coming under pressure both at the national and the international level and had just announced it was cutting its price for sales to South African public services by 70 percent. In October 1998 the health minister made a decision: the country was unable to bear the cost of preventing mother-to-child transmission, and therefore the trials must be stopped. The health minister's spokesperson indicated that the government did not have the necessary resources to implement a program adapted to all pregnant women in the country and that it would be unfair to do it for just a few. Priority must be given to education and prevention so that fewer women would become infected and vertical transmission would diminish. Little noticed, yet remarkable, is the fact that this choice corresponded at that time to the position of many international institutions, beginning with the World Bank, which feared that expensive treatments would become a burden, and UNAIDS, which asked for further studies leading to more economically realistic protocols.

There were strong reactions to the health minister's announcement. The government of the Western Cape Province, which was the only one headed by an opposition coalition consisting of the Democratic and National Parties, decided to ignore it. A program was set up in two dispensaries of Khayelitsha township near Cape Town, which became a sort of stronghold of resistance by the medical profession and NGOs, starting with Médecins sans frontières (Doctors without Borders). But Minister Zuma intervened to demand that the program remain experimental and be halted after twelve months instead of being extended to all the provinces, as its promoters had said it would be. In February 1999 six hundred women had been tested in the two dispensaries and ninety-six who were HIV-positive and close to term were receiving a short treatment. Three babies were born under this protocol, with a theoretical risk of infection two times less than if their mothers had not had the treatment. "The three babies born to mothers on an AIDS treatment project in Khayelitsha have a good chance of life without HIV. Babies born next year might not have the same chance," one reporter wrote (in fact, the risk of transmission is about one in ten with antiretroviral prevention and two in ten without it). Other interventions were more overtly political, as for example when Dr. Costa Gazi, a member of the Pan Africanist Congress, brought a court case against the government for human rights violations. General elections were not far off, and the controversy also naturally served the interests of the opposition.

At the same time, social actors were mobilizing. In December 1998, taking advantage of International Human Rights Day, the Treatment Action Campaign was officially launched, bringing together the AIDS Law Project and other organizations active in the field of AIDS. A few months later TAC was to become the main protagonist in the fight for equal access to treatment. Its first public operations, inspired by Act Up in the United States and in Europe, were spectacular: hunger strikes, die-in demonstrations around Baragwanath Hospital, a petition for the prevention of mother-to-child transmission signed by fifty thousand people nationwide in only a few weeks, a meeting with Nkosazana Zuma during which a platform was agreed on for joint action to address the pharmaceutical industry, especially Glaxo-Wellcome, to make them lower the price of antiretroviral drugs. Contrary to the political opponents who took advantage of the controversy to put the government in an uncomfortable position, TAC tried—at least initially—to become an ally and to find a way out of the crisis. Most participants in the campaign were in fact in profound sympathy with the new regime, and many had been comrades in the battle against apartheid.

In June 1999 the ANC triumphantly won the general elections and Thabo Mbeki became the second democratically elected president of South Africa. The nomination of Manto Tshabalala-Msimang as health minister was supported in professional and activist circles, all the more as one of her first decisions consisted in guaranteeing the confidentiality of information about AIDS and personal consent for testing, an issue her predecessor had dealt with in an authoritarian manner. When the results of a clinical test in Uganda were made known, in which mother-to-child transmission had been cut in half thanks to a single dose of nevirapine, and when an official delegation was sent to that country, it was thought that a national program to implement the new drug, much cheaper and easier to use than AZT, was imminent. On her return, however, Tshabalala-Msimang declared that no program would be undertaken until nevirapine had been tested in South Africa. Even more worrisome, when she spoke of AZT, she now evoked less its problematic cost than its potential toxicity and the risk of causing resistance. The final blow came from the chief of state himself, who in his speech to the National Provincial Council on October 28, 1999, also alluded to the dangers of the drug and asked the minister to evaluate it further. This seemingly minimal shift in the debate, from a financial to a medical argument, was a turning point in the controversy. From a traditional economic discussion, the government turned to questioning scientific certitudes. What the Virodene affair had revealed, although it concerned an unauthorized substance, was confirmed by the fact that AZT—a duly tested and recognized drug—was being criticized for its supposed negative side effects: politics was now meddling in science.

Actually, a new fact had entered the picture: a contact had been established by the government with those in North America whom international AIDS specialists had thought had been sent packing with other losers in the history of scientific progress. These heterodox researchers, who were denying the link between HIV and AIDS and claiming that AZT killed patients, were beginning to find effective outlets among South African media.[23] This brought about a paradigm shift in the evaluation of antiretroviral drugs. As long as it was the cost of the drugs that was put forth as an argument, it was possible to take issue with the government on an equal footing, either to dispute their cost-benefit calculations or, conversely, to say they had made the right choices when deciding on public health priorities or even, as most activists would do, to attack their decisions at home but at the same time support them in their international efforts against the pharmaceutical companies. But when the president and his health minister changed the argument to one of toxicity, the polemic entered a dangerous zone.

In a book denouncing the effects of the drug and the hypocrisy of the researchers, the South African AIDS dissident Anthony Brink exacerbated the situation: on an all-black cover, the word "AZT" is cut out in large white Gothic letters, playing on the symbolism of death and satanism abundantly used throughout the text; for example, the labels on the samples bear the skull and crossbones symbolizing danger. An unwieldy ally, this former lawyer-turned-reporter claimed that his first article, "A Medicine from Hell," published on March 17, 1999, in the *Citizen* had deeply influenced Thabo Mbeki and that he then became one the most active champions of the president when the latter began casting doubt on the safety of the antiretroviral drugs. These new *liaisons dangereuses* were a turning point. The controversy entered a new phase. We were now in the phase that Richard Horton (1996), editor in chief of the *Lancet,* in his analysis of the three books published by Peter Duesberg countering the dominant model of AIDS, has called "heresy." The term is significant. More than simply a change in scientific paradigm, we find ourselves in a territory that lies beyond normal science.[24] Rather than an epistemological break, which might conceivably have allowed the Berkeley scholar to continue participating in the intellectual universe of his peers even while contesting their presuppositions (which is how the heterodox academics describe themselves and the president defends them), the break is sociological in the form of ostracism from the scientific community (which is how the defenders of orthodoxy reject their adversaries).[25] Politically, the AIDS dissidents have not managed to gain recognition as "revolutionaries," as Thomas Kuhn uses the term; rather, in Pierre Bourdieu's sense, they are simply denounced as "heretics," and, indeed, the punishment is excommunication.

HERESY

we were reading Marx,
to define a space
for our craft of details labour
as our dream of the commune

was imminent
on every count
of strikes
we were scientists: paging through census figures to discover why
statistically blacks died from falling objects more often than all others

ARI SITAS

"The 1970s Years"

In an ironic and exasperated opinion column of December 14, 2001, Sipho Seepe of the *Weekly Mail and Guardian* called the South African president "Professor Mbeki (PhD.www)," giving him the title "instant graduate of the Internet Medical School."[26] It was rumored that Mbeki, who suffered from insomnia, spent nights surfing on the net, which is how—a senior member of the United Nations confided to me in April 2000—he learned about the AIDS dissidents. The story was then making the rounds of the press agencies. As a user of the internet, the South African president is supposed to have discovered that for a number of years a group of scholars had been openly challenging the commonly accepted theory of the viral etiology of AIDS, offering alternative scenarios, contesting the role of HIV, denying the very existence of an epidemic, and claiming that the epidemiological pattern of the illness in Africa was due to malnutrition and parasitosis. The anecdote is interesting in that it reveals an unexpected side of the "network society" that Manuel Castells (1996) wrote about: politics, at the highest level, happening live on the "world net," with a president "surfing" to inform himself on the state of the art in medicine. This version of the facts is only partly true, however.[27] Thabo Mbeki's familiarity with dissident circles goes farther back and occurred in a more mundane manner: it came from reading newspapers, from Brink's article on the damaging effects of AZT, which, probably, included a reference to Peter Duesberg's theories, and from personally meeting with South African dissidents' allies such as Anita Allen, nicknamed the "president's muse" because of the way she supposedly influenced his thinking on AIDS. This being the case, the caricature published by the cartoonist Dr. Jack in the same *Weekly Mail and Guardian* of April 19, 2002, gives a humorous perspective: it shows the head of state in his pajamas and slippers facing his computer on whose screen one can see the homepage "virusmyth," one of the main websites of AIDS heterodoxy; leaning languorously on the computer, the famous reporter is smiling down at him. The ways of dissidence are many and diverse. But however the heretical theories about AIDS were born, as soon as the president and his health minister heard about them, they spread almost as fast as the epidemic, to borrow Dan Sperber's (1985) metaphor, suggesting we ask ourselves why certain representations are more contagious than others, an especially relevant question in the present case. In only a few weeks a group was set up that mixed orthodox and heterodox scholars worldwide and a meeting was announced, throwing the national and international AIDS communities into an unprecedented turmoil.

An Unlikely Encounter

The document, a poor-quality fax handed to me by the head of an international agency, surprises by its contents as its form. It bears the date January 20, 2000, and is addressed "Dear President Mbeki" and informally signed "Dave and Charlie." It was sent by David Rasnick, a biochemist introducing himself as a visiting research scholar at the University of California, Berkeley, and Charles Geschekter, a specialist on African history at California State University, Chico. Along with their colleague Peter Duesberg, professor of molecular biology at the University of California, Berkeley, they are the most famous AIDS dissidents. Their moment of glory came at the end of the 1980s,[28] when their theories were discussed in North American media and backed by several associations of activists, homosexuals in particular, before finding themselves gradually pushed to the edges of the international research community. But they remained active in a network called "the Group for the Scientific Reappraisal of the HIV-AIDS Hypothesis."[29] It is easy to imagine, in such conditions, the benefits the group could expect to reap from the publicity afforded them by this unexpected contact. When Rasnick announced it in the media, he did not mince words: Thabo Mbeki had sent him questions, the researcher had answered him by letter, and the president had even telephoned him at home on January 21. "He had read everything we had written, everything that was available on the internet," Rasnick declared with satisfaction, adding, "I think he's courageous." But neither the scientific nor the general international press was ready to see it this way: "Are AIDS dissidents advising South Africa?" the journal *Nature* fretted on March 16; and the *New York Times* headline on March 19 read: "South Africa in a Furor over Advice about AIDS." The global controversy was starting.

In fact, the letter faxed by the two researchers arrived in reply to eight questions that the health minister had put to them on behalf of the president:

1. What means and methods are used in the public health system to test the HIV status of individuals? 2. What definition is used to classify a person as being afflicted with AIDS? 3. Of the people determined to have died of AIDS, what opportunist disease was identified as having been the immediate cause of death? 4. Would there be any record of the treatment that such people have received for these diseases, including their health profile? 5. Has any research been done on the health profiles of populations where allegedly it has been found that there are large numbers of HIV-positive people? 6. Has any research been done on HIV-positive infants, children and orphans with regards to their health profiles, those of their mothers and families, as well as the lifestyles and socioeconomic circumstances? 7. On what do we base the statistics we publish occasionally on the incidence of HIV and AIDS, and how do we arrive at the projections? 8. Are there any anti-HIV/AIDS drugs that are dispensed by the public health system on a regular basis, including to medical workers who might be exposed to needle pricks?

Coming from a health officer or even a health minister, the questions obviously are relevant. It is remarkable, however, that rather than address the numerous and competent existing South African specialists, the president had turned to foreign researchers and, what is more, notorious AIDS dissidents, handing them between the lines the weapons to defend their heterodoxy and to combat orthodoxy, not even forgetting a description of the miserable state of South African populations that would further give the basis for an alternative explanation of the epidemic.

The answer given by the Californian biochemist and historian is obviously in line with the positions they have frequently voiced: what is called AIDS is a syndrome comprising various pathologies known previously by other names; serological tests are not reliable and are not correlated to any clinical condition; the virus is only an innocent passenger in the body, and the antibodies present prove only their immunological encounter; sexual transmission of the virus is practically impossible and statistically nonexistent; what children and adults on the African continent are dying of and that people call AIDS is in fact a combination of malnutrition, tuberculosis, and illnesses caused by parasites, all connected to poverty; antiretroviral treatments are not only inefficient, since they attack an inoffensive microbe, but dangerous, because of their toxicity; governments and medical agencies use these treatments only because they have a vested interest in the international pharmaceutical industry.[30] Astutely rhetorical, the text mixes references to scientific publications (in the most authoritative international journals) with sentences taken from manufacturers' leaflets (about the possible mistakes in the tests and the potentially negative secondary effects of a medicine), pictures of the South African locations they visited (recalling the social and economic havoc wrought by apartheid), and quotations from the health minister's talks (which back up their demonstration). Their statements are categorical: "We know of no study that shows that AIDS is sexually transmitted. Furthermore, we know of no study that shows that AIDS is contagious at all. All the evidence, on the contrary, shows that AIDS is no more transmissible than alcoholism." Cynicism is not absent: "The only blessing of poverty is that it may protect poor Africans from the highly toxic anti-HIV drugs that have already killed thousands, perhaps tens of thousands of Americans." The letter ends by expressing "support and admiration" for the South African president for his "courage" to confront "the world HIV/AIDS establishment and the drug industry." The link is now solidly established with the dissidents' network.

A few weeks later, following a suggestion by Tshabalala-Msimang, Mbeki put forward the idea of a "panel" that would include the top world specialists, both orthodox and dissident, to make available the most up-to-date information and propose strategies for the African continent. Tshabalala-Msimang's plan, once again, was to reach a "consensus." At least that is what she claimed in a long communiqué dated March 6, 2000. What was to follow showed—it was of course predictable—that it was intellectually and humanly impossible for the two sides to come together. Therefore, a year later, in March 2001, the Presidential AIDS Advisory Panel Report published not one but two series of preventive measures: those that expressed "the point of view of the members of the panel who do not see any causal link between HIV and AIDS" and who prescribe general measures for improving sanitary conditions, reducing poverty, and improving the health system; and those that expressed "the point of view of members of the panel who do see a causal link between HIV and AIDS" and who insist on sex education, condoms, and antiretroviral drugs to prevent mother-to-child transmission. It could hardly have been otherwise.

In the widely publicized confrontation between orthodox and heterodox scientists, name-calling is part of the power struggle. Since a scientific norm exists—which defines the orthodox stand—so must deviancy, with which heterodoxy is associated. Sam Mhlongo, professor of family medicine at Pretoria University, together with the British biologist Andrew Herxheimer, both members of the heterodox group, drew up some "critical remarks on the orthodox biomedical science."[31] In it they oppose the "true believers" (thus whittling down orthodoxy to belief in a "dogma") and the "so-called dissidents" (thus placing themselves in the position of victims whose adversaries make them out to be "heretics"). Their description of the champions of the official position abounds in religious vocabulary. The International AIDS Conference in Durban was stamped with "the hallmarks of faith, belief, and orthodoxy"; the opening ceremony that "featured Christian choirs" was placed under the auspices of "the pioneering missionaries of the Victorian age—David Livingstone and Robert Moffatt." By contrast, those who defend a critical reappraisal—the authors themselves included—are presented as preferring scientific references. A quote from Thomas Kuhn to the effect that science cannot exist if there are no "counter instances" allowing for criticism is used to justify the existence of the AIDS dissidents, who appear as the bearers of a new paradigm and the precursors of a future revolution. When the panel met, the "orthodox believers were not prepared to have a real discussion," just as, in what was to follow, they refused to pursue the scheduled debate on the website, to which "only the dissidents posted contributions." For the authors, this silence definitively condemned the official science.

Of course, one gets an entirely different view from the diary of an anonymous member of the panel belonging to the orthodox camp. Large excerpts of it were published in the *Weekly Mail and Guardian*.[32] The author opposes the "round-earthers" and the "flat-earthers." This time, it is no longer a question of belief versus science but of true versus false (which does not preclude another, more moral distinction between the "good guys" and the "denialists"). Bringing up the polemics about the shape of the earth that raged at the end of the Middle Ages is of course ironical, since AIDS dissidents constantly claim an affinity with the historic figure of Galileo, persecuted for his disturbing discoveries.[33] According to the orthodox panelist, AIDS dissidents are irrational; he even describes them in psychiatric terms. For instance, about the New York specialist in internal medicine and infectious diseases Roberto Giraldo, he writes, "He puts forth a borderline, incomprehensible and basically embarrassing amalgam of paranoid observations and pseudo-scientific jargon." Frequently, too, mockery is used to disqualify. For example, about Peter Duesberg and Harvey Bialy, specialist in molecular biology: "They started to act out a little, gesturing to friends, acting a lot like little kids in school." It is therefore easy to understand why any sort of dialogue becomes impossible: "Most round-earthers decided that to play with their new friends was a waste of time and made them feel intellectually compromised by even entertaining their half-baked ideas." Whence the refusal to continue the debate on the internet.

There are thus two quite different ways of reading the issues in the confrontation between the two sides. Some—the dissidents—contrast their critical approach to what they see as a dogmatic stand on the part of their adversaries. The others—the orthodox—repeat a scientific truth that according to them can only be contradicted by pathetically irrational people. Those are basically the classic modes of legitimation used by the social actors in all controversies, the ones trying to participate in the game, the others trying to keep them out—what Joan Fujimura and Danny Chou (1994) call "styles of scientific practice," which include not only ways of providing evidence but also ways of acting in public. Were one to be satisfied with that, however, one would have the impression that the dissident movement that had shaken the scientific and militant circles in the United States as reported by these two authors was being reenacted a decade later. But something else, something completely new, was happening on the South African stage. The affair was not limited to medical and activist circles, as was the case when it first appeared in North America: in South Africa, it invaded the public arena and infiltrated civil society for several years. The unprecedented acceptance of theories that many thought had been discarded once and for all, that many no longer even want to discuss, is due to the fact that the nonviral theory of AIDS mirrors a specific historical configuration. If responsible politicians, beginning with the head of state, are so taken with the heterodox model, it is because, even before they ever heard of it, it reflected their own preoccupations. The AIDS dissidents were quick to understand this and to come up with an alternative, ad hoc explanation. For if the virus is not responsible for AIDS, how can the epidemic be accounted for? In the West the hypothesis most frequently put forward was that of "recreational drugs," substances used by homosexuals and heroin addicts; it was replaced by the antiretroviral medicines as soon as they came into use, giving birth to the iatrogenic model. Concerning Africa, it was necessary to find a different interpretation, one that would be plausible given the economic and health situation of the continent: malnutrition, repeated infections, and poor conditions of hygiene. It is remarkable that in all their arguments Rasnick and Geschekter systematically return to the historical context of South Africa, explaining the epidemic by misery resulting from the politics of inequality and segregation of the past half century. Black South Africans cannot help but feel concerned by such talk.

From that perspective, the document drawn up by Mhlongo in collaboration with Herxheimer must be read less as a repetition of the theory developed over the past ten years by the group of North American researchers than as a way of making it into a local or even continental outlook, in which the question of race occupies a central position. Contesting the viral hypothesis is political before it is scientific. Or rather, its success can be accounted for by the encounter between a deception and a hope, a sense of injustice vis-à-vis the biomedical discourse and a sense of recognition through the alternative theory. The anonymous author describing the panel's daily life obviously does not understand this when he writes, for instance, that the economist Alan Whiteside's claim that during the last census in Malawi two million persons were declared missing "clearly did not affect the dissidents." This assumption is both unlikely and unfair, at least insofar as African AIDS dissidents are concerned.

The title of Mhlongo and Herxheimer's text could hardly be more transparent: a virus is being made responsible so as to avoid naming poverty and what this does is absolve apartheid and its racist remains. After quoting official statistics from the 1950s and 1960s showing that tuberculosis and infant mortality were considerably more prevalent among blacks than among whites, after recalling the results of several surveys carried out during the 1980s, particularly the Race Relations Survey that showed levels of malnutrition unequaled even in the rest of the continent, the authors conclude: "What is amazing today is that orthodox health professionals and to some degree HIV/AIDS dissidents ignore this information—hence they claim that they are seeing a new disease (AIDS). We would suggest strongly that all those who are involved in AIDS research should visit this history which is still very relevant since nothing much has changed as regards the daily disabilities that black Africans face in their lives. It is difficult in the light of the evidence and the history of South Africa to accept that a retrovirus is responsible for the disease which doctors encounter in their practices or hospitals." This is a far cry from the dissidents' discourse that is so often caricatured and mocked. Coming from the person considered the President Mbeki's main counselor on AIDS, this opinion cannot be simply brushed aside as the anonymous author did in his diary: "Sam Mhlongo: a very confused person who seems to be on the dissidents' side." Analysis is needed here. One thing in the document deserves special attention: the importance of the discussion surrounding the statistics produced during the meeting of the panel by the president of the Medical Research Council, Malegapuru William Makgoba.

A Quarrel about Numbers

"DEAD." On Sunday, July 9, 2000, opening day of the Thirteenth International AIDS Conference in Durban, these four letters, in large black type, were emblazoned across the front page of the *Sunday Times*.[34] The full title of the article, "Young, Gifted and Dead," referred cruelly to Nina Simone's song "Young, Gifted and Black." The article was subtitled "Horrible Truth: In SA, Young People Are Dying before Their Parents." Neither the participants who had come from around the world to attend the conference nor the regular South African readership could ignore this brutal revelation.[35] There were four diagrams, two for males, two for females, showing the numbers of deaths at each age—in light blue for 1990, in dark red for 2000 (in fact, they were clearly figures for 1999). Whereas a decade earlier, the number of deaths rose regularly and predictably between ages 15 and 74 for both sexes, the mortality rate had become higher for the young than for the old—with an astonishing plateau and even a slight decline from 30 to 99 years for men, and a curve showing two peaks for women that indicated as many deaths between ages 25 and 39 as between 64 and 79. Such a situation, practically unprecedented in the world, drew from Malegapuru William Makgoba, president of the Medical Research Council, in his speech before the conference, the remark, "If we had been involved in a major war that would be the only other thing that could explain the high number of young men and women who are dying in our country." In the language of public health, war no longer serves as a metaphor; instead it is a comparison. Makgoba added forcefully, "This is the first data presented that actually gives South Africa a picture of what is really happening. These are not projections. These are real figures. . . . These statistics show that something is decimating our population. If you look at changes in death patterns, you can see what used to happen before AIDS became an issue in South Africa. That's the reality. In any normal population you would expect the old to die, not the young. But here you have young people dying and young women dying, which is unheard of in biological terms. It can only be explained by the peak incidence of AIDS." This speech was not only meant as a warning; it also sought to convince. Makgoba first delivered it to the members of the Presidential Panel whom he had addressed a few days earlier when opening its second meeting. In front of his colleagues and the health minister, he wanted to establish the truth about the epidemic, its origin, its cause. As one reporter put it, Manto Tshabalala-Msimang was "stunned" on hearing him.

The Department of Home Affairs reacted the very next day. It released the data, which thus looked as if they were giving arguments to the president's opponents. It published a communiqué: "The department is merely responsible for recording deaths and determining trends falls outside the ambit of its functions." However, making a stab at interpreting the trends described in the newspapers, it set the record straight: "Statistics SA confirms that South African adults overwhelmingly die of accidents and violence. The profile of deaths can therefore not be solely due to HIV/AIDS." The rising death rate was thus attributed mainly to social problems. In the government's view, the problem of violence had been inherited from the apartheid regime. Above all, the official response injected a totally new reasoning into its critical appraisal: "The two sets of figures for 1990 and 1999 quoted in the report could not be compared directly. The 1990 figures were provided by Statistics SA and excluded the deaths of people of the former TBVC countries, while the 1999 figures reflected the total number of deaths in South Africa in that year."

Statistics SA is the official institution that had already existed under apartheid. "TBVC" corresponds to the four former homelands, Transkei, Bophutatswana, Venda, and Ciskei, where the supposedly ethnically homogenous African populations had been confined and to which the South African government had granted independence between 1976 and 1981, a decision never acknowledged internationally. The white government of Pretoria, little inclined to produce dependable statistics on the African populations on the whole, could thereafter completely and legally wash its hands of those extraterritorial zones. Thus the comparison between the two series of statistics made no sense to the Department of Home Affairs. In the days following this discussion, both arguments were repeated by the president himself, condemning the ethical and scientific irresponsibility of the researchers of the Medical Research Council, whom he accused of having proclaimed information liable to induce fear among the population without sufficient prior verification. Simultaneously, the satirical magazine *noseweek*'s editorial concentrated on this new affair and, picking up arguments close to those of the Department of Home Affairs, expressed astonishment at the confidence with which Malegapuru William Makgoba had interpreted the controversial and unreliable data.

This polemic was neither the only nor even the first one to be kindled by AIDS statistics. For example, also in 2000, in the columns of the *South African Medical Journal,* a dispute occurred between Medical Research Council researchers and Health Department civil servants that was set off by the yearly antenatal clinic survey carried out in 1999.[36] The slight incidence decrease—from 22.8 to 22.4 percent—which the Health Department saw as a significant change in the progression of the illness, was considered by the others as likely a result of the sample's margin of error. The first were getting ready to publish some good news at last that would check the attacks against the government; the second did not see anything to rejoice in. Behind an apparently inoffensive skirmish, it was just one more episode in the permanent war between scientific circles and official services over AIDS. However, beyond the specific issues related to a pessimistic or optimistic reading of the epidemiological facts and its evolution, the quarrels over numbers often represent interests that have nothing to do with science but reveal the more general questions being put to society at large.[37] The controversy surrounding mortality statistics is illustrative. It recalls a recent past and asks history to explain the present. True, in so doing it has an ulterior motive, since it means denying the seriousness of the epidemic, thus arming scientific dissidence. But once again, it is the reference to apartheid that keeps it going.

The arguments cannot be too easily dismissed, as many have done by seeing in them only a sign of the bad faith of the head of state and his entourage. A year later a more complete and detailed study of the mortality statistics published by the Medical Research Council offered a more thorough analysis.[38] First, the study's authors explained, death caused by violence, accidents, and homicides are particularly frequent in South Africa, varying from one-fifth to more than one-half of the cases of male mortality in the 20 to 39 age bracket. They thus account for an important part of the excessive number of deaths of young adults. The increase in the number of natural causes is a new phenomenon, however, that can only be related to AIDS. Second, death reports are very unreliable in the health information system, to the point that it is estimated that only 54 percent were recorded in 1990 against 89 percent in 1999. The difference concerns almost exclusively the African populations of the former homelands and the townships, which confirms the critique addressed by state officials. The demographic techniques used to correct these distortions nevertheless allow the statisticians to verify the rapid increase in the number of deaths of young adults, especially among African men, which again can only be caused by AIDS. The report's conclusion can thus be drawn relatively prudently as follows: "While there is inevitably some degree of uncertainty because of the assumptions underlying both the model and the interpretation of the empirical data, we estimate that about 40% of the adult deaths aged 15–49 that occurred in the year 2000 were due to AIDS and that about 20% of all adult deaths in that year were due to AIDS" (2001: 6). These conclusions, quite in accordance with scientific methodological prudence that is sometimes forgotten, indicate that the Department of Home Affairs' discussion was not totally without basis. For researchers, discussing the data is once again a throwback to a time when statistics were an integral part of the politics of segregation.[39] If numbers speak, they do not speak about AIDS alone; they also speak about history, a history made of resurgences but also of repetitions, as the list of court actions involving AIDS illustrates.

Two Trials

"The last time the TAC and [the] government were in court together they were on the same side against the Pharmaceutical Manufacturers' Association in the pursuit of cheaper drugs. This time the national Department of Health and eight of the nine provincial Ministers will be in the dock facing the TAC." This statement, taken from an article in the September 14, 2001, *Weekly Mail and Guardian,* perfectly captures the shift in alliances that took place within just a few months.[40] In April 2001, when the government and AIDS associations together had triumphed over the attempt by the thirty-nine largest international pharmaceutical companies to impose their drug policies in South Africa, they congratulated each other on the steps of the Pretoria courthouse not only for this victory of the African David over the multinational Goliath but also for this hoped-for reconciliation between the state and the civil society. In September of the same year optimism was no longer on the agenda. This time, and in the same place, the Health Department was facing a court action brought against it by yesterday's ally, the Treatment Action Campaign, which accused the health minister of not making nevirapine, an inexpensive, easy to use antiretroviral drug whose effectiveness in reducing mother-to-child transmission had just been demonstrated, available to public health services. In fact, instead of seeing in the second trial an unexpected reversal, it would be more accurate to say that the first trial had been a fortunate parenthesis in a conflict that had begun several years before. Between the government and the activist organizations war is the rule, peace the exception.

After the wave of emotion stirred up by the invitation to AIDS dissidents to participate in the Presidential Panel just before the Durban conference, and after the virulent exchanges surrounding the mortality statistics released by the Medical Research Council, the end of 2000 saw the president and members of the government under siege by the press, which relentlessly pursued the same question: do you believe HIV is the cause of AIDS?[41] In his answers, Thabo Mbeki ran hot and cold: sometimes, as when he addressed Parliament in an official speech, seeming to distance himself from the polemic; at other times expressing doubts, for example, in the *Time* interview. Under similar fire, his ministers showed embarrassment, and most refused to answer, except for Minister of Research Ben Ngubane and Minister of Labor Membathisi Mdladlana, both of whom declared, no holds barred, that a cause-and-effect relationship did exist. In this context TAC brandished its weapons for the trial scheduled in September 2000, first as a way to put pressure on the government and then as a real threat to forcibly impose prevention of mother-to-child transmission. At the same time the Democratic Alliance launched an offensive against the government in the form of aggressive attacks in Parliament but also through an exchange of correspondence between its leader, Tony Leon, and President Mbeki, the fifty-four pages of which were made public in October 2000. As for the South African press, it actively pursued its campaign of criticism, soon joined by the most prestigious international papers, the *New York Review of Books* first and foremost, which dedicated several long articles to the "AIDS mystery in South Africa," to use the phrase coined by Helen Epstein in an article published on July 20, 2000. Meanwhile, the *Presidential Panel Report* was being prepared most discreetly: when it appeared, toward the end of March, it was eclipsed by the preparations for the first Pretoria trial. The journalist Belinda Beresford announced, "Drug Giants Prepare for War."

Indeed, for three years, the thirty-nine major drug companies constituting the Pharmaceutical Manufacturer's Association had been fighting the South African government in the courts, preventing it from implementing its legislation in matters of public health. The law known as the Medicines and Related Substances Control Amendment Act, or Act 90 of 1997, stipulated in Article 15c that the parallel importation of drugs would be permitted. This meant that the state would be able to buy foreign products when they were being sold at lower prices. The example given by the health minister concerned a malaria drug that sold for 0.40 rand in Mozambique as compared to 15 rands in South Africa. Clearly, this legislation would allow the public health services to cover a far wider range of treatments with the 2 billion rands budgeted by the government to buy medicine. As new Director General of the Health Department Ayanda Ntsaluba has pointed out, what is at stake is political: "We are about 0.6% of the global market and 1.2% in terms of value. We are not going to cause difficulty to major pharmaceutical companies. The issue for them is not South African markets. It's the precedent that it sets. That is the biggest threat to them." On top of the legal actions undertaken by the multinationals, the United States also brought pressure to bear on the South African government, placing the country on its "watch list for potential trade sanction" and announcing that a complaint would be lodged with the World Trade Organization. One reason for this is that preparations were then under way to negotiate the new Trade Related Intellectual Property Rights (TRIPS) agreement, to be signed during the Doha Conference in November 2001. The pharmaceutical multinationals, finding the existing rules too vague and too flexible, wanted them reinforced, in particular in developing countries by protecting the patents more efficiently and limiting parallel imports.

The Pretoria trial thus became the symbol worldwide for defense of "the public health exception." This slogan allowed for specific procedures in international legislation controlling intellectual property in cases of "national emergency or other circumstances of extreme urgency," which include "public health crises," to quote what was to become the Doha Declaration, a limited concession accepted by multinationals for compassionate reasons. The TAC, which wanted to testify in support of the South African government and whose "Drop the Case" petition collected 250,000 signatures, in association with humanitarian organizations, in particular Médecins sans frontières, and AIDS agencies such as Act Up started a campaign denouncing the pharmaceutical industry and damaging its image even among its shareholders. "Even the horror of AIDS does not stop the thirst for profit," declared an editorial signed by Ebrahim Harvey in the March 16, 2001, *Weekly Mail and Guardian.* Harvey was echoing the position of many in the North American press. Without naming it directly, he also repeated the South African government's two-year-long attacks against the "big pharmas." On April 15, 2001, the first day of the long-awaited trial, the Pharmaceutical Manufacturers' Association dropped its court action. On the steps of the Palace of Justice in the South African capital, the president of TAC, Zachie Achmat, declared, "Every South African can be proud, we stood firm against the most powerful lobby in the world, the drug companies." "But," he added, "now another struggle begins."

For as soon as it became known that the case had been withdrawn, the health minister declared this would not change her policies one iota: in particular, the clinical tests on nevirapine for the prevention of mother-to-child transmission must continue in the eighteen pilot sites where its use had been limited exclusively to experimental purposes. TAC decided to take her to court, and a long legal battle got under way. On December 14, 2001, the

Pretoria High Court ordered the government to implement the prophylaxis of mother-to-child transmission by using nevirapine. On January 4, 2002, the government lodged an appeal against the ruling, which was postponed as a result. On January 25, the activists interfered again to force the Health Department to implement the court's decision without waiting for the result of the appeal. On March 11 Judge Chris Botha ruled in favor of the activists and ordered the immediate implementation of his first decision. On March 22 the government filed a request to suspend the order, but the case was dismissed two days later. On April 4 the appeal before the Constitutional Court confirmed the decision to make nevirapine immediately available to all the public health services in the country. Finally, on April 16, without waiting for the ruling that the Constitutional Court was to make in early May and, probably informed as to the foreseeable outcome of the trial if she pursued the case, the health minister issued an instruction authorizing the distribution of the antiretroviral therapy. "AIDS Drug Gets OK" was the front page headline of the *Sowetan* the next day.

In the ensuing weeks the program got off the ground in the maternity wards and hospitals, not without logistical difficulties, however. It was a victory for the activists and undeniably a defeat for the government. A tragic coincidence occurred, however. On March 14 Sarah Hlalele, the young mother living with AIDS who had brought TAC's case to the court and had become the icon of the struggle for the right to treatment access, died from a rare side effect of her antiretroviral therapy. The public announcement of her death and its cause was made only a few days after the decision of the change in government policy had been communicated. Many feared that the health minister would use this affair as evidence that her reticence towards the drugs was well founded. But she did not. A "martyr" to the cause of AIDS, according to her friends and family, Sarah Hlalele was protected by the respect and compassion she had inspired.

Thus spring 2002 looked like the beginning of a new era. The moment was perhaps ripe to overcome the violent antagonisms and simplistic dualities of the South African AIDS scene. With Helen Schneider, who directed the Center for Health Policy of Witwatersrand University in Johannesburg, I began working on an article in which we tried to account for the historical meaning of, and the political stakes in, the recent polemics. Published on March 1, 2003, in a leading international medical journal,[42] the article was generally well received in the scientific and political circles of South Africa; it stressed how the epidemic of today made sense only in light of a past too quickly forgotten. Our initiative elicited encouraging approval from senior officers in the Health Department who were close to the government as well as from their vigorous opponents, leaders of TAC. Within a few months, however, the electronic page that the *British Medical Journal* had opened on its website so that a debate over the article could take place turned into a tribune for AIDS dissidents the world over, which in turn incited the keepers of the temple of medical orthodoxy to reply. During the year that followed the publication of our article, no less than 232 responses could be read on the page. Except for a few during the first month that discussed the perspective we suggested, almost all the rest dwelled on the heterodox theories, to criticize or defend them. David Rasnick, the first to react, denounced the "expansion of AIDS Inc., an American monopoly"; Claus Köhlnlein, another dissident Presidential Panel member, reaffirmed that AIDS did not exist and was only a "test epidemic," that is, an artifact linked to the use of serological tests; Eleni Papadopulos Eleonopulos got her famous "Perth group," named after the Australian university where she worked, back in the act, to put to pieces the viral interpretation of AIDS; finally, Sam Mhlongo accused us of "remaining ourselves firmly anchored in the controversy," since we accepted the link between the virus and the illness. Most of the responses, however, no longer even referred to our original article and were only eager to continue their uninterrupted conversation. Originally meant to reach "beyond the controversies," as its title indicated, our article had on the contrary given them an excuse to pursue their verbal battle in the virtual arena that had always before provided them with a resource for the debate.

PROPOSITION 2: THE CONFIGURATION OF THE POLEMICS

The political history of AIDS in South Africa since 1996 is a chain of disputes rather than the endless solitary controversy that has often been described. This is the thread I have tried to follow and the chronicle I have attempted to piece together here. I show below that to comprehend this, however, requires that we go further back in time. But let us for a moment take all the episodes together. At first sight they appear heterogeneous. A mundane scandal around the financial and political mishandling of an educational program turned into a musical comedy. A false discovery unduly validated and proclaimed, with suspicions of corruption amid the party in power. A decision concerning public health questioned by doctors and activists who pit the value of a human life against the cost of treatment. A scientific meeting that includes the champions of heterodox ideas to review the state of the art of knowledge on the epidemic considered as a provocation just before the worldwide official event on the matter. The publication of dramatic statistics criticized by public authorities for scientific and political reasons. A court case won by the government against the pharmaceutical industry, another one lost against partisans of the prevention of mother-to-child transmission.

In this astounding list, we naturally find the same actors: the government, especially the head of state and his two successive health ministers; health professionals, mainly researchers in biomedicine; political parties, especially the parliamentary opposition; AIDS activists and also human rights activists; scientists and journalists who are part of the intellectual dissidence. We also find the same general set of problematics: the relationship between science and politics, the autonomy of research, the government's responsibility. But in this representation of the field of controversies to which I shall return later, an argumentative and narrative framework has been woven into the background: justifications are put forward, stories are told. The skeleton of these constructs shows through in public discussions as well as in private commentaries, in the general press but also on the internet. Scarcely visible at first, it becomes clearer and clearer as we look. Let us attempt a comparison. The short story occupies a central place in South African literature. When discovering the collections, the reader is impressed by the diversity of themes, then, often, little by little he or she becomes aware that they share a thematic structure. This is typically the case in the work of Nadine Gordimer.[43] The same may be said for the collection of disconnected polemic episodes that progressively form a meaningful frame. In hindsight, it provides the ideological structure of the controversies and, if one hypothesizes that controversies of this scope touch the most sensitive points of society, in the end it reveals the ideological structure of South African society. I want to mention three elements in particular.

The first one is national identity. The question of the nation and its construction, institutional as well as symbolic, is not new, as one often supposes. It was central throughout the twentieth century, that is, from the end of the Boer War when former enemies, British and Afrikaners, were reunited in one and the same union. From the outset, but more and more markedly as the nationalistic Afrikaner ideology infiltrated white society, the concept of nation became racially exclusive and excluding, especially insofar as the so-called African or native populations were concerned. With the end of the rule of apartheid, the theme of national regeneration became central to the new project of living together. A new form of nationalism, multiracial but ambiguously African—in other words, socially inclusive but historically determined—arose. Appeals to Africanity must be understood in light of this relationship to that past and to that future: *Sarafina II* was intended to be a culturally adapted communications technique, though it was borrowing from a very cosmopolitan genre; Virodene was presented as a local discovery, though the inventors originated from eastern European countries; Thabo Mbeki's letter to the world leaders called for specific answers; the first Pretoria trial proclaimed South Africa's resistance to the multinationals. Conversely, AZT symbolized Western control over the drug, and biomedical science seemed alien to the realities of the country. The biological threat of AIDS, along with its predicted demographic decline, attacked the process of national reconstruction in its very flesh and blood, making all discourse on the theme especially sensitive.

The second issue is race. Like all the colonized societies on the continent, South Africa has known all along that its economic, political, and social relations were defined along color lines. However, from the end of the nineteenth century, the process of racial segregation began to be more and more actively implemented. Under the rule of apartheid, it became tantamount to an intrinsic dogma and official doctrine. The advent of democracy confirmed a project that broke radically with the racist ideology but was caught in a double bind: on the one hand, one must deny the racial categories and their concrete consequences; on the other hand, one cannot help but see that they persist in representations, practices, and social institutions, so that they must be recognized in order to be combated, notably through affirmative action. AIDS, though it is repeatedly said that it affects all groups, is so much more prevalent among the black populations that it revives racial divisions. The polemics surrounding it are ever more influenced by racialist readings and, furthermore, in ways that are ever more radical. In the *Sarafina II* affair, some said the criticisms by political opponents had racist overtones. When the medical authorities refused to permit clinical trials of Virodene, they were accused of lacking compassion for patients because they were black. When the debate on AZT began, in particular over its supposed toxicity, there was suspicion that someone intended to harm the African populations. At the Durban conference mutual accusations of racism became more and more radical as they were publicized through the bitter exchanges between Thabo Mbeki and Tony Leon. Simultaneously, the racial explanations of the origins of the African epidemic, supposed to have been provoked accidentally or willfully by whites, entered into the shared repertory of interpretations.

The third issue is the conspiracy theory. It, too, delves into history and especially into the history of apartheid. One has only to think of the argument used to justify the toughness of the regime—the risk of destabilization, the besieged fortress syndrome that plunged the country into economic and political isolation—but also of the threats leveled at opponents of apartheid, whether at home or in exile. South Africa after 1994 was seemingly freed from that widespread suspicion of the others, be they distant or close. Yet the polemics surrounding AIDS have progressively rebuilt a double barrier of danger, internal and external. During the debate that raged around *Sarafina II,* the enemy was inside, the political opposition of course but progressively activists as well. The Virodene episode extended this interpretation, but health professionals had also by now become the new adversaries. The AZT case was nonetheless a turning point, especially from the moment when AIDS dissident networks entered the picture, for the plot appeared a global one, dangerously connecting the Western world, science and capitalism: the pharmaceutical firms were suspected of wanting both to test their molecules on African patients and to enrich themselves at the expense of the continent with the blessings of the wealthy nations. If Thabo Mbeki's radical heterodoxy clashes with the consensual atmosphere during the Durban conference, largely financed by the international drug companies, conversely, the fact that during the Pretoria trial activists rallied to the government's cause against the "big pharmas" dazzlingly confirmed in his eyes the correctness of his interpretations. From this perspective, the withdrawal of the case in April 2001 would seem to indicate that the plot had been finally thwarted. But, aside from the fact that the theme does not easily disappear from the public arena, even more disquieting rumors began to be heard in South African society, beyond the political circles, about a government-led plan to exterminate the poor.

These three elements that are part of the polemical framework and more broadly of the historical fabric of South Africa constitute the ideological configuration of postapartheid. It would be possible to reread J. M. Coetzee's books in the light of this triptych, finding at least for the novels from the apartheid period a sort of ideological prefiguration of the present scene: *In the Heart of the Country* in 1977, for the impossible national construction; *Age of Iron* in 1990, for the racial definition of social relations; *Waiting for the Barbarians* in 1980, for the besieged fortress syndrome. The three elements are intimately intertwined, the racial question undermining the national edifice, the conspiracy suspicion feeding on racist experiences, the construction of the nation being threatened by external as well as internal enemies. Though they are not absolutely specific to South Africa, as we shall see, these elements stand out with exceptional violence there. Picking them out of the proliferation of discourses and the emotionality of the debates surrounding AIDS means putting the present in line with the continuities and ruptures of history, where the same patterns constantly recur under new rubrics.

THREE

Anatomy of the Controversies

The African potato was said by some to work much better than Virodene (which was then the latest pharmaceutical invention for the treatment of AIDS), providing the disease was caught in the initial stage. It was also rumoured to be far more powerful than Viagra, for men whose performance in bed was less than sparkling. The African potato was said to outperform all other pharmaceutical inventions.

PHASWANE MPE
Welcome to Our Hillbrow

"AIDS TRAGEDY TURNS TO FARCE." Thus the activist Timothy Trengrove-Jones reported on the latest episode in the South African AIDS chronicle in the September 15, 2000, issue of the *Weekly Mail and Guardian.* The object of Trengrove-Jones's comment was Health Minister Tshabalala-Msimang, a favorite target of editorials and cartoons. The star journalist John Robbie, famous for his bluntness, had managed to pin her down during his Radio 702 talk show on September 6. Robbie began by mentioning the book she was said to have distributed at a meeting of her provincial colleagues. *Behold a Pale Horse* was the work of William Cooper, a former U.S. CIA agent who after quitting the CIA had exposed several plots organized by secret societies in touch with space aliens and held responsible among other things for having assassinated John F. Kennedy. According to Cooper, one of their purposes was to "target the undesirable elements of society for extermination" and "specifically . . . the black, Hispanic and homosexual populations" who would be infected with AIDS through a project called MK-NAOMI that in Africa uses the smallpox virus.[1] After this surprising public revelation, the journalist asked Tshabalala-Msimang point-blank, "Is HIV responsible for AIDS?" When she avoided the question, he became more insistent, even addressing her by her first name. When the health minister reacted indignantly at his rudeness, Robbie exploded, "Go away! I cannot stand this rubbish any longer." Tshabalala-Msimang left. The incident caused a stir in South Africa. It was generally admitted that the journalist had been out of bounds—in fact, he was obliged to apologize—but for many people the interview confirmed that the cabinet members' denial of the link between HIV and AIDS was due to a deeply entrenched irrationality combining strange beliefs and shameful sources. Combined with the suspicion that a worldwide plot was being hatched by Freemasons and extraterrestrials, the accusations leveled against the pharmaceutical industry by the government could thus easily be discredited. The pseudoscientific authorities they supposedly relied on could be portrayed as cranks, moreover cranks connected to racist organizations. This was a reassuring picture that made heterodoxy look absurd and ludicrous in a context in which no opportunity was missed to cast doubts on the sanity of Thabo Mbeki and his health minister. Orthodoxy thus spared itself the trouble of having to prove the truths it propounded or to question its blind spots or biases.

One has but to read several of the commentators on the South African controversies over AIDS—journalists, politicians, activists, scholars—to realize that the intellectual landscape of the AIDS epidemic has been reduced to simple terms: on one side, medicine and science, people of goodwill and good sense, efficacy and truth; on the other, a president and a few dissidents, corrupt politicians and quack scientists, incompetence and error. In other words: here, a consensually established theory, dictating coherent choices in terms of solutions for AIDS and limited only by a lack of funds or political will; there, groundless theories attracting a few marginal characters who appear driven by a dangerous paranoia and whose inconsistencies spell danger for the population. The first know; the second believe. That dichotomy affects even the shape of discourse. When speaking of the orthodox community, its viruses and medicines, observers use a calm tone and sound arguments and provide objective statements. When speaking of the dissident universe, its social interpretations and fight against poverty, indignation is second only to irony, and subjectivity invades every line they write. The orthodox position is presented seriously; the dissident position is described with irritation or mockery.[2] The reader or hearer of these analyses can only join the party of truth, unless he or she wishes to be categorized as a disbeliever. As for the anthropologist or sociologist who wants to explore the matter further, he or she will be exposed to the doubly disqualifying accusation of denialist relativism and criminal irresponsibility.

If we go along with these analysts, things are clear. The only problem, as they themselves admit, is that it is quite hard to understand. Hard to understand that a head of state that most observers agree is intelligent and honest should adhere to this old-fashioned nonsense promoted by a group of marginal scientists. Hard to understand also that his declarations should unexpectedly be so well met by various segments of the South African population. One then finds oneself resorting to what Geoffrey Lloyd (1990) has termed the "hasty diagnostics of irrationality," that is, interpretations intending to explain scientifically representations or acts that one actually considers reprehensible and illegitimate. Such diagnostics thus presuppose an analytic asymmetry permitting one precisely to place everything that appears rational on one side and everything that seems irrational on the other. Edward Said (1978) is a pioneer in this critique of the prejudices toward others. What he writes about Orientalism applies as well to Africanism. The case of AIDS is typical in this respect. Over the past twenty years many speakers and researchers, including those affiliated with international institutions, have put forth a litany of "beliefs" that are presented as "obstacles" in the fight against the pandemic.

The South African version, however, presents one major original feature. Irrationality is not on the side of tradition but of modernity, or, one might be tempted to say, of postmodernity. What emerges is not a set of ancestral representations (though these are not completely absent from certain theorizations) but contemporary phenomena stemming from both scientific dissidence and conspiracy theory. These phenomena have a global dimension and stem in part from what Robert Merton (1968) calls the "organized skepticism of the scientific attitude" and in part from what Richard Hofstadter (1964) calls the "paranoid style in politics." In other words, they belong to the present scientific and political activity that is common if not normal. The situation in South Africa is thus not entirely unprecedented, whether in regard to heterodoxy in science or to conspiracy in politics: the history of epidemics shows on the contrary the long-standing existence of such phenomena. The South African example is not limited either to the continent but represents a global reality, as, for example, in the United States, where the duo of dissidence and conspiracy often first makes itself heard: both Peter Duesberg, representing the scientific world, and William Cooper, representing the political realm, are Americans. We will thus have to demonstrate, first, how the present configuration differs from past ones and, second, how the South African figures are distinct from others elsewhere—in what way the controversies are both contemporary and specific.

To do this it may be necessary to recognize that the object of the controversies is not what it seems to be or rather that it is not exactly what we think it is. What fundamentally is at stake may not be, as is usually claimed, knowing whether the virus is or is not the cause of AIDS. Nor is it, as is more subtly suggested, a rivalry between authorities disguised as a scientific debate. It is of course a question of knowledge and power, of confrontations of scientific theories and struggles in the public sphere, but it is not only that. The parallel with the controversy that shook AIDS circles in the United States during the second half of the 1980s and that Steven Epstein (1996) studied at length is instructive from this standpoint. The content is practically the same: the viral etiology of AIDS versus an innocent passenger virus. The protagonists also are similar: the international scientific community versus the West Coast dissidents joined by a few Australian and European researchers. Yet the stakes are completely different. First, in terms of content, the theories vary significantly. The heterodox theory, heretofore polyphonic, relatively technical, and readily anecdotal when it attributed the development of AIDS to "recreational drugs" (heroin, cocaine, and poppers), now is propounding a coherent theory that would seem almost self-evident if one considers the social realities of South Africa: poverty among the African population and the concomitant problems of insufficient hygiene, chronic malnutrition, and multiple infections. In other words, political economy has entered the scientific arena in the debate over the causes of AIDS. Second, on the side of the protagonists, the quarrels have brought new actors on the scene. With the appearance of the South African president and his ministers, the polemic has shaken free of the specialized circles of science and activism. Public administration is now meddling with scientific knowledge. So, rather than an ancient controversy surging up afresh, quite a different story is being played out and other stakes are being played for. But before trying to explain, let us look at what the controversy is made of and who its prime movers are.

Two facts make the controversy surrounding AIDS in South Africa different from those usually studied by sociologists of science. First, though bearing mainly on scientific matters (biomedical in this case), the polemics run in all directions to the extent that beyond academia where scientific polemics usually take place, all of society has been drawn in, albeit to varying degrees and in different ways. Second, though they concern knowledge and its modes of production and validation, the controversy triggers immediate action. Beyond the debates about the etiology of the virus or the assessment of a drug, it is the programs for prevention and the protocols for treatment that are being challenged (with foreseeable consequences in terms of human lives saved or lost). Because they take place in the public sphere and because they question public intervention, the controversies must be seen as political even though their object is scientific.

This qualification is justified by another, deeper reason. Controversies can also be said to be political because they bear on the government of human beings. In her study of the phenomenon of ufology in the United States, the political scientist Jodi Dean (1998: 6–8, 225) declared that the widely shared belief in the existence of space aliens and flying saucers, in the plotting of secret societies and manipulations in the political sphere, stems from the widespread notion that scientists and leaders are hiding things from us: "Given the political and politicized position of science today, this attitude toward scientific authority makes sense. Its impact, moreover, is potentially democratic. It prevents science from functioning as a trump card having the last word in what is ultimately a political debate: how people will live and work together." Furthermore: "The pleasure that conspiracy theory provides has less to do with coherence and meaning than with power and contestation." From this perspective also controversies are political, and they are "political because they are stigmatized." The same is true in South Africa. The AIDS debates show that the suspicion surrounding medicine and politics, whites and Westerners, has infiltrated the entire political project that society has been trying to construct. Thus, to govern means making do with this reality, for if one wants to change it one must first acknowledge its existence.

From this perspective I want to follow two directions. The first line concerns the ordeals to which social actors are subjected. This means examining the very stuff the controversies are made of, the truths being defended and the arguments employed, so as to shed light on the underlying efforts at social construction. I therefore attempt to find a way to surpass the Manichaean oppositions true and false, good and bad, not to pit those who defend viral etiology against those who furnish social explanations but to make it possible to detect the doubts behind the confidence, the ambiguities behind the absolute opposites, the shifts behind apparently stable positions. I tackle these problems (expressed here in terms of authority and ethics) in this new light but show, too, that the social sciences themselves cannot be overlooked. The second path leads to the arenas where these disputes take place. It corresponds to what might be called an external approach to the controversies, in the sense that it examines the individuals and their logic, the different social worlds in which they act and live. I would like to show that, rather than with alliances for or against legitimate science, as is generally claimed, we are dealing here with principles and persons in coalitions relatively independent from the subject of the disputes. They are strategic coalitions, not intellectual alliances. In fact, it is incorrect to say there is an orthodox camp and a dissident camp. I use a Proustian representation of society and speak of two sides to describe the various forms of attachment to the cause of AIDS. At the end of this exploration, I look at the possibilities of getting beyond the simplistic duality implied by the accusation of denial.

ORDEALS

Who said mankind has one great song,
Who said the great ones are those whose songs belong to all men.
MAZIZI KUNENE
"Two Wise Men"

In an article titled "Leave Science to the Scientists, Mr. Mbeki," published in the *Sunday Independent* in June 2000, three professors at the prestigious University of Natal, Ahmed Bawa (physicist), Daniel Herwitz (philosopher), and Hoosen Coovadia (pediatrician), begged President Mbeki to "allow science to maintain the autonomy it requires to function as the knowledge system it is." The response appeared in the same paper one week later, from no less than three ministers, Manto Tshabalala-Msimang (Health), Ben Ngubane (Research), and Essop Pahad (Cabinet), whose jointly written article was titled "Mbeki's Stand on AIDS Was Dictated by African Realities." The authors declared, "Responsible leader that he is, our president has decided that he too must familiarize himself with all aspects related to this tragedy so that he can occupy the front trenches in the fight against it." How long can science remain autonomous when a major crisis obliges the government to intervene? How far can politicians' search for information go when the scientific community considers that some of its members no longer respect the basic tenets of science? It is clear that the three academics believed the government does not have the authority to settle a debate for which it lacks both the most elementary scientific know-how and the rules of the game, whereas the three ministers felt that politicians must do their duty to the nation and the people even if it means overstepping the boundaries of its domain. And that is indeed the point: the government and the AIDS specialists were disagreeing over the principle that defines the relationship between scientist and politician.[3] This relationship was now being tested anew by the South African protagonists. The government feels it is necessary and legitimate to inquire into the very content of science in order to make a more enlightened decision: setting up a panel is precisely intended to allow politicians to settle what is seen as a scientific conflict. But for the AIDS specialists biomedicine is too complex to be entrusted to politicians, however well intentioned they may be: decisions must be made independently in the scientific sphere by the researchers themselves with no outside interference. Two conceptions of society are thus at odds: the first asserts the supremacy of the body politic and demands the right to interfere anywhere in the social arena; the second aspires to autonomy and claims that science obeys only its own laws in a field that belongs to it alone. The two conceptions can be reconciled only if the polemic is resolved in scientific circles (whether by agreement or unilateral exclusion) and if its terms are accepted in the political sphere (by validating the agreement or approving the exclusion). In the present case, the crisis had in fact been resolved in scientific circles (by marginalizing the dissidents) in the early 1990s, but this outcome was challenged a decade later by the government (which put the heterodox and the orthodox scientists on the same plane as if the matter had not been settled). However, the binary representation that holds that scientists, as owners of knowledge, oppose politicians, as owners of power—or, in more polemical terms, that the truths of the first oppose the errors of the second—does not do justice to the facts. It does not provide a basis for understanding, unless one wants to get into psychopathology or accuse politicians of extreme cynicism. Medical authorities' declarations presented as bona fide facts, ethical demands elevated to the rank of unquestionable models, anthropological interpretations provided as if obvious—all three need a critical appraisal.

The Intermittences of Medicine

In early 2002, first by the Pretoria High Court, then by the Constitutional Court, the South African government was ordered to make nevirapine available without delay to all HIV-positive pregnant women.[4] These court cases and their outcomes were seen as a triple victory: for public health, because prescribing the antiretroviral drug to parturient women and their newborns meant reducing the statistical risk of "vertical infection" and thus saving thirty-five thousand children a year; for human rights, because the judges ruled that it is the state's constitutional obligation to respect, protect, promote, and implement the right of every individual to access to health care. Moreover, the courts' decisions were a victory for democracy in the sense that the "New South Africa" had demonstrated its capacity to accept the fact that members of civil society could legitimately attack the authorities even in an ordinary court of law. In the weeks that followed, despite its protests, the Health Department complied. The program to prevent mother-to-child transmission was implemented nationwide. Until then it had only been carried out experimentally in eighteen hospitals, two in each province, a restriction the government had imposed for three main reasons. First, the innocuousness of nevirapine was not ascertained, as serious secondary effects had been described and five out of forty women had died in the South African sample during the initial multicenter trial. Second, its effectiveness had not been sufficiently demonstrated, especially in real situations in which women breast-fed, which meant a high probability of contaminating babies that the drug might otherwise have protected. Third, it was suspected that the virus became resistant when antiretroviral drugs were administered only over extremely short periods, which could weigh heavily on the future of the infected women and children treated under this protocol. The three arguments had been brushed aside.

When I became vice president of the National AIDS Council in France in spring 2004, our first task—to my surprise—was to prepare an official opinion titled "Promote access of pregnant women living with HIV/AIDS to antiretroviral drugs in Third World countries." Taking recent data into account, we were supposed to make recommendations for the prevention of mother-to-child transmission. After having listened to ten international experts, among them representatives from the World Health Organization (WHO), the text was written up, discussed, and then adopted on June 24, 2004. The main point concerned the revision of protocols being used in Third World countries and notably in South Africa, in particular, nevirapine in monotherapy. These protocols were now criticized by the experts for three main reasons: the drug's proven liver and skin toxicity for the mother and the not well understood mitochondrial dysfunction in the child; the relative lack of effectiveness because of breast-feeding but also because of unsatisfactory practical implementation in the field; and finally and above all, the high incidence of viral resistance not only to this drug but also to its entire therapeutic class, among which are the most frequently used treatments. The document asserted, "Generalizing treatments using nevirapine monotherapy seriously compromises the chances of therapeutic success for the tritherapies presently available in the South [i.e., developing countries] and therefore, in the long run, the survival of these women and their children."[5] The final recommendation was to replace these protocols by "efficient, prophylactic multitherapies." This official opinion incidentally included several of the recommendations published by the WHO on its website in January 2004: the "revision" was presented as provisional and —remarkably—the public was encouraged to write in their reactions and comments. The arguments used to criticize the dangers of nevirapine in mother-to-child transmission were thus very similar to those invoked by the South African government a few years before.

The new recommendations were confirmed during the Fifteenth International AIDS Conference in Bangkok in July 2004 by a series of scientific papers warning about the risks of short-term monotherapies with nevirapine. But they went nearly unnoticed among the new subjects of controversy raised by AIDS policies in Asia, caught in turn between denial and authoritarianism. The South African health minister, Manto Tshabalala-Msimang, recently reconfirmed in office after the general elections were largely won by the ANC, tried to rekindle the polemic by being ironical about the dangers of the drug she had been forced to make available to all the health care facilities in her own country, but she was hardly heard.[6] In South Africa itself, the new state of the art also ended up setting new norms that medical authorities discreetly advocated. Single-dose nevirapine, the efficient, low cost, and simple to use wonder drug for preventing mother-to-child transmission in poor countries thus quietly began its descent into the purgatory of clinical tests.

Two aspects of this almost complete shift in the norms established for the prevention of mother-to-child transmission must be stressed. First, it shows that biomedicine is capable of being critical and reactive: protocols are under constant evaluation, data are thus being continuously updated (criticism), and revisions are followed by updated recommendations (reactivity). Second, it shows that the new recommendations obey the double principle of equality and accountability: there is no question of introducing a different norm a priori for certain countries or groups, even if certain adaptations might be justifiable a posteriori depending on context, and what is good for the first world must also be good for the third world (equality); international as well as national authorities must work toward making practices uniform (accountability). In a way these two series of elements define the practices and ethics of biomedicine.

What poses a problem, however, is the absence of memory and its consequences. That the South African government was publicly accused of genocide and condemned by the courts for having applied what could have been described as a precautionary principle (keeping the program experimental, given the scientific doubts of the moment) and for having prevented the widespread use of prevention treatment because of its potential dangers (uncertain at the time but established today) remains unsaid. For medical professionals, the state of the art at a given moment determines the norms. The evolution of knowledge, at the heart of scientific activity, is what will guide the normative changes. When new discoveries are made, the norm changes. Seen this way, biomedicine is always right. At the time when it makes a definitive statement—and to the extent that it has mobilized all the scientific resources immediately at its disposal—it is speaking the truth, even when it declares the contrary of what it had asserted previously. One might of course consider this position from a Popperian perspective: *biomedicine* is a science precisely because it makes statements that are falsifiable (Popper 1959). The argument is not wrong as regards the *bio,* that is, the scientific component of medical knowledge: the respect of *ex ante* protocols and *ex post* peer evaluation confirmed by scientific publications follow the same logic, even if the definition and the application of "gold standards" in clinical trials is still a subject of discussion and debate (Marks 1997). But, compared to biology, for instance, the specific nature of biomedicine comes from the fact that it is also *medicine.* It has effects on persons and on society, through diagnoses and treatments, through individual counseling and collective pronouncements, through the production of norms that in the end turns doctors into "moral entrepreneurs" (Freidson 1970). Thus, contrary to science, when biomedicine speaks the truth it also speaks morals and, in so doing, becomes socially vulnerable. Though it can always claim it has done its best at any given moment, it is accountable to the public in the long term. And though it may forget, the public will remember.

Applying a distinction familiar to moral philosophers, one might say that biomedicine carries out its self-evaluation in the light of a "deontology"— its conformity to the obligations and duties it has set for itself, especially its practices and ethics—whereas society also evaluates it from a "consequentialist" perspective—in reference to the totality of its effects, which calls for a diachronic approach (Pettit 1996). As far as prevention of perinatal transmission is concerned, biomedicine may well judge that not only has it not failed, it has functioned perfectly by radically revising its norms when new information becomes known. In the social world, however, the different moments of truth appear as just contradictions, especially upsetting as the assurance of speaking the truth was redoubled by the claim it was doing good—and that the adversary was wrong and doing evil. When one questions AIDS specialists today, they are not surprised at the changes in rhetoric and say that they always knew there would be risks, especially of toxicity and resistance. But they did not say so at the time, and later they no longer remembered they had not. Perhaps this historic inconsequence should be discussed in health circles, precisely because of its inevitable social effects. For lack of being taken into account, it often leaves the public and sometimes the policy makers disoriented and suspicious.

The medical truth produced—or what is presented as such at any given time—is thus the result of a double mechanism that unfolds simultaneously: consolidation through the formation of a temporary consensus; translation that goes from the scientific circles to the public. At first there are observations and experiments, clues followed or dropped, debates and doubts. In the present case the best strategy for the prevention of mother-to-child transmission was still in 2000 at the stage of being discussed, evaluated, and warned against by AIDS specialists.[7] Little by little the truth came out: its name was nevirapine, and its ease of use and low cost made it a "magic bullet" (Brandt 1985), ideal for poor countries. A preventive procedure seemed to exist that was both pragmatically adapted to the economic and medical situation of the third world and ethically satisfactory since it reduced by half the number of transmissions at birth. An excellent cost-effective compromise for public health: what was lost in terms of results (not as good as those obtained by the tests carried out in rich countries) was gained in terms of easy implementation (and thus, in the end, of lives spared).[8] Very quickly, therefore, the new doctrine "set," as one would use the term to refer to cement. At the same time, and this was part of the hardening process, it was translated for a larger public, simplified for the purpose of communication. It is remarkable in this respect that every time biomedical assertions were pronounced by health professionals or AIDS activists, without also mentioning the need to view them with caution, they were in sharp contrast to the prudence that still prevailed in the journals and even in scientific symposia. Two regimens of truth for two distinct social worlds, and the general public does not necessarily get the best one.

The consolidation of new facts into truths and their translation from scientific circles to the public arena are mutually reinforcing. Hesitation gives way to certainty and margins of error disappear. Truth solidifies. During a lecture given in July 2000, Dr. Glenda Gray (one of the scientists responsible for the South African Intrapartum Nevirapine Trial [SAINT]) thus announced "good news for South Africa and for the world": "We have a vaccine to prevent mother-to-child transmission. The data are clear, both from the South African and Ugandan trials: Nevirapine is safe and effective." And as far as resistance was concerned, she asserted the matter was "irrelevant." Trengrove-Jones commented, "The government's response is shameful. Predictably enough, there was the call for more research. Then the issue of resistance was raised. It was hard and remains hard not to feel there is massive intransigence and obstructionism."[9] For him, there is no other explanation than bad faith.

The double operation of consolidation and translation thus has two corollary ways of excluding contradictions, on the one hand, and dismissing opponents, on the other. First, anything that does not fit in with the truth in the process of consolidation tends to be pushed to the margins: the effectiveness obtained under specific experimental conditions is extrapolated to ordinary health care situations in the third world; deaths observed are not related to the toxicity of the drug but to the poor implementation of the trial; the resistance of the virus, though by then one knew that all monotherapies produce it, is not presented as a problem. Second, everything that risks slowing down the national protocol is dismissed as being due to bad faith or ill will: asking for additional investigations becomes systematic obstruction; doubts expressed by the Health Department are ascribed to the health minister's shady connections with the dissidents; delays in implementing the national plan are seen as criminal negligence. In the end, every trace of the collective attempt to check the facts has been erased. Only the naked truth remains, without memory—and will remain so until the advent of a new truth.

In writing these lines, I am well aware of leaving myself open to criticism by those researchers or activists, doctors or administrators who are working honestly to advance medical knowledge for the benefit of the greatest number and to implement it despite great resistance. Some may well think I am using arguments that may be taken up by scientific heterodoxy. But it seems to me that one cannot construct a public health policy—or a democracy—by simplifying facts, rejecting critiques, and, finally, denying history. When one makes contradictory statements only a few years apart without acknowledging the contradictions and without considering that this might have social consequences, one does a disservice to the cause one is supposed to be serving. Medical science would probably be more credible if it did not appear to function as a creed. It is much harder to publicly confront a patient's death due to the secondary effects of an antiretroviral drug when one has accused the government of inventing them than if one had acknowledged its potential dangers in the first place. This happened to the Treatment Action Campaign, several of whose members died from just these effects,[10] and the organization had the courage not to hide the facts.

In the South African case, the way that an unchallengeable truth had been hammered out and the fierce attacks on the government left many people shaken. When it became known that the U.S. Food and Drug Administration had not given the green light to nevirapine (which thanks to the Uganda tests had become the basic drug for preventing perinatal transmission), many people started to wonder. However, while admitting that "if the worst-case scenario is true and if in their enthusiasm the researchers did interpret the study in a more positive light than other scientists would have, they should be punished for any break of ethical or scientific standards and the consensus on nevirapine reassessed," journalists nevertheless continued to criticize the health minister for using this argument "to justify the government's lethargy in providing the drug."[11] As if, no matter what information is brought to the debate, politicians can only be wrong and insidious. At a certain point in the history of the epidemic and the controversies, it became impossible to question the way in which medical knowledge was produced. Any opposition was called denial. The passions involved in the battle against AIDS had made the complexity of things inexpressible—and inaudible. But if one looks closely, that complexity is very much there—and troubling.

The Frontiers of Ethics

"Furor over Testing on Humans." On April 7, 2000, in the midst of the growing polemic surrounding AIDS dissidence, the *Weekly Mail and Guardian* devoted a full page to three articles on AIDS.[12] The first article was about the interruption of the clinical tests of nevirapine for the prevention of mother-to-child transmission in South Africa, following the deaths of five patients. To justify her decision, the health minister had gone before Parliament to raise the "problem with the proliferation of clinical trials in South Africa," remarking that the country seemed to be "a fertile source of trial subjects for international drug companies" and "that South Africans are unlikely to benefit in the long run from being guinea pigs for the rest of the world." The doctors in charge of the clinical trials protested against this political interference, declaring that the problem was "the trials, not the drugs"—that is, the way the clinical research was being done. The second article reported on a survey done in Uganda by a team from Johns Hopkins University that had been challenged by the editors of the respected

New England Journal of Medicine for having infringed the code of ethics. It transpired that to study the conditions surrounding HIV transmission, the research team had observed couples of whom one partner was seropositive and the other seronegative without proposing treatment and prevention, with the result that there were "90 new cases of contamination that might have been avoided." According to the article, "the ethical standards were indeed different from those that would govern research in developed countries." The third article referred to a memo written by the CIA about the dangers AIDS presented to the "democratic transitions" in sub-Saharan countries and the social burden that this illness of "catastrophic proportions" would represent in the next two decades.

Reading about people dying in South Africa as a result of clinical trials with drugs produced by international firms, about lowered ethical standards in an epidemiological study in Uganda, and about the investigation by the U.S. secret services on AIDS in the third world, all on the same page, leaves one with a strange feeling. The suspected or verified use of human guinea pigs, the presumed complicity between the pharmaceutical industry and the academic community, the dramatic scenarios produced by supposed intelligence experts—all these seem to corroborate the climate of suspicion and lend credit to the conspiracy theories that unfolded at the same time in the social arena.[13] Indeed, this information was being disseminated by a reputable newspaper that can hardly be suspected of supporting the president in the present controversy. Thus it is not the reflection of reality in the media that is disturbing but the reality itself that the media is trying to render to the best of its ability. To add to the confusion, it should be noted that the clinical trial, which for the first time established the effectiveness and innocuousness of nevirapine (regarding which the South African minister spoke about "guinea pigs" in the first article) was carried out in Uganda by a team from Johns Hopkins University (the team challenged for having treated the test subjects like "guinea pigs" in the second article came from that same academic institution). The same vocabulary, the same country, the same university. If we are given the impression in the first case that the health minister's interpretations are part of a general paranoia, what we discover in the second case is that the suspicion has been confirmed scientifically by an international medical journal. The borders between the imaginary and the real, between conspiracy theories and disturbing facts, are beginning to blur.

Scandals surrounding ethics in research on AIDS in Africa are as old as the epidemic or at least the discovery of the disease. As Nicolas Dodier

(2001) demonstrated, they cast doubt on the universal nature of norms in "transnational medicine" and oppose two approaches: one in which it is necessary to adapt codes of conduct to the local contexts and one that holds that the same principles must apply everywhere. The historical trend is a shift from the first to the second, which is what the nevirapine story illustrates: starting from a position little concerned that the benefits of this drug were lesser compared to the protocols used in rich countries (but of course also taking into account the facility of application and the lower costs, supposed to suit the local situation better), one has arrived at a series of recommendations explicitly in line with the protocols approved for Western populations (with the opposite risk this time that they turn out to be unrealistic, particularly in Africa). These ethical debates are crucial because they show that what is at stake in public health is not only a question of truth or falsehood, as the medical discussions usually have it, but also a question of good and evil, or sometimes fairness and lack of fairness. The accusations leveled against the government are basically moral condemnations. Letting children die whose lives might be saved was for four years the most serious reproach addressed to the head of state and his cabinet. If the government was accused of passive infanticide and scientific heterodoxy, the former was much more socially reproved than the latter. In the moral competition engaging the two camps, the activists and doctors (supported by a large majority of the press) were certainly the winners by far, having imposed a clearcut separation between good and evil, between those who save lives and those who sacrifice them. They won at least in the global and national public spheres, since important segments of nonwhite society saw in it an ideological manipulation. However, the strictly Manichaean construction of the moral arena, equivalent to the radical polarization in the political field, leaves unexplained two points essential for the understanding of what is at stake in AIDS.

First, medicine is far from being exempt of all ethical criticism, especially where its activities in the third world are concerned. A long article signed by David Rothman in the *New York Review of Books* (2000) had as its title "The Shame of Medical Research." The author reviews a series of clinical trials and epidemiological surveys carried out in the second half of the 1990s in developing countries that posed serious ethical problems. Most of these studies bore once again on the prevention of mother-to-child transmission. Analyzing them thus throws some light on the South African debates. Marcia Angell, editor in chief of the the *New England Journal of Medicine,* was the first to raise these questions in a rigorous editorial.[14] After stating that the fundamental rule of all random testing comparing two treatments is, "there be no good reason for thinking one is better than the other," a rule that obviously when one of the two products used is a placebo, she looks at the way it applies in work done in the third world. Since 1994, she writes, thanks to the trial called ACTG 076, we know that zidovudine, or AZT, reduces mother-to-child transmission at least by half, and thus all studies concerning North American subjects systematically include such prevention. However, in their review of the clinical trials conducted in developing countries, published in the same issue of the journal, Peter Lurie and Sidney Wolfe reveal that fifteen of the sixteen research programs used a placebo, thus exposing the children of this group to a natural risk of contamination. Nine of these trials were financed by the National Institutes of Health in the United States and all of them referred to a WHO work group for recommendations on the use of a placebo. Nine of the eleven countries were African: Ivory Coast, Burkina Faso, Ethiopia, Uganda, Tanzania, Kenya, Malawi, Zimbabwe, and South Africa.[15] Angell concludes that "these fifteen studies clearly violate recent guidelines designed specifically to address ethical issues pertaining to studies in developing countries" by making the risk of contamination one or two out of five. What can be the rationale behind this "general retreat from the clear principles enunciated in the Nuremberg Code and the Declaration of Helsinki as applied to research in the Third World"? Angell wonders.

In her answer, the editor in chief of the medical journal rejects the two most frequently given reasons: it is not because the standards for treatment are any lower in the third world (or at least that reason is unacceptable); nor is it because the results obtained in rich countries are not applicable in poor countries (at least one cannot make this an a priori principle). In fact, it is the very way that scientific activity functions that makes this deviance possible, both because of the reference to the gold standard of treatment and because of the international competition between researchers even in their access to subjects. She concludes: "To survive, it is necessary to get the work done as quickly as possible, with a minimum of obstacles. When these considerations prevail, it seems as if we have not come very far from Tuskegee after all." *In caude venenum.*

The reference to Tuskegee is central to medical ethics and crops up again and again during discussions in South Africa. Let us reprise this infamous case. A study was carried out under the auspices of the U.S. Public Health Service from 1932 to 1972, consisting in comparing two samples representing a total of 616 poor American blacks, some infected by syphilis and the others supposedly healthy, in order to uncover the illness's "natural history." If at the outset one could rightly consider that since there was no known effective treatment for syphilis, observation without intervention was justified, after the discovery of penicillin in the early 1950s knowledge of antibiotics' benefits should have led to modifying the protocol. But it did not. It is only after the scandal provoked in the early 1970s by the revelation in the press of the existence of this study that the U.S. government decided to put an end to the research after forty years (Jones 1981). The fact that the people tested were "African Americans" gives special meaning to the scandal in the South African context of today. For the journalists or officials who refer to it publicly, it is the key to an obvious continuity in racially differentiated, sometimes openly racist practices in medicine. That is more or less the backdrop against which the actors on the AIDS scene talk today about "human guinea pigs"—meaning black people exposed to undue risk in unethical trials.

Second, the position defended by the South African government cannot be whittled down to a kind of cursed side of ethics. Even if the use of antiretroviral drugs in the prevention of mother-to-child transmission and in the treatment of patients was indeed controversial and curtailed by the health minister, the fight against AIDS cannot be limited to that single aspect, crucial though it was. In this respect, the title that Catherine Campbell (2003) chose for her book on AIDS—*Letting Them Die*[16]—is somewhat unfair to the government's achievements on behalf of South Africans during its first decade in power. It is common to see health problems exclusively from a medical perspective, in particular the use of drugs. Yet we know that, especially given the existing inequalities in South Africa, social interventions that improve living conditions and reduce economic disparities often have a much more decisive effect on heath status (Marmot and Wilkinson 1999). Even in the case of AIDS patients, the chances of being infected and the length of survival are closely linked to the material and human environment in which they live, as we will see further on. Acting on living conditions and economic disparities may be as important for the survival of poor patients as administering antiretroviral drugs; moreover, the two are not mutually exclusive as the two "sides" of the controversy tend to claim.

In a balanced analysis of ten years of health care reform and AIDS policies in South Africa written for the *New England Journal of Medicine*, Solomon Benatar writes:

Given the importance of the social determinants of health, the new government can be proud of its many achievements that have improved health among the nation's approximately 45 million people. These include stabilization of the economy, substantial economic growth, reversal of discriminatory legislation, and rationalization of the complex bureaucracy associated with the policies of apartheid. In addition, the government has provided access to clean water for 9 million people, built 1.5 million houses, and installed electricity and telephone connections to more than 1 million homes. It has also constructed hundreds of new clinics that provide primary health care, desegregated medical services, made health services free to expectant mothers and children under five years of age, and developed new food programs that reach 5 million children.[17]

The health budget has tripled over an eight-year period, and $1.7 billion have been dedicated to setting up antiretroviral treatments over the next five years. In addition, one of the most important changes for poor patients has been the homogenization of the welfare system (which before was unevenly divided according to "racial" groups) as well as the extension of criteria and grading, representing a considerable increase in social expenditures as this budget now amounts to $4.3 billion.[18] The point here is not to assess the social programs the South African state has conducted in order to justify the delays in the provision of prophylactic antiretroviral drugs but simply to reintroduce yet another ethical dimension rarely considered in the moral debates dividing South African society: the question of social justice. It may be added that this is not necessarily to the government's advantage, and though it is generally recognized that the government has allowed large parts of the population to gain access to basic necessities (water, electricity, and medical care) and minimum resources (through social grants and food parcels), it is also generally admitted that the inequalities, concomitant with the forcible integration of the country into the global economy, have grown over the past ten years.

The simplification of the ethics involved and the polarization of the moral question about AIDS point once again to a double process of minimizing the dubious practices of certain scientific projects and of highlighting beneficial government policies. Such a selective memory fires the sense of injustice of those who do not forget. On the local just like on the global scale, the "double standard" is an essential mechanism that stimulates resentment in unequal human relations.

The Uses of Culture

The lecture on witchcraft and AIDS delivered by Adam Ashforth at the University of Witwatersrand in April 2001 is the sort that provokes reactions among the South African public.[19] His thesis was that in Soweto, where he has done research, the patients dying of AIDS are usually considered victims of witch attacks (*isidliso* in Zulu, *sejeso* in Sotho). The omnipresence of the "witchcraft paradigm" thus conveys a general sense of insecurity and creates a twofold problem for "public policy": acknowledging the practices involved (diviners and healers) and managing the punishments inflicted on the accused (which can include murder). For the postapartheid government, Ashforth concluded, this is a challenge insufficiently dealt with. At the end of his speech, there was a flurry of criticism from African students and researchers. Once again, they said, blacks were being represented as locked in tradition and beliefs, magic and rituals. Cultural modernity and political conflict in the townhsips were covered up by a stereotyped image. Presenting witchcraft as the major political issue implied that social, economic, and racial issues were of secondary importance. They denounced this analysis as one more example of the symbolic violence inflicted by the ethnographer, telling them once again, You think you know yourselves, but I know better.[20] Indeed, Ashforth defended himself by referring to his research and its empirical results. He spoke of what he had seen and heard in Soweto. He had even lived for some time in the township. In response, his young audience protested that they were born there and knew it too.

Beyond its anecdotal interest, this event reveals the problems that analyzing culture and reporting on it pose today. As we know, the "politics of representation" have become a central issue in South Africa, as they have more generally in what Stuart Hall (1996: 441–442) calls "black cultural politics."[21] For a long time that approach focused on racial disqualification and discrimination (i.e., Africans seen as inferior); today it tends to shift toward cultural essentialism and exoticism (i.e., Africans seen as different). Many see this as simply a new version of Eurocentric, usually white, discourse. Here, the two discourses—the ethnographer's and the "subject's"—do not overlap, however. But let us return to Ashforth's thesis. Witchcraft related to AIDS does correspond to an empirically observable reality. It is possible, though, to interpret it somewhat differently, in a less culturalist manner,[22] more deeply inscribed in social and political dynamics, and following two modalities that I will simply call sociological and anthropological.

Applying a sociological grid points to the fact that the witchcraft paradigm is not only compatible with the viral explanation, as it is rightly stated by Ashforth, but also competes with it in terms of stigma, accusations, and general social effects.[23] In other words, the two discourses do not emerge indifferently from a circulating flow of meanings but are part of a stock of interpretive resources into which the agents delve according to certain tactics. For instance, a young female patient from Alexandra whose husband had died of AIDS a few months before tried to impose the viral explanation of her own declining health against her family-in-law who claimed it was caused by witchcraft in order to take possession of her child. The point was thus a matter of managing a conflict between allied families, and the different interpretations were being used to serve opposing interests. Conversely, a man I met in Tickyline, also ill and whose wife had also just died of AIDS, asserted that she did not have AIDS (which would have made him responsible for her illness) and explained instead that she had been bewitched by one of her cousins after a quarrel over unacknowledged debts. Here again, the explanation served a family power struggle. As Peter Geschiere (1997: 214) wrote, "As long as the family remains the basis of social security, the enigmatic discourse on witches and their secret forces will continue to mark people's reactions to modern changes in Africa." Without succumbing to functionalism, one might say that witchcraft fits in with the social dynamics, on which it confers a certain meaning and even legitimacy. Whence the second argument that can be brought into the discussion.

An anthropological perspective may go beyond a strictly political science analysis postulating that the increasing number of witchcraft accusations would have become problems mistakenly abandoned by the government to the courts and communities.[24] Because it makes sense to an important fraction of African society, witchcraft somehow provides a shared reference that simultaneously allows for local individual interpretations and national or international explanations. In other words, rather than think in terms of the practical management of sorcery, we might be better off considering that witchcraft theories are a general matrix of interpretation of social relations in which the ideology of persecution allows both victims and perpetrators to be represented. That is the direction taken by Clifton Crais (2002: 5) in his historical study of the problem of evil in the Eastern Cape: "Where there is power and all the emotions it unleashes, there is the occult. The moral discourse of magic has been a central and historical feature of the African political imagination, a way of understanding the inequities of the world, the tyranny of the hatred, but also the way the world should be." Thus witchcraft becomes the language of misfortune and memory: "The pervasiveness of magic in people's daily lives speaks of a world and a past that is rarely disclosed, a history of deadly important whispers that concern the most basic of issues: life and death; jealousy, hatred and selfishness; agriculture and the rains; the persecution of the state; the exploits of the powerful and the exploitation of the powerless." It is within this interpretive framework that witchcraft shows its true political nature.

Generally speaking, one has to recognize the public success of the interpretations of AIDS—scientific or profane—that have attributed the main role to culture either to explain how the illness started to spread or to analyze the obstacles to prevention and treatment.[25] The director general of USAID made a memorable statement when he claimed in June 27, 2001, *Boston Globe* that Africans were incapable of taking antiretroviral drugs because their traditional conception of time would not allow them to absorb their doses at regular intervals. The way the French daily *Le Monde* reported the difficulties of controlling the progression of the illness on September 14, 1999, is also well worth noting: "The cost of treatment and cultural tradition prevent the epidemic from being halted in Africa, where medicine men prescribe to penniless patients to make love with young virgin girls to purify themselves of the virus." The "virgin-cleansing myth"—the belief that male HIV carriers can purify themselves by having sex with young virgin girls—blossomed in South Africa, but it gained worldwide popularity quite rapidly.

It is difficult to reconstitute the genealogy of the belief, or, rather, of the discourse about the belief. One can only observe the ease with which it was repeated and accepted. It is clear that it validated a whole set of prejudices and fantasies about African sexuality, adding to it a Conradian note of violence, even of barbarity, and of magic, even of Satanism. The myth rapidly appeared on the web site TruthOrFiction, among the "urban legends that kill," which describes the new "eRumor" in the following manner: "It talks about an epidemic of infected males violating virgins, including children, because of the belief that the younger the virgin, the more potent the cure." It also became the subject of a petition that used it to counteract the threat that a child protection unit was to be closed down: "There is a myth in South Africa that having sex with a virgin will cure AIDS. This has led to an epidemic of rapes by infected males, with the correspondent infection of innocent kids. Many have died of these cruel rapes. The child abuse situation is now reaching catastrophic proportions and if we don't do something then who will? Please forward this on to as many people as you know and after the 120th name on the petition mail it to childprotect pca@saps.org.za. Don't be complacent, do something about the kids of South Africa!"[26] At the same time, it was being analyzed by ethnologists such as Suzanne Leclerc-Madlala (2002), who, on the basis of data collected in KwaZulu-Natal, linked it to the "notions of 'dirt' and women's bodies" and to "metaphors that inform the local interpretations of AIDS." She concluded her study by declaring that "closer attention paid to the shaping influence of cultural schemas is critical to better understanding belief-behaviour linkages in the context of rape and AIDS." In the same vein, psychology, medicine, public health, and social work have seized on the myth and turned it into a commonplace of their surveys on rape—especially of underage children—and venereal diseases, particularly AIDS: henceforth, one can write that "attempts to explain baby rape include virgin-cleansing myths" without questioning this reality.[27] Rachel Jewkes, director of the Gender and Health Group of the Medical Research Council and a specialist on violence against women, has often denounced such a culturalization of rape, notably in a letter addressed to an international medical journal and published under the significant title, "Child Rape Is Not Exotic."[28] In my own surveys, I encountered a reference to that belief in a case of rape only once; I mention it below, and its interpretation remains problematic. A psychologist specializing in sexual abuse in the province of Limpopo told me he had never heard such a story in his professional activity. A survey carried out in neighboring Mpumalanga Province only found it mentioned by the interviewees because they had read it in the newspapers. In fact, if one considers that violence in relations between the sexes is so common—in couples, families, school, the workplace—and that so many surveys confirm it, then referring to this myth seems like a deception that rape offenders can always resort to in order to justify the unacceptable—for culture is a better attenuating circumstance than barbarity before a judge—but it says less about real practices than about the reality of representations. Considered from this perspective, this discourse adds a new chapter to what Leonard Thompson (1985) labeled "political mythology."

ARENAS

If I could turn all this
Into poetry

Would they forgive me?
—for getting it all wrong;
the subject, the characters, the issues;
the wrong class, the wrong race . . .
given this time and place—

MICHAEL CAWOOD GREEN
"Ethics"

The idea that individual positions in South African society do not simply depend on whether you believe or not in the causality of HIV and the benefits of AZT occurred to me in October 2000, during several meetings with public health specialists and social scientists at the University of Witswatersrand. We were working on a research project, and several times, during formal discussions or informal exchanges, there were references to *the* controversy. Usually they were allusions rather than real comments. I could not help noticing the irritated reactions of certain scholars when hearing the bitter or amused remarks that their colleagues made about Thabo Mbeki's declarations. Raising the subject again later in private circumstances, I became aware of the fact that for the latter seeing Mbeki's views as related to insanity and bad faith totally discredited the national fight against AIDS and made South Africa an object of ridicule in the international community, whereas for the former Mbeki's discourse held elements of truth but was systematically being twisted, as poverty was an essential factor in the spread of the infection and rolling out antiretroviral drugs was not presently realistic given the resources and structure of public health. Yet both were indisputably operating under the banner of science and had no doubts about the viral etiology of AIDS or about the benefits of nevirapine. Their opposition was political rather than scientific. But there was a difference immediately noticeable—although embarrassing to admit—between these two empirically constituted groups: all those who criticized the government were "white" researchers, among them some foreigners; those who defended it were mostly, but not exclusively, in the categories "Africans," "Coloured," and "Indians" (two persons in this group were in fact "white," and I knew they had been and still remained politically involved). I observed the same coincidence several times in different contexts and environments: sarcastic comments on one side, reserved attitudes on the other; little jokes versus embarrassed silence. Often the exchanges were muffled; sometimes they erupted into quarrels. At first I was tempted to see in this only the color line that so consistently resurfaces but that some refuse to see while others call it racism. In hindsight, it seems somewhat more complicated. More than just a question of "race" or again of "race and class," to use the usual categories, it reveals a different relationship to time that expresses itself by distinctive postures. On one side there is a direct connection to the present that implies everything is taking place here and now; on the other side, an indirect connection to the present mediated by the past, meaning that one does not forget so quickly. Thus "public arenas," to use the concept coined by Stephen Hilgartner and Charles Bosk (1988), are much more complicated to describe and analyze than the simplified versions to which they are usually reduced. I propose here to approach them from two angles: their system of actors and their grammar of action.

The President's Side

Our President who is in Parliament
Elected was your government
Its Constitution rules
Development will be done
in the rural areas
As it is done in the urban areas
Give us each day our antiretrovirals
And forgive us for wanting to live
As we survived the Boers
Who discriminated against us
And lead us not into complacency
But deliver us from
opportunistic illnesses
For you have the power to implement a treatment plan
To achieve the African renaissance
Forever and ever
Amandla!

This parody of the Lord's Prayer addressed to the head of state by Krisjan Lemmer in the February 14, 2003, issue of the *Weekly Mail and Guardian* is a humorous rendition of most people's perception that the AIDS controversy centers on individuals.

The extreme personalization of the debate over AIDS—largely a result of the way the protagonists themselves act—has led to a focus on two figures— South Africa's President Thabo Mbeki and Health Minister Manto Tshabalala-Msimang—and, to a lesser extent, Nkosazana Zuma, the previous health minister. The media have greatly facilitated this view, usually presented as pathological or political. Whatever one might think of these alternate explanations, neither allows one to understand why so many people in South Africa have gone over to the government's side on the subject of AIDS, especially with regard to its connection to poverty, but also because of the doubts raised by affirmative medical statements and the accusations brought against the pharmaceutical industry; nor do they allow one to grasp why even more people have found the repeated attacks on Mbeki and his colleagues unfair. A survey carried out among three thousand South Africans during the first semester of 2004 by Harvard University and the Kaiser Foundation showed that after four years of uninterrupted polemics, noisy denunciations, and lost trials, 42 percent of respondents approved of the government's AIDS policy; of the whites, 16 percent were of this opinion, compared to 48 percent of blacks. A U.S. anthropologist who attended the International AIDS Conference in Durban in 2000 made the following disillusioned remark to me: "No African doctor has criticized the government, nobody wanted to play the informer." She supposed nobody would dare to publicly oppose Mbeki. There is certainly some truth in her comment, but I am nevertheless struck by the fact she did not consider the alternative possibility that these doctors were sincere and convinced Mbeki was—at least partially—right.

The many interviews and informal discussions I have had with African colleagues and with people in health circles generally have made me realize that in private (i.e., without the social control of others) many of them either saw things the same way that their president did or did not share his views but defended him nevertheless against his adversaries. This last point is crucial. Supporting the government and its actions, including its AIDS policy, does not necessarily mean agreeing with what Mbeki says. It is enough to look at the September 2000 survey conducted by a group of journalists who asked the ministers what they thought of the etiology of AIDS to be convinced. Though several refused to answer and though all expressed their solidarity with the government, real differences in opinion existed, from the skeptical "HIV may cause AIDS" (Minister of Education Kader Asmal) to the positive "Of course, HIV causes AIDS" (Minister of Labor Membathisi Mdladlana). In reality, most of the ministers refused to let themselves be locked into what they felt was a "nondebate," a term employed during one of our discussions by William Pick, then director of the School of Public Health at the University of Witwatersrand.

Consequently, if one wants to understand what is being played out "on the president's side," one must—contrary to most of the commentators on the polemic—accept two premises: first, that this side really does exist, in other words that it is not made up of merely a few individuals caught in an incomprehensible error but of a substantial portion of the population, albeit unevenly distributed across society; second, that it is heterogeneous, meaning that it is made up of people who do not defend the same theories on AIDS but nevertheless belong to the same side. That is the sort of political typology I want to develop. While indicating that they only constitute ideal types and that intermediate conditions exist in the real world, I distinguish three main groups: the "heterodoxes," the "socials," and the "faithfuls." Like all typologies, this one naturally simplifies reality.

The "heterodoxes" can be plainly defined as those who reject the body of knowledge endorsed by the vast majority of the scientific community. The crux of the matter here is the link they refuse to recognize between HIV and AIDS. This objection is also the hard core of the dissident theses developed by the groups in California (around Peter Duesberg) and in Australia (around Eleni Eleopulos), which also include more radical factions that challenge the very existence of the illness (such as David Rasnick, who claims that it would be enough to stop testing to put an end to the epidemic) and more marginal elements (such as William Cooper, who believes that AIDS is the work of secret societies aided and abetted by extraterrestrial forces). Several alternatives to the virus have been suggested: first, "recreational drugs" (famous poppers used by homosexuals); then, "AIDS by prescription" (antiretroviral drugs, initially AZT). These ideas are different from and even opposed to the criminal conspiracy theory (popularized by Erich Segal who charged that U.S. laboratories, where the microbe is supposed to have begun its career, orchestrated a biological war), precisely since they believe that a virus does exist. The South African version of heterodoxy is doubly original compared to the previous ones that arose in the industrialized countries. First of all, it introduces poverty and more broadly the socioeconomic conditions that prevail in the etiology of AIDS (which certain California dissidents, Charles Geschekter for one, willingly make their own). Second, it accuses Western science of being racist, only capable of imagining stigmatizing scenarios to explain the havoc wrought on the African continent by the epidemic (a thesis already developed in the case of Haiti by the quite orthodox researcher Paul Farmer).

An underground document was making the rounds of the ANC in March 2002 and appeared to many commentators typical of what they saw as the denialist infamy. It sums up this position in a particularly striking manner: its sixty-six pages include quotes from Frantz Fanon, John Le

Carré, Mark Twain—and Thabo Mbeki. Bearing the enigmatic title *Castro Hlongwane, Caravans, Cats, Geese, Foot and Mouth and Statistics: HIV/AIDS and the Struggle for the Humanisation of the African,* the text is anonymous and opens as follows:[29]

> This monograph discusses the vexed question of HIV/AIDS. It is based on the assumption that to understand this matter, it is necessary to study it. It does not accept the assertion that only scientists and medical doctors are capable of understanding this medical condition. It recognizes the reality that there are many people and institutions across the world that have a vested interest in the propagation of the HIV/AIDS thesis, because they have too much to lose if any important element of the thesis is proved to be false, and these include the pharmaceutical companies. It recognizes that there are many well-meaning institutions and individuals in our country and the rest of the world who have innocently accepted and propagate the positions advanced by those who share these vested interests. It accepts that these have to be exposed to the truth, in the conviction that their consciences will enable them to side with the truth against the untruth. It also accepts that the HIV/AIDS thesis, as it has affected and affects Africans and black people in general, is informed by deeply entrenched and centuries-old white racist beliefs and concepts about Africans and black people. At the same time as this thesis is based on these racist beliefs and concepts, it makes a powerful contribution to the further entrenchment and popularisation of racism.

Unfurling its own hypothesis, the document goes on:

> The monograph accepts that our people, and others elsewhere in Africa and the rest of the world, face a serious problem of AIDS. It accepts the determination that AIDS stands for acquired immunodeficiency syndrome. It accepts that a syndrome is a collection of diseases. It proceeds from the assumption that the collection of diseases generally described as belonging to the AIDS syndrome has known causes. It rejects as illogical the proposition that AIDS is a single disease caused by a singular virus, HIV. It accepts that an essential part of AIDS is immune deficiency, that this immune deficiency may be acquired, that there are many conditions that cause acquired immune deficiency, including malnutrition and disease. It therefore argues that, in our situation, many and varied interventions have to be made to protect and strengthen the immune system of our people. It accepts that these include attention to our nutrition and the eradication of the diseases of poverty that afflicts millions of our people.

The rest of the text develops this argument at length.

By its mix of literal interpretation and ideological argumentation, this long creed, far from being anecdotal and marginal as it is often said to be, is at the heart of the dissident theory in its African variations. It has even been said that it was inspired or even partly written by President Mbeki. Whatever the truth may be, it is clear that some of those in Mbeki's circle propound this thesis. Physicians such as Sam Mhlongo, politicians such as ANC representative Peter Mokaba, and presidential spokesperson Parks Mankahlana, Health Minister Tshabalala-Msimang and members of provincial governments, such as Ngoako Ramatlhodi in Limpopo, constitute Mbeki's first circle of support.[30] These figures, all of them African and all of them involved in the battle against apartheid, applied a historical and political grid to AIDS and the controversy, thus differing in their approach from the foreign dissidents and even from white South African journalists such as Anita Allen and Anthony Brink, whose interpretation is mainly scientific or ideological.

The "socials" represent the second circle of President Mbeki's followers. They are not attracted by the dissident thesis and therefore do not question the viral etiology of the epidemic, but they are sensitive to the social dimensions of the illness. They feel that Mbeki is asking the right questions when he puts forward historical and political interpretations but that he is not giving the correct answers when he espouses dissident theories. Though they do not interfere in the debate, which they consider useless, over the role played by the virus, they take sides on the social causes of AIDS and the practical possibilities offered by treatment. As to the first point, they agree that measures to relieve poverty and reduce inequalities are a priority. As to the second point, they feel that living conditions among the poor and the structure of the health system make it particularly difficult to implement costly and complex therapies. The idea that giving antiretroviral drugs to patients who do not even have enough to eat constitutes a real problem; it is not just a diversionary tactic for confronting a badly intentioned government. Nevertheless, many of them have more recently become convinced that despite the difficulties involved in implementing multitherapies, it has become unavoidable to develop access to treatment. This was typically the position of the more progressive circles of public health and social work at the beginning of 2000. It also corresponded to the analyses defended internationally during the same period.[31] To mention but one example, as the Global Fund for AIDS, Tuberculosis, and Malaria was being set up, there was a head-on clash between the curative and drug-dependent approach (defended especially by the French) and the social and preventive approach (represented primarily by the Canadians).

David McCoy, technical director of the Health Systems Trust, an important South African institution that analyzes public health policies, thus explained in 2001 how the implementation of the prevention of mother-to-child transmission in the context of his country was up against a triple obstacle: lack of infrastructure, lack of trained personnel, and lack of efficient health care organization.[32] Referring to a nationwide survey, he declared, "There is no reason why areas providing a sub-standard level of basic health care should be any more successful with a mother-to-child transmission programme. This is specially the case when hundreds of front-line health workers in poor and isolated working conditions are stressed, undervalued and burdened by excessive demands and expectations." Reversing the accusation of denial usually hurled at the government, he concluded, "It is hard to understand why, but one does get the impression of a state of denial about South Africa's Third World realities and a fixation with its First World capacity." Here, denial has changed sides. For these public health specialists as well as for many development experts, the activists and physicians are so far removed from the realities prevailing in poor rural areas where most of the African population of the country lives—but where they themselves rarely go—that they have no inkling of the implications of antiretroviral drugs programs in terms of equity. However, for those who defend the "social" position, the question is not only one of cost-efficiency but also of justice: actions that may be generous in principle but unapplicable in many parts of the country will generate even greater disparities than those that already exist. That is the worry that National AIDS Programme Director Nono Simelela voices in all her speeches. Similar arguments can be heard among the civil servants from the Departments of Health and of Social Development.

The "faithfuls" make up a vast group, less unified on the AIDS issue than the two previous groups but basically united on the political level. Independently of all specific positions on AIDS (they do not generally adhere to the heterodox ideas on the epidemic, and they do not necessarily have a social theory about the illness), they stress historical solidarities. Although many see serious faults in their president's declarations that could be costly for the country's parliamentary majority in terms of national trust and international image, they insist—and often remind others—that, regarding this "democratically elected" government, loyalty must come first. For them, the poor management of AIDS is part of the mistakes inevitably connected to the exercise of power, and it is at any rate a lesser evil compared to the considerable progress accomplished in terms of civil rights and social justice. Temporality figures in their judgment. Their analysis takes the form of a diachronic comparison that weighs on the moral scale what they lived through yesterday and what they are experiencing today, most of them as Africans or more generally as "non-Whites." In this respect, their loyalty also translates into a deep identification not only with a party (generally the ANC) and a struggle (against apartheid) but also with a condition (dominated people) and a group (racially defined by others). This identification transcends the cleavages concerning political options.

During the Pretoria court trial brought against the government by the Treatment Action Campaign over mother-to-child transmission, the Human Rights Commission had at first agreed to testify as *amicus curiae* and give evidence in favor of the AIDS organization. But in November 2001 its president, Barney Pityana, withdrew his statement from the court case, though he had made it under oath. He was accused of giving in to government pressures.[33] Notwithstanding the reality of intimidation, it is not possible to disregard the strength of the sense of solidarity and loyalty. Nevertheless, these too have limits that the divisions within the ANC make abundantly clear, especially the rebellion of the provincial governments against the obstinacy of the national health minister in the nevirapine case. The tension was at its highest in February 2002 when Gauteng premier Mbhazima Shilowa generalized the prevention of mother-to-child transmission to all the public health structures of his province, ignoring Tshabalala-Msimang's decision to restrict the use of nevirapine to the experimental centers. The central committee of the ANC sided with the government, while the provincial committee of the party assured the premier of its support. The affair blew up at the very time Nelson Mandela had distanced himself from Thabo Mbeki on that issue.[34] Shortly afterward, the rulings of the Pretoria High Court and Constitutional Court fell one after the other, putting an end to the quarrel by obliging the health minister to apply nationally what Gauteng Province had announced locally.

Beyond these often violent events and against the reduction of the presidential camp to dissidence, it must thus be pointed out that above all the president's camp is a coalition of shared memory and identity, that is, a union of perspectives fundamentally united by history. This is true whether we consider heterodoxy, built on the remnants of apartheid and the permanence of racism, or the social perspective, focusing on inherited inequalities, or loyal support, expressing the solidarity to a past of common fights and aspirations. The truths about the epidemic are all different. But one truth is the same for all: time and its mark.

The Orthodox Side

"To found a party of HIV-positive people" was the project announced by the strange visitor who discreetly came to meet a young man living with AIDS from Soweto. As he told us afterward, this young man did not at first understand for whom the politician was working. Later, he realized that he belonged to the Democratic Party. His project—or what he remembered of it—was to create an apolitical party bringing together HIV-positive people in order to better defend their cause. With a potential membership of five million members, he thought, this was no small constituency. But the project fell through. Besides, though the young man said he was a member of the ANC, he also declared he had no illusions about the "fat cats" who thrive on poor men's backs, and as far as he was concerned, he was more attracted by the AIDS organizations than by the political parties, which he felt were too corrupt. In Johannesburg he was active in the Treatment Action Campaign, whose famous T-shirts he wore and never missed a single demonstration. But back home in rural Limpopo, he turned to the competition, the National Association of People Living with Aids (NAPWA) for a job because it was the only association active in that region.[35] The AIDS scene is crowded and hotly fought over. The NGOs struggle for it, as do the political parties and, of course, the international institutions.

The "orthodox side" is no more homogeneous than the "president's side." The latter unites people around a certain relationship to history, but the former proceeds from a consensus on the topic of AIDS. Where the president's men and women brought together people and groups believing in the same political project and sharing the same worldview (often circumscribed by color), the second brought together actors united in their desire to assert their truth and implement their treatment (sociologically and ideologically, they differed on all other issues). Within this framework and using the same ideal-typical grid, I will define three subgroups: the "activists," the "experts," and the "opponents." The alliances among them sometimes seem unnatural and remain fragile.

It has been said of the activists and more particularly of TAC members that their leaders were "old left-wingers, illiterate inhabitants of the townships and marathon runners."[36] They are moved by a moral conviction rather than adherence to a scientific doctrine: their cause is to save lives, the lives of those whose infection could be avoided—children yet unborn and victims of rape—and the lives of those for whom treatment could mean a longer life span. Because of his official position, his militant involvement, and his personal history (homosexual and ill, he was the first major figure in South Africa to reveal his double condition), Justice Edwin Cameron is in a way the movement's conscience. He puts it quite simply: "Of all the contextual realities which define the epidemic those which determine access to life itself are certainly the most critical."[37] As crusaders in the war against the epidemic, TAC activists are without pity for those who oppose their mission, as the often-insulted and mocked ministers and senior civil servants have good reason to know. Once the militants have been won over to a truth, they do not waste time discussing ways to put it into practice: if a preventive measure or treatment exists, implement it. Principles must be applied; problems will find a solution. This voluntarist strategy has permitted some real progress in the fight against AIDS, especially following the court case against the government. It probably also created deadlocks by causing the government's representatives to toughen their stand when they were forced to the alternative of capitulation or intransigence.

The activists have an important trump card: the experience they have acquired in the resistance movements against apartheid. They know how to mobilize instantly, organize street demonstrations, bring lawsuits in the courts, sway the media on their side, and establish contacts with international networks. Above all, that experience provides a legitimacy they fall back on if confronted by accusations of racism: Zachie Achmat, chairperson of the organization, has been a longtime member of the ANC; Mark Heywood, its spokesman, often refers to his contribution to the struggle against apartheid. Even more decisive is the backing of the Congress of South African Trade Unions, which belongs to the Tripartite Alliance in power. Its support is due to real and historical connections between the two organizations. Of course, for many of these old militants who fought against apartheid, the decision to combat the democratic government in which they had placed so much hope was a difficult, sometimes heartbreaking one. They are nevertheless determined today in their fight against AIDS, which means taking a position against state officials but without compromising themselves with the parliamentary opposition, though it has tried to win them over many time. Conversely, their relations with the scientific and medical community are remarkably peaceful. At the end of his study on the history of AIDS in the United States, Steven Epstein (1996: 343) wonders "what approaches to, or conceptions of, science activists would like to promote." He asks, "Are AIDS activists really just trying to 'clean up' science by eliminating biases that academic researchers are introducing? Or to supplant 'clean science' with something that answers to different epistemological and ethical aspirations?" In South Africa, things are clear. The TAC militants have never put themselves in a position to compete with or criticize biomedical science. On the contrary, they have become its best allies and have not challenged its results or methods.

The "experts" are the clinical scientists and research scholars. Most AIDS specialists are both; that is, they are medical practitioners who also do important clinical research in their fields, especially because of the ongoing therapeutic trials. Physicians are what could be called natural experts on AIDS. For historical reasons, most are white and, except for a few notable exceptions, were not very critical of the apartheid regime and are today not very favorable to the presidential majority: since the ANC came to power, threats of expatriation have often been voiced and in fact a large proportion among them have left. Of the thirty thousand practicioners in the country, over two-thirds are in the private sector, a tendency that has grown over the past ten years; the public sector, understaffed in the poor rural and urban areas, is largely dependent on foreign physicians, especially in the most deprived northern parts of the country where they represent 50 percent of the profession.[38] These figures suggest that for a majority of doctors social involvement is quite limited and secondary compared to the classical professional stakes and that their engagement in the AIDS problem, as a group but also as individuals, has rarely been important. Nevertheless, there have been some courageous, usually isolated cases of physician-activists, who sometimes run the risk of incurring disciplinary action; for example, Matthys von Mollendorf, head of Nelspruit Hospital, was fired for having backed an organization that delivered prophylactic antiretroviral drugs to rape victims.[39] Generally, the way professionals deal with AIDS depends less on compassion, although it is present in the rhetoric of justification, than on what might be called a clinical ethos, which consists of establishing a strictly medical relationship wherein it is taken for granted that somebody who is ill must receive care and treatment, without any concern for the social conditions of the patient.[40] Clearly, their individualistic approach differs from that of public sector physicians ("the socials" discussed above), who privilege the general good (how to improve a community's health status and reduce inequalities) over the private concerns of the sick person.

AIDS has thus garnered support on a relatively small scale in medical circles, aside from important figures such as Jerry Coovadia (professor of pediatrics at the University of Natal), who presided over the Organizing Committee of the Thirteenth International Aids Conference, Quarraisha Abdool Karim (virologist at Durban Hospital), who led the National AIDS Programme, or Glenda Gray (pediatrician at Baragwanath Hospital in Soweto), one of the initiators of the clinical trial SAINT for the prevention of mother-to-child transmission. As far as researchers are concerned, their participation in the controversies is limited to the Medical Research Council's determined engagement in the fight against AIDS in the sensitive area of demographics, with Rob Dorrington and his Actuarial Research Center, Rachel Jewkes and her Gender and Health Group, and especially its former president, Malegapuru William Makgoba, one of the leaders of the research on a vaccine.[41] A longtime comrade-in-arms and personal friend of Thabo Mbeki, Makgoba publicly challenged him in scientific circles as well as in the national newspapers and finally broke with him.

Finally, the "opponents" are members of several small political parties, for which the side effects of the AIDS polemics clearly have been beneficial. Through their controversial choices and brutal reactions, the South African president and his health minister created a gap into which the leaders of the opposition wasted no time rushing in. That was the case with the Democratic Alliance: the day after the 2000 elections it reunited the Democratic Party (the "liberals" of the previous regime) and the National Party (the "conservatives" who had laid the foundations for apartheid). Simultaneously the controversy erupted on the international scene and the political crisis worsened nationwide. At the head of the coalition, Tony Leon made AIDS his battle cry in the fight against the ANC, hoping to win the votes of the fraction of African voters disappointed with the present administration. In a dispute widely echoed by the media, he was then able to appear as the president's only serious contender. The letters they exchanged mixed scientific arguments, mutual accusations of racism and racialization, references to the past, and perspectives on the future.[42] He was, however, not the only one to have built his political career on AIDS.

At the same time, Costa Gazi, a member of the Pan Africanist Congress of Azania and a physician in the public health sector, jumped into the fray, again widely publicized in the press. After lodging a complaint before the Human Rights Commission against the health minister for negligence and accusing her in an interview of assassination, he offered to pay for the treatment of patients in the nineteen dispensaries he was in charge of out of his own pocket but was turned down.[43] More recently, Patricia De Lille, a renegade from the same party and the ebullient founder of the Independent Democrats, also used AIDS in her campaign, not only to discredit the ANC and its president, but also to dramatize her own serological test, the sick child whose treatment she was sponsoring and the inclusion of HIV-positive candidates on her national list.[44] Thus—without wanting to prejudge the sincerity of those political actors in this so-called humanitarian and therefore potentially consensual cause—it is obvious that AIDS has become a resource in the political arena and an argument in the electoral market. In this context, the government finally announced in April 2004—after four years of resistance and only three months before the national elections—that antiretroviral treatments would be made available in all the public hospitals across the country.

Battle Scenes

Between the two "sides," the president's and the orthodox's, confrontations are a daily occurrence. They take place in political institutions such as the Parliament, where the verbal jousting around AIDS has attained a rare level of violence; in spaces not intended for that purpose, for example, during the 2003 TAC civil disobedience campaign when public buildings were occupied; in more traditional places such as the streets, where demonstrations take the cultural form of *toyi-toying,* a collective foot-stamping accompanied by chants inherited from the struggle against apartheid; or in new venues such as internet web sites, which have become particularly efficient tools for the communication of theses and countertheses. Department meetings or newspaper offices, general assemblies or professional encounters may in this way become caught up in fights or arguments related to the AIDS issue. I have thus been confronted with a number of such episodes either directly or indirectly. I will give two examples that I experienced personally and that seem significant regarding how people choose to put themselves onstage. The first took place in an auditorium at the University of Witwatersrand in April 2001 during the closing session of the Aids in Context Conference. The second took place in a villa in the residential quarter of Johannesburg during a reception in honor of the Global Fund for AIDS, Tuberculosis, and Malaria delegation in April 2003.

"It's a holocaust against the poor," TAC president Zachie Achmat said on April 7, 2001, in an attack on the South African government's policies.[45] He was addressing an auditorium of academics and militants on the last day of the first South African meeting of the social sciences on AIDS, and the accusation was aimed specifically at two government representatives, Nono

Simelela, head of the National AIDS Programme, which coordinates actions against the epidemic, and Helen Rees, executive director of the Medicine Control Council (MCC), who signs the authorizations allowing drugs to be marketed. Nevirapine, the antiretroviral drug whose effectiveness had just been established by international trials, had been awaiting national approval for several months so as to be used in the prevention of mother-to-child transmission. The MCC had stipulated that the laboratory marketing the product must guarantee follow-up for viral resistance and had not yet given the green light. After the death of several women during clinical trials, the health minister had just announced that these trials were dangerous and were being interrupted *sine die*. Furious about the delays, Achmat brought up the case of a seropositive mother of three infected children who had written to him before she died, and he charged the two doctors on the podium with being "accomplices in the deaths of all these children." Tension was palpable in the audience.

Nono Simelela took the floor. Visibly shaken by the attack, she spoke through tears: "It is unfair to suggest that I have delayed the programme and am responsible for the death of children. As a mother and as an obstetrician, I have chosen this profession and I have got the love and energy to do it. It is easy to criticize and to judge, but for us who have this political commitment, there are constraints and realities we have to face." She continued: "In this country, the average white person has always known freedom. As far as I am concerned, I went to bed one night with no right to vote and I woke up in the morning as a free person. But we still have to deal with the legacy of the previous regime, which is embodied in the lack of resources in health facilities and the lack of capacities among health professionals. It takes time not because we don't want to do things but because we need to learn and we know it is costly in terms of lives." Returning to the dilemmas she was confronted with in the making of health policies, she added, "How must the government decide between the different possibilities offered to combat AIDS? This is an important question—a question of equity and ethics. The need for treatment for people with AIDS must be balanced with other needs of other people. Moreover, in a country where five million people are living with HIV, the problem of selecting those who will receive antiretrovirals is a major challenge." She ended by calling the intellectuals, academics, and activists to join the government to take the most urgent steps. Silence fell over the hall. Nono Simelela left and did not return for the debate. The emotion in the audience was not only provoked by the tears we had seen her shed during her talk—though that was remarkable enough for a senior civil servant. It was also due to the special accent of truth in her words—which belied the accusations leveled against her.[46] Everybody I met in the following months, including those most hostile to the government's policies, told me that the director of the National AIDS Programme was a responsible and competent person, a courageous and devoted official, that she played a major role in the battle against the epidemic and that she managed to do so in a most delicate context. The words she spoke quietly and with conviction in these circumstances were all the more powerful. The same cannot be said of her minister, who, in another context some time later, chose other weapons.

With the title "The Madness of Queen Manto," the April 11, 2003, *Weekly Mail and Guardian* squarely hit its mark—the health minister.[47] The article commented indignantly on the content of the speech she had delivered during the welcoming ceremony a few days earlier in honor of Richard Feachem, managing director of the Global Fund for AIDS, Tuberculosis and Malaria. She had accused "the white man"—TAC spokesman Mark Heywood, who stood in the audience—of "manipulating those Africans" who belonged to his movement and spent their time criticizing the government. Reporting this surprising incident, the journalist mentioned the embarrassment of the other members of the Health Department's delegation, the consternation of the guests, and the anger of her visitor at her "racist comments." In fact, it had all been set up. When I arrived at the reception attended by about fifty "diplomats, academics and captains of industry," to quote the reporter, I was met by a small group of TAC demonstrators bearing billboards with a red and black "Wanted" poster complete with photographs of the health minister and her colleague, the minister of commerce and industry. They were accused of "not preventing 600 deaths a day from AIDS." As Manto Tshabalala-Msimang explained at the beginning of her talk, when they heard of the posters on which she appeared "like a criminal," her security people had instructed her not to use the main door; she had thus entered the Hyde Park pavilion where the reception took place through the "back entrance." She then mentioned the recent events initiated by the activists at the civil disobedience campaign: "They come with two buses and go to the commissions where they wait for the white man to tell them what to do. . . . Our Africans say: What should we do now? And the white man tells them: You must do this, you must say that, you must go there, you must *toyi-toyi* here." At this, Mark Heywood shouted at her, "You are lying, Minister. You are a liar." While a bodyguard asked the activist to keep quiet, Tshabalala-Msimang continued her speech. She attacked in particular the Global Fund whose executive director had just begun working on an important project with an organization from KwaZulu-Natal, sidestepping the official institution for the coordination of cooperative programs, and reminded him that "the democratically elected governement" alone had the right to conclude such agreements. The atmosphere of the event was somewhat tense.

During cocktails after the ceremony, several of the people I spoke with said they were shocked or embarrassed by the minister's declarations. In the following days, the small world of AIDS hummed with disapproval at the violently racist attack. Having just returned to South Africa, I indeed found the attack surprisingly virulent. However, I was to learn later that three weeks before, while delivering the inaugural speech at a Public Health conference in Cape Town, she had had to make her way through cordons of activists who wanted to prevent her from speaking and she had been interrupted by the whistles of TAC militants who had insulted her with shouts of "Murderer!" "Coward!" "Manto, shut up!" "Go to jail!" Without allowing her to finish, TAC president Zachie Achmat read an especially aggressive statement against her, and, as she proffered her handkerchief to wipe his sweating brow, he had pushed it away disdainfully, asking the audience, "Does someone decent have a tissue?" to which the minister, under police protection, could only reply, "That is democracy in South Africa." A complaint had been lodged against her by TAC for "culpable homicide" a few days earlier.[48] This episode was only one of the many moments of low-intensity warfare that the organization had initiated against the government and particularly against the health minister three years before. Having this context in mind, Tshabalala-Msimang's attitude was, if not justifiable, somewhat more understandable to me.

Let us return for a moment to the interpretation of these two scenes. The arenas where social issues are debated can be apprehended not only through the description of the systems of actors involved, the president's side and the orthodox side. Their meaning can also be apprehended through what one might call their grammar of action, that is, the codification of language rules and usages by which actors enter the scene, arguments are displayed, and conflicts finally crystallize. Social scientists are certainly indebted to Charles Tilly (1986) for the notion of "repertoire of collective action"—the stock of all the possible forms of public intervention among which actors pick and choose with the purpose of influencing the course of events. More than the description of the relatively conventional forms that this notion brings to light (demonstrations, petitions, happenings, etc.), the possibility of analyzing actions as they recur and their transformations over the long term (in Tilly's case, the second millennium in Europe) is what makes it useful. In South Africa, AIDS activists were not content to use the rhetoric of the parallel between the fight against apartheid and the fight against AIDS; they also looked in the repertoire of action of the former to enact the latter. This indicates a mutually shared referent as much as a tactical mode of legitimation.

Using the past as a resource probably attained both its heights and its limits during the "civil disobedience campaign" launched by TAC in April 2003, because though it expanded TAC's former modes of intervention, it clearly introduced an element of discord within the movement.[49] At the time the first episode reported here took place, in 2001, the activists were still limiting their actions to relatively classic forms: street demonstrations, newspaper articles, public statements; the first court trials against the government were to open several months later. At the time of the second episode, in 2003, a new repertoire was being inaugurated: civil disobedience. Considering traditional protest inefficient, the activists had decided to return to what had been one of the important modes of intervention under apartheid.[50] It meant undertaking a series of barely legal actions, excluding violence but using provocation: bursting in on paragovernmental bodies such as the Human Rights Commission, noisily interrupting all the public events involving the health minister, lodging accusations of homicide against the health minister and her colleague, Minister of Trade and Industry Alexander Erwin. Though largely symbolic and not really risky (there was neither scuffling with the police nor any arrests of demonstrators), choosing this mode of public intervention estranged TAC from some of its sympathizers and a segment of public opinion. Engaging in this form of action indeed implied putting Thabo Mbeki's government and D. F. Malan's politics (previous mobilization of this kind had been organized against the architect of apartheid) on the same level.[51] According to COSATU, "civil disobedience" was an unfortunate expression because it meant "breaking unjust laws, mainly against unjust illegitimate governments." The activist Nonkosi Khumalo could well justify his movement by saying it is "not protesting against an illegitimate government but the government's illegitimate politics related to AIDS." But the harm was done. In playing with the symbols of the fight against apartheid, this time TAC had gone too far.

To complete the analysis of the grammar of action, I want to add the notion of repertoire to the concept of style. Repertoire corresponds to the morphology of an intervention in the public arena, style to its syntax. In her study of the letters written by convicts to the king to plead for mercy in sixteenth-century France, Natalie Zemon Davies (1987) speaks of "genre"—in her case, supplication. Style, as I understand it, is what one feels to be the correct manner to behave in an aim-oriented interaction so as to best succeed. Using this concept, one can study the way AIDS is being debated in South Africa and in particular how TAC as leader of the protest addresses members of government but also how the latter reply. The purpose is not to give formal clues of a specific rhetoric but to grasp what is at stake politically. From this point of view, continuity of style between the two sides seems more stable than continuity of repertoire, as if it were anchored in more permanent structures. The extreme verbal violence that typifies that continuity resorts, on the one hand (from the activists' side), to the register of criminalization and, on the other (from the government's side), to the vocabulary of racialization. Accusations of being "accomplices in the death of children" expressed on "Wanted" posters, in trials for "culpable homicide," and through references to "the holocaust" are answered by blaming the contempt of "the white man" and insinuating that he has enlisted "our Africans." It is remarkable that the commentators' indignation is usually fueled by racialization discourse—and the polemic use of race by the South African president or his partisans certainly deserves criticism—but never by its criminalization counterpoint employed by the activists, who yet aim equally at disqualifying the adversary.[52] It is true that as regards history, the two positions once again are not symmetrical.

Protests against TAC methods now and then crop up in readers' columns or in what certain African leaders confide to the press, usually giving cultural arguments: it is contrary to traditional values. For instance, one reader wrote indignantly to the *Sowetan* on April 4, 2003, after the newspapers had printed a picture on their front pages of the activist Zachie Achmat pointing a threatening finger at the health minister: "In African culture it is rude to point a finger at an older person, no matter how much you disagree with them. Achmat's behaviour is un-African and as a result cannot be left unchallenged by the media." Similarly, in an interview in 2000 published on the web site www.hsf.org.za, then president of the Medical Research Council, Malegapuru William Makgoba, complained about the attacks against the government in the following terms: "My own understanding is that South African leaders get better advice confidentially rather than publicly. Unfortunately, Western civil society makes its pronouncements publicly. African leadership understands advice given confidentially, behind the scenes. That is a fundamental difference. My son or daughter doesn't criticise me to the neighbours before he or she talks to me." In reality, the problem is less cultural than political or even historical. Several times I heard people say, "They can't help it, they just talk to us the way they did during apartheid," or, "They don't even realize things have changed." Gestures of avoidance such as not wanting to touch the handkerchief proffered by the health minister, shouts of "Shut up!" or "Go to jail!" and insults such as being called a murderer or a liar are not only considered ordinary acts of incivility, they are inevitably interpreted as unconscious resurgences of the past.[53] Even if Achmat claims his longtime membership in the ANC and even if Mark Heywood insists on the years he fought against apartheid, both in the sincerest and most truthful manner, that impression lingers among many of those who suffered from being treated in a similar way under apartheid.

PROPOSITION 3: THE FIGURES OF DENIAL

The history of AIDS is always told as a story of denial, especially in the third world: unacknowledged illness, rejected causes, refuted origins. Nowhere, though, has this discourse taken on such a depth of meaning as in South Africa. The question of denial is at the heart of the controversies developed there: denial as the negation of a truth (that the illness is caused by a sexually transmitted virus) with deleterious consequences (the refusal to use medication considered at best inefficient, at worst dangerous). The word *denial* itself is usually presented by those who use it as being merely factual, but it is both prescriptive and polemic. Prescriptive, because it establishes one side for truth and one for falsehood, proclaims one's own truth and casts out the other one as error. Polemic, because it also constitutes one side for good and one for evil and thus always amounts to an accusation. Both dimensions become evident in the fact that people are constantly slipping from "denial" (the empirical observation that reality and truth are being denied) to "denialism" (an ideological position whereby one systematically reacts by refusing reality and truth). This is a shift that is all the more significant, as denialism is usually reserved for the most morally sanctioned forms of denial, in particular those that concern genocide. In the case of South Africa, the accusation of "denialism" applied to the doubts expressed on the etiology of AIDS goes hand in hand with the accusation of "genocide," referring to the delays in implementing prophylaxis and therapy with antiretroviral drugs. The government's opponents have constantly repeated this accusation, turning these two historically significant and deeply disqualifying words—denialism and genocide—into commonplaces. Understanding what is being played out in—or beneath—what is called "denial" thus supposes that we leave the logic of polemics for the time being and perhaps even avoid the matter of who is right and who is wrong—at least in terms of method, not of evaluation. Let us proceed step by step.

To begin, let us accept the complexity of the question of denial as seen by the heterodox, that is, by those who are taken to be the denialists. Of course, the South African president publicly challenges the causality of the virus and wonders why specialists insist exclusively on sexual transmission. But his government has also financed the most explicit information programs on sexuality and the distribution of condoms is among the most generous in the world. For sure, the complicated way in which he states his position is not only an exercise in diplomatic rhetoric but also probably the result of deep doubts, causing him to say that the virus cannot be "the only cause" and that the specificity of the South African scene is its "extreme poverty." Yet the discourse of many of his collaborators is not strictly one of denial: they are sensitized to the argument of inequality and to accusations of racism; or they consider that poverty, malnutrition, insufficient resources, and the risks of increasing inequalities make the use of antiretroviral drugs problematic; but they do not refute the link between HIV and AIDS. In this respect, aside from a small nucleus of real "heretics," none of them function in the intellectual universe of the dissidents who, on the contrary, have very firm convictions. Acknowledging this cognitive haziness is really the only way to account for the paradoxical fact that, in this context of constant polemics, actions are constantly being developed "as if" one adhered to the unanimously accepted scientific doctrine.[54] Notably, during the controversy, health care policies continue to operate.

Next, we must acknowledge the symmetrical existence of forms of denial on the orthodox side too, that is, on the part of those who are considered to be speaking the truth, the whole truth, and nothing but the truth. In the history of AIDS, the early identification of groups at risk followed by the rapid discovery of a virus led to a double interpretation, behavioral and biological, grounded, of course, but partial. This perspective led to restricting action to certain areas in research (surveys of so-called knowledge-attitudes-beliefs-practices, immunology and virology studies) and intervention (trying to change risk behaviors and prescribing antiretroviral therapies). However, the political economy of the illness, as a possible interpretation, and social health policies, as a complementary response, were not considered, at least up to the time when "human rights" and "women's vulnerability" entered the picture. It is likely that this nearsightedness had direct negative effects on the efficiency of the actions undertaken and indirect negative consequences for the way society accepted them. We must therefore consider that there is a blind spot in denial, which is the denial of those who accuse the others of denial. Let us push this argument a little further. If biomedical research continues to challenge its temporary truths about the illness and the treatments, which is a reasonable way of considering scientific activity, conversely, communication of its results in the public sphere works as if these truths were definitive and indisputable. In clinical practice as in the activists' battle, knowledge is transformed into belief, making any critique a matter of bad faith. Of course, physicians and militants themselves do not fool themselves and adopt this attitude of certainty in order to affect opinion.[55] However, when the progress of knowledge forces a heretofore accepted truth to be reexamined or even shows that the opponents were right, as we have seen with nevirapine, rather than give rise to critical reflexivity, it is followed by the public affirmation of a new dogma.

But the use of symmetry as an instrument to analyze the controversies does not mean that the content of the truths in the two camps are symmetrical. Methodological relativism—which consists in treating both points of view in the same manner—is in no way intellectual relativism, which would mean considering both perspectives as equally valid. This working rule not only illuminates the relationship to knowledge by revealing that, on the president's side, certain of the arguments given by the "socials" are quite relevant and that, on the orthodox side, certainties hammered out by the "experts" are sometimes later discarded. It also allows one to analyze the role of action differently, showing that, on the one hand, the controversy did not prevent health services from functioning almost normally, since they are much more influenced by the momentum of institutional and professional histories than by unrest in the public sphere, and that, on the other hand, simplifying the terms of the debate was a necessary tactic to make public intervention all the more forceful. In both cases, there is a common pragmatic logic irreducible to cognitive and ideological factors that brings the two camps closer together rather than keeping them apart.

To delve more deeply into this reflection, it is not possible to remain with the dichotomous and static view of two truths face-to-face. First, there are more than two truths: orthodoxy, dissidence, and a third way that is politically on the side of heterodoxy (because it defends the president) but scientifically closer to orthodoxy (it recognizes the existence of the virus but injects both a historical and a social dimension into the debate). Second, there is a dynamics of interaction between the different truths and the groups defending them that produces rivalry and exasperation. The model through which Jon Elster (1990) distinguishes between two forms of negation may be useful here.

Take a proposition claiming to truth, Elster explains. One can agree or disagree. But the disagreement can take two very different shapes. Either the proposition is rejected: it is negated from within; or its modality is disproved: it is negated from without. In religion one thus has the believer (God exists), the atheist (God does not exist), and the agnostic (uncertain about or indifferent to the existence of God). Similarly, where AIDS is concerned, we have the orthodox (AIDS is caused by the virus, and antiretroviral drugs are effective), the dissident (poverty is responsible for AIDS, and antiretroviral drugs are toxic), and the third way (the question is wrongly addressed, the two etiologies are not mutually exclusive, and implementing treatment presents the risk of increasing inequalities). As we can see, the binary opposition is not workable (one could naturally examine the differences in even greater detail). Up to now, we have stayed with this rather static interpretation. Let us introduce movement by following our philosopher and use two paradoxes borrowed from the field of religion: On the one hand, the religious may have difficulty accepting the distinction between atheism and agnosticism, which they criticize equally. On the other hand, the atheist may have difficulty understanding that by alienating the religious they actually comfort them and even perpetuate the religious mentality. In both cases, there is a radicalization of the opposition; the religious might change the agnostic into an atheist, and the atheist may reinforce the beliefs of the hesitating religious. If we apply these two dynamics of mutual reinforcement and of partisan polarization to the field of AIDS in South Africa, many of the tensions and contradictions become intelligible.

It would, however, be overly simple to stop there—with a problem that might be solved through logic alone. By using this method, I want to show that what one usually sees as irrational and incomprehensible could be elucidated by applying simple intellectual methodologies. But the problem of AIDS in South Africa is not solvable through logic. Once the disputes have been dissected and the multiple truths interacting with one another identified, we must face that which resists: beyond the socio-logics, we must confront the anthropo-logics, to use Georges Balandier's (1974) expression.

What resists is the instability that escapes all efforts at systematizing truth and introduces uncertainty and doubt beyond dissidence. Nobody can precisely explain why the virus has progressed so rapidly in South Africa, why we discover today that the drug recommended by everyone for the prevention of mother-to-child transmission has a high probability of becoming resistant, why international organizations have just reduced official AIDS statistics by one-third in Kenya, why we hear one day that AIDS was inadvertently brought in Africa by the polio vaccine (and this fact is later rejected) and the next day that the epidemic of hepatitis C on the continent is due to vaccinations against schistosomiasis (and this reality is today scientifically proved). This very particular configuration of the facts and their exposure in the public sphere derives from what one might call the system of confusion in the real.[56] It is thus this situation of "knowing and not knowing" that must be accounted for. It is the heart of what is called denial, that special figure by which one doesn't know what one knows.

Schematically, this figure can be examined from two theoretical standpoints. The first is Sartre's bad faith hypothesis, which leads to lying to others and often to oneself: "I know but I don't want to know." According to this hypothesis, the South African government, beginning with the president, is consciously refusing to tell the truth in the name of a political project: for example, as his spokesperson abruptly said, preventing mother-to-child transmission would produce a number of orphans that the state would not be able to support; consequently, one can think that the government would have people believe antiretroviral drugs are inefficient and toxic so as to avoid having to prescribe them. This sort of argument has been widely used in the polemics, but I will not consider it here seriously, because it is difficult to accept the conscious duplicity of such a large part of the South African population, but also on the basis of evidence from my interviews, conversations, and observations, which have illustrated the sincere involvement of many. The second interpretation is the Freudian hypothesis of the unconscious denial that does not permit acknowledging something one rejects: "I know, but I can't accept I know." The South African government and maybe society as a whole push away the untolerable, for example, that sexuality which has been the object of so many racist representations and so much discrimination should be responsible for the transmission of the illness that is decimating the nation at the very moment it finally achieved democracy and a deracialized identity. In my view, this interpretation is the only one that seems capable of expressing the experience of AIDS, simultaneously historical and ontological, capable of touching the accusers as much as the accused. To use the distinction proposed by Alain Cottereau (1999) between "denial of reality" (it's not true) and "denial of justice" (it's not fair), I suggest that it is exactly because reality is too unfair that it is denied. Denial, in its deepest sense, signifies the intolerable.

"Alas! Alas! how terrible it is to know when knowing is worthless to he who knows," cried Tiresias upon refusing to reveal to Oedipus the awful truth of parricide and incest that the latter both ignores and rejects. South Africa discovered in a progressive and contradictory way, in the confusion of truths and the violence of controversies, an evil that was gnawing away at it and which she could only handle in an imperfect and uncertain manner. Some—on the president's side—have seen in this the heritage of the past, at the risk of becoming paralyzed in their fight against the epidemic. Others—on the activists' side—have only wanted to see the realities of the here and now, putting all their hopes on treatments, even if they are limited and unjust. As Stanley Cohen (2001) writes, there is something "tragic" in the human condition that leads us perpetually to turn a blind eye all the while perceiving that this blindness leads to a dead end. Common sense, he adds, teaches us to get through daily life in spite of this double bind. The South African AIDS tragedy, because of the history that produced it, probably exceeds such ordinary competence.

FOUR

The Imprint of the Past

History is this disc whispering to an end,
and, on the remote, someone's finger
starting it up again,
from the beginning.

DAN WYLIE

"Tuesday"

"YOU MAY BE UNAWARE OF the desperate attempt made by some scientists in the past to blame HIV/AIDS on Africans, even at the time when the United States was the epicentre of reported deaths. To me as an African, it is both interesting and disturbing that the signatories of the so-called Durban Declaration return to the thesis about the alleged original transmission of HIV from African animals to humans, given what science has said about AIDS during the last two decades. I accept that it may be that you do not understand the significance of this and the message it communicates to Africans, hence your queer observation that I seek to silence your critics, without responding to their arguments." This is how, in a letter dated July 27, 2000, the South African president addressed opposition leader Tony Leon. The epistolary exchange between the two men, publicized by the press in October of the same year,[1] lasted several weeks and adds up to fifty-four pages of arguments and counterarguments concerning AIDS, anti-retroviral drugs, and politics. Echoing the head of the Democratic Alliance, for whom "it is far easier to dismiss a person as 'racist' than to argue issues on the merits, or even acknowledge that your opponents just might be right, every now and then," most commentators saw it as just another attempt to "racialize" the AIDS issue. For them, it was a purely rhetorical game in which bad faith and tactical calculations combined to disqualify the opposition and rally the black electorate. All the critics were indignant and ridiculed Thabo Mbeki's semantic extravaganzas. Their favorite piece was the speech he gave at the University of Fort Hare on October 12, 2001, honoring the memory of Z. K. Matthews,[2] the first black man to graduate from college in South Africa, at the beginning of the twentieth century (when any educated African was said to be a "miseducated Negro"). The president spoke of the educational system of the time that justified and perpetuated the racist order, of those "medical schools where they [black people] are convinced of their inferiority by being reminded of their role as germ carriers," of those "schools where they learn a history that pictures black people as human beings of the lower order, unable to subject passion to reason." His comments segued into the AIDS controversy: "And thus it does happen that some who consider themselves to be our leaders take to the streets carrying their placards, to demand that because we are germ carriers and human beings of a lower order that cannot subject their passion to reason, we must perforce adopt strange opinions, to save a depraved and diseased people from perishing from self-inflicted disease." Once again, people were scandalized by the president's words. To quote the journalist Drew Forrest in October 26, 2001, *Weekly Mail and Guardian,* raking up Africa's history and the racial stakes of her public health care policies was only a "smoke screen" to cover up the mistakes of his own dissidence: "It apparently means that those who advance a viral explanation of AIDS believe that black people are unclean, uncivilised and sexually promiscuous." This protest against the confusion of scientific arguments and racial ideologies was no doubt sincere. A careful perusal of the history of South African public health, however, shows how recurrent the same racist "stereotypes" have been over a century, as Joseph Oppong and Ezekiel Kalipeni (2004) have shown. Reminding South Africans of that historical fact, even if it is done for political reasons, does not make it any less real. Therefore, this past has to be explored on both sides—the facts and how they are being exploited—in order to understand how it is influencing the present.

In the view of people living in today's world, the past has indeed developed in two dimensions. It has become history and memory. On one side are the archives, documents, the history of historians—what looks like an exercise in scientific objectivity searching for the verifiable traces of the past. On the other side are the memories of individuals, peoples, places, which resemble the subjective and mundane workings of a quest for the festering wounds of the past. The symptoms are many, from museographic elaborations constructing "memorials" to political devices fashioned on the model of "truth commissions," from polemics on the uniqueness of the Shoah to controversies surrounding demands for reparations for the slave trade, from the French rediscovery of the crimes committed in Algeria to the Vatican's acknowledgment of the Church's historical errings. Naturally, the divide is not all that clearly delineated, and memory feeds on history just as history is built up around memories.[3] In fact, one might define the politics of the past for any given society or era as being both the source and the product of the collective act of distinguishing history from memory, on the one hand, and of making the connection between them, on the other. Naturally, too, the contemporary period has not invented this diptych; memory has always forged the identities of groups and individuals; history has long been considered an instrument for keeping time at a distance.[4] But never have history and memory been so publicly confronted in a competition to impose an interpretation of the past.

From an anthropological point of view, the two interpretations rest on two different representations that often interact, sometimes mix, but are founded on different systems of truth. It is possible to spot signs of them in speeches referring to the past, in narratives reconstructing history, or when people talk about their memories. But how can we infer the existence of a lived link between the past and the present? How can we read the mark left by events that took place years, decades, even centuries ago in the experience of people today, some of whom confronted them directly, others through what they heard from parents or friends, or yet again imperceptibly or surreptitiously when memories are triggered by images or words? Of course, there is what people say, but everyone knows that reference to history or memory does not necessarily tell all the truth about what really happened. Conversely, there is what is left unsaid, and we also know that repression allows one to cover up the most painful traces of the past. Anthropologists must thus avoid over- or underinterpreting the data as well as restricting themselves to what they are told or ignoring what is being kept back. As we have seen, in the South African controversies over AIDS, bringing up the past is a common strategy among the protagonists. They all in their own way refer to apartheid, some to recall its lasting imprint in today's social relations, others to deny yesterday's systematic remembrance. That, however, does not suffice to reconstruct the reality of the link between the dark years and the postapartheid years, in the sense that argumentation and narration are rhetorical strategies used in the polemic as much as symptoms of the marks of history. But is it not precisely just such an uncertainty that lays bare the truth of the politics of memory?

By digging into the past to find the key to the present, by deliberately choosing supposedly meaningful facts, by probably also leaving aside other facts considered less significant, by thus striving to communicate their own interpretation of the world (which cannot simply reproduce that of the agents), social scientists are wielding scientific authority, of which they must be aware and which they should be able to criticize. At the end of his research on the deciphering of the genome, Paul Rabinow (1999: 172–174) warned anthropologists against succumbing to two forms of hermeneutics. The first is the commentary based on the model of biblical exegesis to explain the oral texts produced by interviewees or the written documents found in the archives as if they were a sort of revealed truth.[5] This is what I would be doing were I to take literally the letter Thabo Mbeki addressed to "world leaders," or any of his other speeches on AIDS, Africa, or racism, as a final evidence of the mark of the past on contemporary political life. The second is an unveiling, meaning that what was obscure to the informants is transparent to the researcher whose talent allows him or her to unearth the illusion, or, in Marxist terms, to unmask the ideology.[6] In the present case, this would lead me to consider that Puleng, or any other person whom I met in the townships or the former homelands, does not know she is a product of the history of apartheid and that it is my role to discover it in her stead.

This is a useful lesson, and one must try to listen to it. I am not sure, though, that unless one goes in for depicting the social universe like an impressionist painting or unless one lets oneself get carried away by the purely aesthetic consideration of a literary work, it is really possible to completely avoid interpreting. As Johannes Fabian (1995: 41) put it, "Ethnographers report what they understand. If what is reported is not to be dismissed as mere recording or description, it must be recognized as understanding." It seems to me that, on the one hand, the speeches of the South African president on AIDS do say much about the violence of history but that, on the other hand, the stories told by AIDS patients and collected in the townships and former homelands deserve to be reread in the light of a past they do not themselves mention. Perhaps this means that rather than seek to escape the dangers of hermeneutics so rightly warned against, one must accept the consequences of interpretations inherent to any undertaking that aims to account for what men and women do and think; in other words, to carry it off in full recognition of one's preconceived ideas.

How, therefore, must we interpret the practical relationship of individuals and groups to their past? Michel de Certeau (1987: 97–99) draws a fruitful parallel when he discusses the ways psychoanalysis and history have construed that relationship with respect to time and memory: "Psychoanalysis is articulated around a process at the heart of Freud's discovery: the return of the repressed. This 'machinery' brings into play a conception of time and memory, the conscious being both the deceptive mask and the effective trace of events that have organized the present." According to this interpretation, "the dead haunts the living," and though we often deny it, the past is always and everywhere at work on the present. Two contradictory mechanisms thus join together to form the space of memory: "forgetting, which is not a passivity or a loss but an act against the past," and "the mnemonic trace which is the return of the forgotten, i.e., an act of the past now forced to appear only in disguise." One's conscious being in the present is thus built up on the unconscious play between what has been excluded and what is returning. "Historiography on the contrary develops according to a fracture between past and present. It is the result of the relationship between knowledge and power in two supposedly separate locations: on the one hand, the present workplace (scientific, professionnal, social), the technical and conceptual apparatus used for studying and interpreting and the descriptive and/or explanatory act; on the other hand, the locations (museums, archives, libraries) where the materials being studied are kept and, secondarily, the past systems and events that these materials permit one to analyze." This distinction between two sorts of objects transpires in the very principle of the historiographer's activity, in "the will to be objective" and in its ultimate actualization in the form of a "scriptural staging." Scientific discourse consequently supposes that a certain discontinuity in historical time has been established. The conflict between psychoanalysis and historiography is in fact one between "two time strategies," especially to "confer an explanatory value to the past and/or to make the present capable of explaining the past." Anthropology does neither. It no more has the tools to explore the unconscious than the intention of reconstituting the past. Yet its work on interpretation makes it similar to psychoanalysis and its concern with distanciation likens it to historiography. More fundamentally, perhaps, it finds itself in an in-between where like the first it enters into a dialogue with living subjects and like the second it tries to turn them into scientific objects. If that be the case, it is indeed in the present that anthropology searches for the imprint of the past, without, however, allowing itself to access any interiority whatsoever. That is to all intents and purposes the frailty but also the demanding specificity of its methods.

Having been actively involved in the fight against apartheid and having written extensively about it, André Brink (1998: 30) has suggested yet another no less stimulating duality that can serve as a model when dealing with the past: law and literature. "The Truth and Reconciliation Commission is intent on effecting reconciliation through establishing, as fully as possible, the truth, the whole truth and nothing but the truth, about human rights infringements during the apartheid years—'truth,' in this context being equated with 'facts.' The enterprise of fiction, on the other hand, reaches well beyond facts: inasmuch as it is concerned with the real (whatever may be regarded as 'real' in any given context) it presumes a process through which the real is not merely represented but imagined." Here again, anthropology finds itself in an in-between. From legal procedures, totally specific since they concern an immanent justice without any sanction, it borrows the quest for facts. From literary and more generally creative activities, it adopts the reconstitution of facts through imagination. However, acknowledging the ambiguousness and the limits of an investigation that claims to respect the canons of positivism but actually functions like a narrative does not mean giving in to the textualist temptation.[7] What the agents say and what the anthropologist will make of it belong to a hybrid species in which facts are constantly being subjected to interpretation. Such reworking is what we call writing.

The studies carried out on AIDS in South Africa generally testify to a remarkable "presentism," to use the expression coined by François Hartog (2003), who has made it the privileged regime of historicity for the contemporary world. On the one hand, studies of politicians and especially controversies limit their chronology to postapartheid, thus falling in line with the common perception that occults all reference the country's dark ages. The implicitly explicative or at the very least illustrative series begins with the *Sarafina II* scandal and the discovery of Virodene and ends with the revelation of Thabo Mbeki's affinities with the dissidents.[8] On the other hand, studies of actual practices, particularly those said to be at risk, seem to consider that representations and behavior patterns in matters of sex and prevention, of violence in gender relations, and of modes of protection used against the infection are only determined by the realities of the here and now. The increasingly numerous surveys done by standardized questionnaires or semidirected interviews on people's knowledge, attitudes, beliefs, and practices have thus been captured in instant, not necessarily trustworthy photographs.[9] None of them yield any understanding of the relationship to the past as it is expressed in politics and in private life, as it appears in the speeches of the South African president, and as it is experienced daily by the inhabitants of the townships and former homelands.

The past, with its cortège of violence and injustice, cannot be completely contained in the only place where it is officially being staged and narrated: the Truth and Reconciliation Commission. Certainly the controversies surrounding AIDS create a privileged framework for the expression and recognition of this violence and injustice.[10] Let me risk a hypothesis. In the enthusiastic albeit perilous period immediately following apartheid, the commission managed to contain the rush of the past into the present by building up an official history and producing a legitimate memory. The facts nonetheless resist this meritorious accomplishment, as do the experiences that the protagonists had and continue to have of that period. The AIDS epidemic, through its powerfully elusive epidemiological reality as well as through the verbal inflation surrounding it, represents the overflow that the Truth and Reconciliation Commission was unable to channel. To try to grasp what is being played out on this new stage through this new narrative, taking into account the contradictions and scheming it entails, may be a way of allowing the "burden of memory" and the "muse of forgiveness," to use Wole Soyinka's (1999) felicitous expressions, to finally meet.

LONG MEMORY

whites shall not be drowned
nor will they be tanned
or banned
only humanised.

SANDILE DIKENI
"Whites"

Our interview with the director of the health service subdistrict and her collaborator in charge of infectious diseases programs is coming to an end. It concludes a survey we just carried out in the rural area the two women are in charge of, Greater Tzaneen. With them, we have discussed the problems that crop up during the implementation of HIV counseling and testing and the practical difficulties encountered in implementing the recent government instructions concerning the prevention of mother-to-child transmission by the use of nevirapine. They have provided us with tables and figures, public health diagnoses, and determined solutions to mobilize the agents. The explanations given to account for the subdistrict's relatively modest accomplishments (though it is held up as a model to the rest of the nation) have been very technical and well argued. But the director does not seem completely satisfied with this vision of things. Somewhat embarrassed at leaving her bureaucratic interpretation of public health aside, she continues with a near-confession: "It's difficult, you know. It will take years to change what we have inherited from before 1994. Years. You've got to understand where we come from to be able to address some of these issues." And she concludes: "It's a postapartheid issue." Visibly, as far as she is concerned, this remark means interpretation. We are in Limpopo, until recently called the Northern Province. The nominal presence of the past has been erased by the change in name but not its physical mark in the geopolitics of the region. With a population that is 97.5 percent African according to Statistics SA, this province is indeed one of those on which apartheid leaned the most heavily: three of South Africa's ten homelands had been set up there, surrounded by vast territories that had progressively been "cleansed" of their "black spots," in other words lands that were still owned at that time by black farmers.[11] The present subdistrict of Greater Tzaneen thus unites three demographic ensembles: the white area that included the small town of Tzaneen but also the huge plantations of white farmers; and parts of the two former homelands of the Lebowa (the population of which is Pedi) and of the Gazankulu (the population of which is Shangaan); both of these African territories include rural townships and villages surrounded by microproperties. According to the official principle of "the self-governing state," each homeland had its own administration. There were also the Transvaal Provincial Administration and National Health and Population Development, in charge of the programs for the "white areas," while the Tzaneen Local Authority only took care of that locality and the Peri-urban Services of the District Council operated in six little white towns. Thus, on this relatively small territory, the apartheid bureaucracy had invented six racialized, parallel, and uncoordinated systems. As of 1994 the three territories fused, implying the reunification of the six administrations responsible for 484,000 inhabitants.[12] Beyond the complex organizational problems it posed, the restructuring revealed once more the wounds of the past. As the director explained, requalifying Shiluvana Hospital as a health care center in 1997 was experienced by the local population as deeply humiliating and followed by bitter protest. From a functional point of view, the proximity of the larger C. N. Pathudi Hospital, only three kilometers away, made its smaller neighbor a superfluous and costly double. But under apartheid the first relied on the Shangaan authority of the Gazankulu, while the second in the Lebowa operated under Pedi tutelage. Today the nurses displaced from Shiluvana to the C. N. Pathudi Hospital are accused of mistreating Pedi patients, especially when they suffer from AIDS, and the Shangaan social worker of this institution is suspected of following up only on requests for allocations filed by patients of his ethnic group. The barbed-wire fence that the apartheid government had put up to separate the two territories has today become an invisible border permanently consecrating the rancors and discriminations between two entities that, sixty years ago, were largely mixed. As an old Shangaan woman told me, "When I was a child, we used to go sometimes to our Pedi neighbors and we had friends there. But after they made the Lebowa and the Gazankulu, that's when problems started." She remembers the violence between the two groups. She herself was a member of the Assembly of God but had to change her religious affiliation under apartheid because her place of worship was in the Lebowa: she then joined the Presbyterian Church. Concluding our interview, the director of the subdistrict said sadly, "There is a lot of trauma here." Her observation is valid far beyond this local health scene. Public health is not an impartial government technology; it is an integral part of a social and political history.

In the Name of Hygiene

"In cases of urgent necessity arising from the prevalence or threatened outbreak in any district of infectious disease, it shall be lawful for the Minister to make and proclaim such regulations to be in force within such districts as may be required by the outbreak, or check the progress of, or eradicate such disease." Thus read the sanitary legislation of 1897, known as Public Health Act (no. 4 of 1883 amended as no. 23 of 1897). Basing itself on this text during the 1901 plague epidemic, the Cape government took the first authoritarian steps of urban segregation according to a logic that Maynard Swanson (1977: 387–395) has termed the "sanitation syndrome;" that is, justified for hypothetical reasons of public health. Those measures consisted in displacing the African populations from the poor, overcrowded parts inside the city to the newly created "native locations" on its outskirts. A few months later, Cape Town's medical administrator Barnard Fuller accounted for the brutal intervention of the public authorities with these words: "Rest the blame where it may. These uncontrolled Kafir hordes were at the root of the aggravation of Cape Town slumdom brought to light when the plague broke out. Because of them, it was absolutely impossible to keep the slums of the city in satisfactory condition."

Yet the statistics taken from the *Mayor's Minutes* clearly highlight the fact that during that epidemic, there had been only 172 cases recorded among Africans against 204 among Whites and 431 among Coloured.[13] Thus, far more than the epidemiological data, social prejudice against the black populations is what led to the first displacement of almost 7,000 Africans from the center of town to the shacks, huts, and barracks hastily built at Uitvlugt (later renamed Ndabeni).

This is not an isolated case on the continent. In many African cities, contagious diseases have led to attempts to set up policies of spatial segregation to protect the European population. As Elikia M'Bokolo (1984: 186) notes at the end of his study of the 1914 plague epidemic in Dakar, "The health policy of colonial authorities, often studied from a triumphalist and hagiographic perspective, seems to obey a logic of global domination system rather than dispersed and disinterested initiatives coming from medical doctors only concerned with human development." However, as Philip Curtin (1992) has shown, though all over Africa similar racist arguments are mixed with scientific theories about the risks of contagion to justify segregationist practices, important differences do exist in how the policies are received, depending on the presence of a numerous and often organized native population. In Freetown, Bathurst, Accra, or Lagos, the separation of the city was generally thought out in terms of displacing not the African inhabitants but the white colonizers, fewer in number, toward newly built and supposedly salubrious neighborhoods. The native authorities also often resisted principally because of the takeovers of property that were a consequence of these demographic movements. Such, however, was not the case in the Cape colony, where the White and Coloured presence harks back to the seventeenth century, while native groups remained far from the cities until the onset of industrialization at the end of the nineteenth century. Through a meticulous historiography, Elizabeth Elbourne (2002) has described the colony's society under British rule; filled with contempt and fear of the other, racism was already deeply rooted in their ways of thinking, and the idea of a "race war" had already been expressed, for the first time, during the Xhosa uprising of 1851. The epidemiological threat thus justified a program that had only been waiting for just such a signal. It met no resistance.

The Public Health Act that thus became the legal foundation of the first official segregation policy in South Africa had itself been promulgated following another epidemic (smallpox this time) that had been raging from May 1882 to March 1883 (Swanson 1977: 395–400). The death toll had been far higher then, with four thousand dead, ten times more than during the plague. The deaths occurred mainly among the Coloured and the Malays within the city, rarely among the Africans who had just begun migrating toward Cape Town. The law dictating the exceptional measures consisting in forced displacements was thus accounted for by a sanitary concern, but its orientation against the black populations was due to their being seen as a social menace. A moderate representative, James Rose Innes, describes them as "native hordes, uncivilized barbarians." Prime Minister Schreiner himself, considered a liberal, exclaimed in July 1899: "They lived all over the place. . . . And they were learning all sorts of bad habits through living in touch with European and Coloured surroundings. We could not get rid of them. They were necessary for work. What we wanted was to get them practically in the position of being compounded." The issue there was to justify new legislation (the Native Labour Locations Bill of 1899) to make urban segregation and the surveillance techniques it imposed in order to control people's movements compatible with the job market and the necessary mobility of the workforce. The government leader's discourse became paternalistic: "Keep the natives out of harm's way; let them do their work, receive their wages; and at the end of their term of service, let them go back to the place whence they came—to the native territories, where they should really make their home." They had been expelled for the good of the city they supposedly threatened for sanitary and social reasons. Henceforth it was claimed they should remain at a distance for their own good, to escape the evils of urban life that endangered them.

The entire history of racial segregation and then of apartheid is caught up in this tension between ideology and pragmatism, between xenophobia and interest, between racial prejudice and capitalist logic. The black populations must be isolated but their access to employment must be guaranteed.[14] Public health has an ambiguous role in this complex game. Sometimes it plays on the fear of contagion, thus condoning ideology a priori. Sometimes it legitimates a posteriori the decision to get rid of a social peril. Always it provides arguments used to justify the rejection of the other, mixing strict rules of hygiene and moralistic remarks. Again according to Swanson (1977: 405–406), "sanitation and public health provided the legal means to effect quick removals of African populations; they then sustained the rationale for permanent segregation." However, by a quirk of history, the "native locations" had hardly been set up when they in turn were blamed for prompting contagion and vice. The crowding of black citizens into overpopulated places was indeed an objective danger, as attested by the

130,000 "African" deaths during the 1918 flu epidemic, but also a subjective one, as shown by the anxious declarations of representatives concerning the risks that these pockets of "black misery" constituted for the "white cities." Yet to these new evils the same old remedies were applied. Far from casting doubt on the segregationist project, these dangers reinforced it: if there was a risk of epidemics, it was not due to the confinement of populations in overpopulated, unsalubrious, poorly equipped territories, but because the local policies governing these exclusionary zones were not energetic enough. Separation was therefore to be continued but the means of control made tighter.

The history of epidemics is thus an integral part of the history of racial segregation in South Africa. The risk of contagion has often been the most effective argument to justify the implementation of legal and physical measures initiating or reinforcing the separation of groups that it would have been more difficult politically to justify by strictly biological criteria. If it was necessary to rid the cities of their African populations, it was not because of the color of their skins but because their way of life was incompatible with the constraints of urban prophylaxy. In a word, the problem was not natural but cultural. The contrast between the two terms is nevertheless not so extreme, since the solution consisted in the end in putting the "natives" back in the natural setting of their cultural development, and expediently grouping them in rudimentary places made especially for them outside the towns was but a stopgap measure. The recurrent theme of the "barbarian horde" and the frequent use of the expression "raw Kafirs" illustrate that mixture of naturalistic and culturalistic prejudices in the discourse of prophylactic exclusion. In an article of the *Transvaal Medical Journal* in 1908 titled "Hygiene in South Africa," W. Watkins-Pitchford noted, that "Natives and Asiatics, other than those employed in domestic service, should reside in a specially allotted district of the town is highly desirable. These people have moral ideas and social habits widely divergent from those of educated Europeans, and this fact alone fully justifies such racial segregation. To the hygienist, however, the most convincing argument is the facility which is afforded for sanitary control, more especially in respect of communicable diseases." Segregationist policies in public health thus offer the advantage of being a neutral and technical excuse that can even be presented as beneficial for everybody, some because they are thus protected against contamination by microbes, others because they avoid being corrupted by civilization.

But once it has become an institution, the system of separation boomerangs with deleterious effects on the black populations. Put otherwise, the consequences of implementing a system with a priori motivations serve as a posteriori proof that it was well founded. Prophylactic segregation thus contains the conditions of its own reproduction. For the system is not only differentiated, it is obviously also unequal. Public goods are not equitably distributed among the territories and their populations. The differences are huge to begin with and continue to increase as technologies to control the populations become more efficient, apartheid ending up by establishing considerable disparities. As Cedric De Beer (1984: 57–59) has shown, these exist at two levels. First, living conditions are far more unfavorable in the townships and above all the homelands in terms of access to resources as well as in terms of risk from the environment. At the beginning of the 1980s, infant mortality in Pretoria reached 10 and 53 per thousand in the white and black populations respectively; data for the bantustans, probably far more dramatic, were not even known; but as far as malnutrition alone was concerned, medical estimates made it responsible for the death of about 30,000 children each year, almost exclusively in the homelands. Second, health care structures in the zones of confinement were far more rudimentary and less well equipped, contributing to enlarging the gap with the white zones. Still in that same period, it was estimated that only 3 percent of the country's doctors were working in the homelands, where half of the South African population lived; at the national level, there was one doctor for 875 whites versus one doctor for 232,000 inhabitants in the Qwa Qwa, a homeland situated at the Lesotho border; in the urban centers, where the situation was relatively much better, the daily expense per patient came to 37 rands in the Baragwanath Hospital of Soweto and to 107 rands in the all-white Johannesburg Hospital. A sure sign of the public authorities' lack of interest in these territories, most of the usual indicators of the so-called vital statistics were practically nonexistent there (births, deaths, morbidity, even total number of inhabitants).[15] As we have seen, this historical omission in national demography was used in the July 2000 controversy to reject the validity of data produced by the director of the Medical Research Council on the death rate in South Africa.

The distance covered in nearly a century of institutionalized separate health care systems can be reckoned in the way contagious diseases are monitored. A cholera epidemic arrived in South Africa in 1980 and lasted two years. It is estimated that there were approximately 50,000 cases and 200 deaths. The infection spread first in the recently established little Kangwane homeland, then rapidly to all the other bantustans. Whipped up by alarmist articles in the newspapers, the white population began to panic. Quickly, however, thanks to the efficiency of the racial cordon sanitaire that had been created, it appeared that the illness was circumscribed to the homelands alone. As the danger subsided for the white population, public interest in the problem waned. Soon, cholera became part of the ordinary epidemiological landscape of the bantustans. The president of the Scientific and Industrial Research Council summed it up by stressing that many black farmers "preferred drinking dirty water out of muddy pools rather than the safe chlorinated water supplied by the authorities."[16] Thus, while at the start of the century the statistically unfounded fear of contagion during the plague epidemic had been used to justify the expulsion of the black populations from the cities, henceforth, at the end of a process of segregation and discrimination, and as apartheid seems to have brought it to its logical conclusion, the cholera epidemic could produce its devastating effects on the sole inhabitants of the homelands, the white populations getting away with only a transitory fear.

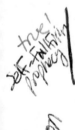

Public health has thus many times served the racist political project of the South African authorities: first, by giving them the excuse of the prophylactic argument, then by confirming it was well founded. One can in this respect speak of a true sanitization of segregation.[17] The fact that in today's context of AIDS it raises suspicion in some segments of the African population and among certain politicians in power should not be surprising. All the less as during the early years of the epidemic, the same reflexes prevailed, with the same racially differentiated programs. As Karen Jochelson (2001: 175) points out, "educational material for Whites emphasized the significance of long-term monogamous relationships, while material aimed at the Blacks focused on debilitation and death."[18] Such discrimination in the messages was followed by a flood of protest from the antiapartheid movements, which immediately called it "typically racist propaganda." Yet it was in direct line with what health education had been for a long time, especially concerning venereal diseases. In the case of syphilis, which received special attention on the part of the health authorities throughout the first half of the twentieth century, they increasingly stressed racial differentiation, not only in the way patients were taken in (it being considered "undesirable" that whites and blacks should mix in specialized hospitals), but also in the prevention campaigns (the former being called upon to combat the epidemic in the name of Christian morals and a national feeling supposed to elevate them, the latter receiving paternalistic advice based on humiliating representations).[19] In other ways and in a different context, pre-

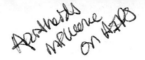
Apartheid influence on AIDS

vention programs for AIDS set up by the dying regime of apartheid kept up the policy of separation, once again based on health arguments since it protected the white population from the perils of "promiscuity," considered an inherent feature of African sexuality. *No one has the patent on purity...*

However, the management of black populations does not obey the logic of separation alone, no more than public health proves its usefulness exclusively in the a priori and a posteriori justification of that policy. Though reputedly a threat to the well-being of the white world, the African body yet represents a workforce that has always been its main raison d'être in South African society. This dialectics of racialism and capitalism has been at the heart of the political system of segregation and later of apartheid. *black body - labor*

The Economy of Bodies

"Although tuberculosis morbidity and mortality rates rose steadily for Blacks living within both the urban and rural areas of South Africa from World War I through the mid-1930s, they dropped dramatically within the country's gold-mining industry." What Randall Packard (1989: 159) affirms here is rather surprising at first sight. It is known that the diamond mines at Kimberley and even more the gold mines on the Rand (minerals whose extractions began in 1867 and 1886 respectively) took a toll on human lives, essentially of African miners, to such a point that the traditional theme of war chiefs' cannibalism has been picked up and reworded in certain narratives and popular songs to stress that particularly violent form of exploitation.[20] According to David Coplan (1994: 7), "at the mines, 'cannibal' *(le-limo)* is a metaphor both for the earth itself, which consumes the miners in its belly, and for overeager black team leaders and white miners, who push black miners to the point of exhaustion in their gluttony for power and higher pay." Almost exactly the same words as the ones E. J. Moynihan, a private consulting engineer, used in the opinion he wrote to a daily in 1910 (quoted by Katz 1994: 3, 213): "This industry about which we brag so much is something to be rather ashamed of, for from the social point of view it is a vampire which battens in the blood of the living and the bodies of the dead." And, comparing casualties during the Boer War and deaths in the mines in the first years of the twentieth century, he added, "Mining is more dangerous than war. But miners get no medals." It may thus be surprising that the mining economy was able to protect its African workers from an illness as socially determined as tuberculosis.[21] The explanation of this paradox illustrates the complex mechanisms that rule over the political economy of health care. *interesting*

As an epidemiological phenomenon, tuberculosis is a newcomer in the history of diseases in South Africa. Though it is likely that the infection had existed for a very long time (perhaps even before the Europeans arrived), its extension to the black populations (characterized by the fact that it spread very rapidly and took on extremely serious proportions) only occurred toward the end of the nineteenth and especially the first decades of the twentieth century. The root causes for this were the massive need for labor in the mining areas (in 1890 already 60,000 men were working in the Rand gold mines; twenty years later they numbered 200,000) and the expansion of the cities following the rapid industrialization of the entire country (during the same period the urban population grew by 200 percent). To these two key factors must be added the living and working conditions of these migrants, in particular being restricted to overcrowded and poorly equipped places—the "compounds" around the mines or the "locations" near the towns—and being exploited in the various industries—the mines in particular—with the intense physical and environmental strain that accompanied small salaries for long hard days of labor. Cold, humidity, dirt, overpopulation, and insufficient nourishment are just so many factors that promote the propagation of tuberculosis; the reports written by government commissions are as explicit about these factors as they were little heeded by the mining industry.

A 1914 document titled *Report of the Tuberculosis Commission* is a noteworthy example of an epidemiological piece that provides not only valuable data on the various pathologies but also comparisons among miners according to their origin, the type of mine they worked in, and the evolution of their physical state. As Alexander Butchart (1998: 95) declared, this sort of production "transformed the previously perplexing mass of bodies into an ordered statistical community" about which administrative decisions could be made. One might think that this is how all such descriptions should be, but in the South African case it takes on special meaning with respect to the racialist project of society, on the one hand, and to the political economy of mining, on the other. Thus one discovers in a study carried out in 1912 that a "basutu" worker had twice as much chance of having the tuberculosis bacillus if he was working in the mines than if he never worked there; the rate of positivity was multiplied by ten for miners from Mozambique. During the first decade of the twentieth century, the risk of developing tuberculosis in the mines grew by 50 percent, representing a loss of about 15 per thousand workers a year by death or repatriation, double if one takes pneumonia into account.

In the mid-1910s the trend began to reverse essentially because the public authorities intervened and obliged the mining industry to take action against tuberculosis. Until then, the industrialists had merely paid attention to the problem for many years (for example, when asked by the health minister of the Transvaal in 1905 to augment the volume of air available to each miner in the barracks, the director general had refused, saying it would be too costly), but now they began feeling the pressure of state authorities. In 1913, tired of their inaction, the government prohibited hiring "North of the 22nd parallel": the road to "tropical workers" was thus cut off. Though the latter represented only 11 percent of all miners, the decision affected a workforce deemed vital for the future development of the mines because of its availability, its supposed vigor, and also its greater docility. But, as Alan Jeeves and Jonathan Crush (1995) have written, it was made more for political than for sanitary reasons, since it was a question of putting pressure on Portugal by making it more difficult for Mozambicans to access the work market. At the same time, a whole battery of measures was taken to improve lodgings and food, physical conditions at the bottom of the mine as well as in the compounds, and bodily hygiene but also medical supervision of the workers.

Though these measures contributed to slowing the onset of tuberculosis, they were not the only explanation for this decrease. Selecting the men allowed to enter the mining work market was also decisive. This was done by controling the hiring agents more closely and being more demanding as to the health status of future workers: clinical exams on the recruitment site, then again when they were hired; more food distributed before being admitted to working in the mine. During the first years of the century, the lack of workers had forced certain mines to accept whoever was available. But with the severe economic difficulties that had been encountered by the farmers after several epidemics had decimated their livestock and several years of drought had reduced their crops, the selection could be carried out efficiently, as could also sending back to their original regions those miners whose physical condition had deteriorated. Thus the low figures for tuberculosis during that period point rather to efficient management of the workforce than to any humanitarian or sanitary preoccupation. Selection of healthy workers and elimination of sick miners were much more effective than hygiene measures. More generally, as Harold Wolpe (1995) has shown, the system of segregation set up during this period allowed the mining industry to find a masculine workforce in the rural zones that could be paid very low wages since the women who remained in their villages could ensure the economic and social reproduction of the family thanks to a subsistence economy.

The logic followed by the public authorities who imposed these changes was equally rational and fits into the "generalised response on the part of the state to the problems wrought by industrialisation," as Saul Dubow (1989: 52) puts it. Contrary to the way certain doctors present it in their writings, the government's action in matters of hygiene in the workplace did not grow out of a sudden generosity toward the black populations. It was triggered by political pragmatism because the local rural as well as urban authorities complained that more and more former miners were returning sick to their "locations" and "reserves," thus contaminating their entourage and potentially the entire community—there again a workforce used by the white population.[22] The Public Health Report of the Cape Colony (quoted in Packard 1989: 93–95) commented as early as 1906: "Noticeable is the general testimonies of district surgeons that the disease is mainly spread by Natives returning from the mines." As tuberculosis "is decimating the Colony's most valuable labour asset," the authors questioned whether "from a human life point of view we ought to waste our Bantus over mine labour." This idea was largely shared by the health authorities across the country. It corresponded in reality to how the mining industry functioned, sending its infected workers back to their towns or villages. In a few years the situation had become as worrisome in the urban and rural districts as it was in the mines themselves. Overcrowding in the segregated zones accelerated contagion in the urban districts, and drought and sick livestock weakened contaminated bodies in the rural districts. From then on, not only did tuberculosis affect a workforce more and more lacking in the factories and farms, but it also endangered the health of the white population both in the cities and in the countryside. The reaction of the administration to both menaces was mainly based on what Packard (1989: 194, 299–300) called "exclusionary policies," based in the mines on "preemployment medical exams and repatriation of miners who developed the disease," and for the rest of the African population, on "a long list of public health acts, urban areas acts, influx control laws, housing legislation, group areas acts, and ultimately, acts establishing bantustans." Medicine itself was deeply involved in this process: "For medical officers working on the Rand and in other urban and industrial centers of South Africa, the struggle against tuberculosis was an exercise in holding back the tide. Sanitary segregation, slum clearance and medical screening were instruments for keeping tuberculosis away from white urban populations and had little or nothing to do with improving African health." Yet the native body was omnipresent in medical discourse.

For in medical circles, tuberculosis was considered a mystery. Doctors wondered why the illness spread more quickly among blacks than among whites. And why was it so severe that many Africans died of it, whereas Europeans generally developed chronic varieties? How can their particular "susceptibility" be explained? One should note, along with Megan Vaughan (1992), that at the same moment in eastern Africa, the opposite question was being asked about syphilis: why are severe forms less frequent there than in Europe? The interpretation most often given by South African doctors to account for the vulnerability of the black populations to tuberculosis was initially based on the idea of a "virgin soil," an absence of previous contact with the bacillus making Africans more fragile. But why? According to Packard (1989), hypotheses diverge on this point. At the start of the twentieth century, when internal migrations were sparse and the first measures of segregation getting under way, the cultural theory (paradoxically naturalistic) prevailed, as we have seen: the native was perverted by contact with civilized life; his true culture was nature. More specifically, where tuberculosis was concerned, Dr. George Turner blamed the bad habits acquired in the city, especially letting damp clothing (from rain or sweat) dry on oneself instead of removing them. During the second decade, an apparently more scientific biological theory gradually replaced the preceding one: in its most radically Darwinian form, expressed by Dr. G. D. Maynard, it turned susceptibility into a hereditary factor that only natural selection might alter; a more optimistic variation, defended and finally imposed by Dr. D. Traill, was that immunity is acquired progressively thanks to the physiological process of tuberculinization. Better than the first model, which presupposed the return of the natives to their original living quarters far from the towns and industries, the second pleased the administrators of the mines, because it justified the policy of intensive hiring of migrant workers for relatively short periods at the end of which they were sent home ostensibly to rest up. In both interpretations, however, the environmental or social factors take a back seat to the cultural or biological:[23] it is always the African body that is "susceptible" rather than the living or working conditions that are wearing it away and affecting it.

Making the history of tuberculosis the backdrop to the more recent history of AIDS thus implies two ideas. First, on a physiopathological and socioepidemiological level, both infections are closely related, to such a point that they sometimes seem inseparable in health statistics and programs, as indeed they are also in the experience of patients and doctors. Tuberculosis in South Africa and on the rest of the continent is the opportunistic disease most often associated with AIDS, but its high frequency even before the latter began to hold sway means that its association with seropositivity does not necessarily make it a consequence of AIDS. On the national level, it is estimated that nearly one out of two cases occurs in carriers of HIV, which is then responsible to a large extent for the fact that tuberculosis has been gaining ground over the past few years. From this point of view, mines have been a good vantage point for AIDS researchers as they were a century ago for doctors working on tuberculosis.[24] As to the dissidents, they point to the close association between the two pathologies and assert that HIV is only an innocent passenger in tuberculosis patients who, when they die, are thus victims of Koch bacillus; that the increasing rate of tuberculosis is above all the result of deteriorating living conditions; and that it is one of the main causes for the rise in mortality. In his declarations, the South African president has mentioned tuberculosis together with AIDS several times. Thus relations of a biological nature exist between the two epidemics; they immediately become the subject of conflicting interpretations and consequently are stakes of a social nature. Second, the histories of both infections are strikingly similar not only in their dramatic evolution in terms of progression and prognosis but also for the interpretations they have inspired and the solutions they have received. In scientific research as in health policies, biological and medical approaches on one side, cultural and behavioral paradigms on the other, have largely dominated the social or economic theories, practically nonexistent in the case of AIDS outside certain limited public health and social sciences circles.[25] True, epidemiological demonstration has become more rigorous and racialist prejudice less acceptable than in the past; but though today the "susceptibility" of African populations is no longer given as an explanation, "sexual promiscuity" is now used to stigmatize them while sidestepping the social conditions that nurture the epidemic.

That bodies are not only resources for labor but also objects of regulation, that the disease not only depends on political but also on moral economies, and that through such representations and actions common racial prejudices and discriminatory practices have been forged, is revealed by the analysis of the ideas and systems concerning so-called African sexuality and personality as they developed throughout the twentieth century and have been brought to the forefront once again by the AIDS crisis.

The Subject of Disease

"Beware of your houseboy, for under his innocent front may be lurking and lying latent the passions of a panther, or worse." This warning (quoted by Butchart 1998: 113) was published in 1893 in a Johannesburg paper, following the attempted rape of a white woman by her black servant. It was the beginning of a long period during which the threatening image of the "black peril" was produced, ending up in a series of laws in all the colonial states of southern Africa, especially Southern Rhodesia where, as Jock McCulloch (1995) reminds us, the first law of the British Empire inflicting the death penalty for "attempted rape" was enacted in 1903. It was claimed that Africans are dangerous but not just in any way: by their sexual drives and irrational characters, or more exactly when the latter liberate the former. In an editorial of 1912 bearing the title, "An Urgent Question of Sociology," the chief editors of the *South African Medical Record* (cited by Butchart 1998: 115) wrote: "We have taken enormous hordes of young adult savages or semi-savages, eminently virile in more senses than one, from their own environment, and have placed them in an environment absolutely teeming with every possible stimulus of the sexual impulse at the same time that they are, necessarily, kept celibate. We have not even tried to put them in the social mosquito-proof house of a reproduction of a native community, but, on the contrary, have freely exposed them to all the stings of a class of human mosquitoes whose interest is to inoculate them with every kind of human vice." Once again it is claimed that civilization depraves human nature by awakening hidden instincts.

In an apparently more subtle manner, the South African psychiatrist B. J. F. Laubscher (quoted by McCulloch 1995: 84) noted in 1937 in *Sex, Custom and Psychopathology:* "The pagan schizophrenic patient in his regression keeps on the whole within the fold of his cultural belief, expressed as ideas, because the archaic and magical forms of thought are as much part of his normal state as they are of his psychotic state. Hence the great difficulty for the normal pagan native to discriminate between the rational and the irrational." After having systematically explored the deviant forms of sexuality in cases collected among the magistrates of the district, he concluded that, in conditions of sexual privation such as the one experienced in city life, Africans have no other choice but to turn to alternatives such as rape. This model, where transgression occurs at the crossroads of drive (desire) and circumstance (bachelorhood), that is, of the inner world of the psyche and the

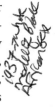

outer world of society, defines the hypersexuality that was to become the common representation of "African sexuality" to this day.

From the end of the twentieth century, these representations have been structured in terms of gender. If the deviant figure of the African man is incarnated in rape, the dominant image of the woman is one of licentiousness. The increase of prostitution provided the sociohistorical framework. It was linked to the double process of industrialization and urbanization that exploded with the discovery of the Kimberley diamond and later Johannesburg gold. While the first contingents of prostitutes were mainly composed of white or Coloured women, the local populations (mostly the Sotho) also began to provide recruits, a majority of migrant women being single and having no other resources. As Jochelson (2001: 28–29) has noted, the category "prostitute" was universally reproved in the 1890s, without racial differentiation: "Prostitutes, both white and black, were part of the residuum—licentious and degenerate." But as of the 1900s prejudice took on an ethnic dimension and Coloured women were all suspected of deviant behavior: "For observers of the time, white prostitutes and respectable poor or middle-class women were worlds apart, but African and coloured women were all promiscuous and potential carriers of syphilis." To account for the presence of this disease among white men, danger had to be extended to black servants as explained in an 1894 article in the *South African Medical Journal* (quoted in Butchart 1998: 131–133): "Properly conducted and careful enquiries will nearly always show a focus of infection. This in nine cases out of ten is the servant-maid; she is generally a church-native, and almost variably wears stockings. She, it can proved, has wantonly kissed the baby; it gets syphilis. The unsuspecting master also inflicts upon his offspring a chaste and paternal kiss and, as a partial consequence, he gets a hard sore on his glands and prepuce. Thus the disease gradually osculates the whole community." Beyond the inventiveness demonstrated to exonerate the white "masters," this description illustrates the most deeply entrenched prejudice toward Africans: civilization (church and stockings) can never permeate the black populations more than superficially; their nature (infection) and their culture (promiscuity) bear the irremediable imprint of a sort of original sin.

At the same time, the editorial writer for the *Lancet* (quoted by Vaughan 1992: 270), talking about an epidemic of syphilis in eastern Africa was contrasting the sexual freedom progressively gained by "women in civilised countries" to the licentiousness brutally imposed on "women whose ancestors had been kept under surveillance": of the latter, he declared they were "merely female animals with strong passions, to whom unrestricted opportunities for gratifying these passions were suddenly afforded." In South Africa, racializing female sexuality had practical implications for the social handling of prostitution. The Contagious Diseases Prevention Act of 1885 stipulated strict control of syphilis by regular medical checkups of prostitutes and therapeutic obligations for the sick. In fact, however, the application of the law was clearly biased: not only were white prostitutes subjected to much less systematic supervision than were African and Coloured prostitutes, but while the discovery of cases among the former were recorded by the medical services, the latter were merely referred to the African police. For Jochelson (2001: 43–45), such differential criminalization of sexuality "reflected the assumption that all poor women, but especially black women, were potential prostitutes and potentially diseased, and so required more stringent control." But also, "in a period when the poverty of the whites was becoming a public issue and racial distinctions were being heightened in civil life, the different treatment accorded to white and black patients and the segregated locked hospitals helped affirm the differences between the black and white poor." During those years, hospitals, asylums, and prisons began to separate out the whites, prelude to the segregation of the entire society.

One would be wrong, however, to perceive the system being put in place through public health since the end of the nineteenth century as a stable and coherent phenomenon. Very much to the contrary, between ideological considerations and pragmatic approaches, it never stopped evolving and contradicting itself. Though syphilis seems to have been brought under control as a result of the requirement of medical checkups and, if needed, compulsory treatment (required for the "passes" needed to move around the country), it became rapidly obvious that such restrictive measures were resisted by the traditional chiefs, who refused to give up the sick for fear they would be imprisoned or deported. Henceforth a different concept of public health began to take shape, more and more attentive to acknowledging "the African as a person"; its effectiveness depended on a double set of measures, some scrutinizing in greater detail the interior of the community and the family to weed out unhealthy practices, others counting on persuasion and the internalization of norms hypothetically propitious for general well-being. In the 1940s, modeled on the pioneering work of the Polela Native Health Unit conceived by Sidney and Emily Kark, social medicine developed in the health care centers: this new practice strove to link prevention and democracy through intensive observation and action, investigating all the African families whether or not they included sick persons and implementing health education in every public place, from schools to meeting halls. The experiment flourished under the auspices of the Gluckmann Commission (Phillips 1993) but was interrupted by the victory of the National Party in 1948 and the instauration of apartheid in the years following. In the field of public health, however, this dual paradigm of constraint and normalization, authoritarian control and moralistic intervention, continued to be operative, with its concomitant violence and prejudices, racial segregation and culturalist interpretations, eugenist theoreticians and social psychologists. On one side, as Shula Marks and Neil Andersson (1992) have written, a segregated and unjust health care system was being put in place: for example, the resources attributed to the General Hospital in Johannesburg reserved for whites exceeded the total amount of means allocated to all the bantustans, increasingly left to their sadly unsanitary fate. On the other side, as Butchart (1998: 121, 167) has shown, sophisticated instruments to realize what in 1953 the psychologist S. Biesheuvel called a "moral attitudes inventory" for African populations as well as humanistic approaches to understand "what your Black patient is thinking," in the words of Dr. A. Barker in 1974, were being developed. Such is the paradox of the African subject of disease produced throughout the twentieth century. The subjection that the politics of "white supremacy" imposed on the black populations by force and separation was accompanied by an ambiguous subjectivization depending on the exaggeration of differences and inequality, especially aggravated by a constant probing into the "African mind," "Bantu society," and the "community." In other words, we are confronted here by the social production of identity and otherness as much as by repression and exploitation, which makes it necessary to bring together Foucault and Marx.[26] Without giving a moral dimension to this idea, we are not dealing here only with a negative process emanating from the sole exercise of abusive power but also a positive one resulting from the application of a disciplinary paradigm. A process that the political opponents of the regime and especially Steve Biko's Black Consciousness Movement paradoxically appropriated for themselves,[27] denouncing its illegitimate oppression by rejecting the logic of racist power, on the one hand, and turning the mechanics of the racialized discipline upside down in demanding a psychological dealienation, on the other.

This is the complex foundation that today's health officers have inherited and that they must make do with when implementing prevention poli-

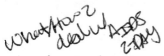

What Ho? dealw/ AIDS today

cies, inventing educational messages, and proposing care patterns, as Duane Blaauw (2004) insists: to combat AIDS means intervening in a field mined by decades of power strategies and resistance tactics, of deployment of techniques of subjection and technologies of subjectification so finely served by public health. It has indeed been the subtlest instrument because it used the principles of domination and segregation all the while resorting to the specific modalities of control of what was a socially valued public good. Thabo Mbeki and the members of his cabinet delve into this heterogeneous set of references when they denounce the prejudice and the discrimination revived by the AIDS crisis: representing Africans as "germ carriers" who live in "sexual promiscuity," however polemical that may be when used to disqualify the opponents' discourse, corresponds to historical realities that, as we will see, have equivalents in the present.

In conclusion, let us return to the words of the director of the Greater Tzaneen subdistrict about the difficulties she runs up against and the problems of access to health care that she faces when administering her zone. The dysfunctioning of the Shiluvana medical center is a long story. Under apartheid, the mission hospital was in a territory claimed by two neighboring homelands. When in 1976 the government took it from the religious congregation that had been in charge, it put it temporarily under the authority of the Lebowa health ministry before relinquishing it five years later to the Gazankulu administration. When the latter began to function, the former withdrew its twenty-four Pedi members from the hospital staff, appointing them to an institution under its control. Thirty patients supposedly of the same origin, some receiving intravenous treatment, were transferred by ambulance. De Beer (1984: 61) observes, "The incident is farcical, its consequences are not." Nor were its causes. Both are still present in the stories that people tell today as soon as they feel confident enough. One day I took an AIDS patient to the C. N. Pathudi Hospital, which is presently in charge of cases that formerly went to Shiluvana. She had a serious lung infection that looked very much like pneumocystosis. Her very poor respiratory condition fully justified her being hospitalized, and I tried to convince the medical and paramedical personnel to do so. When I came back to tell her what was going to be done, she turned down my offer in a weak and breathless voice. The person accompanying her supported her refusal by saying (in front of the nurses) that they, the Pedi patients, were so badly taken care of by these Shangaan personnel that they were better off dying at home than staying in this hospital. A few hours later, after the medical

Pedi treated Bad by whites

exams had been accomplished and with her prescription in hand, I had to take her back home.

BARED HISTORY

This was one of the first pronouncements I remember in which the Truth and Reconciliation Commission testimonies were referred to as stories. Is it not that we often think of stories as imaginary events which we may call tales, fiction, fables, or legends: stories as narratives of some kind or another? Yet, the testimonies we continue to hear at the TRC hearings are the recall of memory. What is being remembered actually happened.

NJABULO NDEBELE

Memory, Metaphor and the Triumph of Narrative

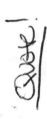

"This sickness, it comes from the white man, because 99 percent of blacks have got it while 1 percent of whites have got it.—What makes you think it is like that?—Every time I look at the newspapers or I watch TV, there is no white man who's got HIV, they're all blacks. I am sorry to say that but it is true.—Never mind.—Even at work, they used to come, these people, and tell us about it, but the rate is always on our side. It's like the white man did it, it's like they want to get rid of us. So that the place can belong to them again, since they say it is their Vaderland, you see." In the living room of her small house in the heart of Alexandra township, the young woman suffering from AIDS has just finished telling her own story. She is now giving us her interpretation of the epidemic.[28] The racial division of the infection as it is presented in the media awakens in her the memory of apartheid. Behind the official discourse on the infection, she imagines a secret motive: the elimination of the black population. AIDS would thus achieve stealthily what the regime had been unable to accomplish by force: build a white nation. People often shared similar views with us during the interviews carried out in the Johannesburg townships or the Limpopo villages, but rarely were they handed to us so openly. For this she apologizes to her white visitors. Yet that reading of the epidemic is quite common. It also seems like a distant echo of Nkosazana Zuma's words that had shocked journalists in 1998 during the Virodene controversy when, referring to her parliamentary opposition, she had declared, "If they had their way, we'd all be dying of AIDS." The doubts expressed by the young patient and the minister's accusations illustrate a social theory of the epidemic that could

Whites gave Blacks AIDS (handwritten margin note)

Quote (handwritten margin note)

be called genocidal, in the sense that it rests on the idea of a project of extermination of an entire people. That theory is part of the ordinary repertoire of interpretations of the epidemic. Can we reassure ourselves by considering we have a phantasmic projection of racism in the first case, a demagogic manipulation of a constituency in the second? Such interpretations, which, once again, cannot avoid the alternative of psychologism and cynicism when accounting for the representations of AIDS, nevertheless fall somewhat short. To apprehend the meaning of what is being said about the pandemic in South Africa—and elsewhere on the African continent—people's words must be reconsidered within their social logics. Recalling the century-long history of public health and management of infectious diseases has provided us with some clues. We must now return to the more recent and specific chronicle of AIDS in which the South African case appears as the extreme example of a continental paradigm.

Sex Again

"An extreme promiscuity is the only element African heterosexuals have in common with homosexuals through whom the AIDS epidemic began in America. In African towns, overpopulation comes with overcopulation." This interpretation of "African AIDS" (as it was named at the time) was not the opinion of a patented racist theoretician or of an extreme right-wing politician. It was Mirko Grmek's (1989: 274) in his famous history of AIDS. A research director at the École Pratique des Hautes Études in Paris and an internationally recognized specialist in medical history, he is the author of the first published general review of the epidemic. Again and again he returns to that explanation, further refining it in a chapter significantly titled "Cultural Incompatibilities," where he means to account for the rapid progression of the infection on the African continent:

> Sexual promiscuity plays a major role. Indeed it has existed from time immemorial among tropical populations, but it recently took new forms. In its process of modernization, Africa tries to accommodate very different and often incompatible cultural traditions. Urban impoverishment, a new phenomenon by its acceleration since the middle of the twentieth century, is associated with an unprecedented development of prostitution and with extended possibilities for sexual contact. One frees oneself from moral and material obstacles imposed by the rural environment and the tribal customs to fall into the trap of an uncontrolled social system. (1989: 279)

All the clichés about Africa, from culturalist essentialism to moralistic incrimination of urbanization, which went into producing a stereotyped view of African sexuality, are in Grmek's book, which was long considered authoritative in the field of AIDS. In addition, the book replicates opinions that were fairly common at the time. Nathan Clumeck, a well-known epidemiologist at the Saint-Pierre Hospital in Brussels who was one of the discoverers of the first African AIDS cases, declared in an interview in *Le Monde*, "We can hardly ask people to stop having sexual contact without giving them a substitute, when we know they live in a society where tragedy is their daily fare and where the main escape is hedonism and pleasure. If we eliminate these, what is left? It is as if we were to tell a population of compulsive and obese eaters: From tomorrow on there's no more food!"[29] And, probably trying to mitigate the responsibility of African societies, he added, "One must remember that colonization and Christianity destroyed the African models where polygamous society had many advantages in matters of birth control and sexuality. We have imposed changes that today, given the local African conditions, have led to a catastrophe. It is too easy to say it's their fault because their sexuality is uncontrolled or because they don't know how to control it." Social sciences themselves contributed to these representations of AIDS.

Daniel Hrdy (1987: 1112–1116), a specialist in infectious diseases and anthropologist at the University of California, Davis, published in *Reviews of Infectious Diseases* a comprehensive survey on the "cultural practices contributing to the transmission of human deficiency virus in Africa." While analyzing in detail a series of ritual scarification, circumcision, and excision practices, he concentrated mainly on sexuality: "Most traditional African societies are promiscuous by Western standards." And here again: "As people leave rural villages and migrate to urban areas, the general level of promiscuity usually increases. This increase may be attributable in part to the relaxation of traditional village values but appears to be due primarily to the destitution of poor migrant women who may become prostitutes and to the greater mobility and rootlessness of young male migrants and soldiers." Curiously, as the author noted in a chapter titled "Contact with Nonhuman Primates," a virus resembling the AIDS virus had been discovered among green monkeys: "There is a striking analogy between promiscuity as risk factor in humans and the 'promiscuous' behaviour of vervets. Typically, female vervets, unlike baboons, are sexually receptive for long periods and during that time mate with multiple partners, sometimes engaging in dozens of copulations on a single day." The comparison between monkeys and humans does not stop there, since during the 1980s there were efforts to imagine how transmission from the former to the latter could have taken place. Animal nature, traditional culture, and modern destructuring therefore mix in an extraordinary overdetermination of "African promiscuity." It is not easy to escape such implacable logic.

This vision of the pandemic is obviously reminiscent of those previously cited texts by early-twentieth-century doctors that tried to explain endemic tuberculosis or syphilis. As Packard and Epstein (1992: 347–349) point out, the same stereotypes are summoned: "difficult adjustment to conditions of a 'civilized' industrial world" for these "dressed natives" in the case of tuberculosis ; "promiscuous sexual intercourse" related to their "natural immoral proclivities" in the case of syphilis. A few decades later, we find the somewhat contradictory dual image of nature corrupted by civilization, on one side, and immorality inherent to their culture, on the other side, practically unchanged, sketching the contours of an immutable picture of Africans, their sexuality, their relation to modernity, and, in the end, the mysterious link between nature and culture. But this way of looking at things, which tells more about our own history than about African societies, makes the epidemic seem inevitable: "Whether it is the image of Africa close to nature (relations with monkeys, sexual desire and promiscuity) and primitive (inflicting the same ritual wounds since the beginning of history) or of Africa 'off to a bad start' on the path of development and given to idleness and pleasure, everything contributes to making this 'cradle of humanity' the ideal accomplice and victim of AIDS" (Dozon and Fassin 1999: 6). One might think that this portrait painted about fifteen years ago was stowed away among the prehistoric souvenirs of the epidemic. Yet it seems not to have aged a bit if one considers recent literature.

In its *AIDS Update* report of 1999, the United Nations Population Fund declared once again that "the problem is promiscuity" and underscored "the primacy of cultural factors."[30] At the end of the second decade of the epidemic, authors could still be writing, "Traditional cultures had strict rules governing sexual relationships. Those codes have broken down and nothing has replaced them." This analysis thus pretends to capture in a couple of sentences the upheavals of social norms and the accumulation of epidemiological risks, reviving the classics of the genre while contributing a few new elements inspired by current events: "The role men traditionally played as head of the family has broken down. Boys grow up without fathers. Wives are left impoverished and unprotected. A South African woman is raped every twenty-six seconds, the highest rate in the world.

Many secondary school teachers sleep with their students and a widespread belief is that sex with a virgin, including girls as young as ten, can cure AIDS." Such a description, mixing empirical facts and unfounded rumors, playing on hyperbole and extrapolation, suggesting relations of cause and effect when they have not been proved, not only draws a catastrophic picture of Africa but also provides a view—legitimated by the international organization label—that is entirely centered on behaviors, explained by social destructuring and cultural determinism. At the heart of this etiological representation: sex—again.

Remarkably, even when AIDS has not struck, sex remains the factor to be explored. In Nigeria at the beginning of the 1990s, for instance, a team constituted by the Australian research couple John and Pat Caldwell (pioneers in the anthropological demography of AIDS) and two Nigerian specialists, I. O. Orubuloye and Gigi Santow, launched a large statistical survey on the sexual networks in a region where seroprevalence barely reached 0.5 percent, compared to more than 10 percent in several neighboring countries in West Africa and especially Central Africa (Orubuloye et al. 1994: 45, 134, 137). In spite of the obvious contrast that precisely should have incited the researchers to look for the reasons this population was apparently protected, they kept invoking instead the same attitudes and behaviors, the same cultural facts and historical developments, the same risk groups and practices. Once again we find a local version of an apparently continental pattern, "the destabilization of the traditional Yoruba sexual system": at the beginning of the twentieth century, the authors explain, polygamy was the rule, and rich men married girls on the average twenty years younger, which in no way prevented extramarital relations among men as well as among women (it should be noted that these three elements are cited today as typical of regions with a high seroprevalence of AIDS, beginning with southern Africa, a fact that the authors seem to be half admitting when they speak of those "surprisingly modern attitudes towards sexuality" of one hundred years ago); with the advent of colonization, Christianization, and urbanization, polygamy was repressed to the benefit of the legitimate couple, but extramarital sexuality developed, including prostitution (whence the description of "extended, overlapping networks" assumed to increase the risk of venereal disease).

Without entering into the ethnographic data, it may be noted that in the present as in the past, in Nigeria as elsewhere in Africa, "sexual activity" is described as dangerous quite independently from any objective epidemiological fact. In a vast historical fresco referencing the European family by Jack

Goody as well as in Robert Murdock's notes on ethnic groups and thus contrasting the "Eurasian system" and the "African system," the latter appears marked by a "moral permissiveness" while the former managed on the contrary to preserve women's "sexual purity" for a long period. This situation is connected to the fact that in Africa there exist "little guilt, substantial permissiveness and scant danger of punishments"—with the result that African society "is vulnerable to all attacks of postcoital affections." The authors eventually enter into details. They pinpoint two groups "at high risk," "truck drivers" and "itinerant market women," because their wandering ways of life seem to expose them incorrigibly to sexually transmitted diseases, even though in their case also no serological data were available. In fact, the actual results of epidemiological surveys are of little importance: their outcome is known in advance, and they are condemned by the weakness and laxity of their moral norms, yesterday to syphilis and sterility, today to AIDS and death. It is therefore fairly surprising to read the Australian scientists' confession (Caldwell and Caldwell 1996) a few years later: "The first assumption we had to scrutinize was the notion that AIDS in sub-Saharan Africa spreads primarily through heterosexual intercourse. We were actually skeptical because elsewhere the risk of acquiring the virus during heterosexual sex is extremely low. If a man and a woman are otherwise healthy except for the fact that one is HIV-positive, then in a single act of unprotected vaginal intercourse, the chance of transmission from the man to the woman is one in 300 and from the woman to the man possibly as low as one in 1,000."[31] If this is the way it is, one can only note that once won over to that idea, the authors became its most ardent promoters, to the point of wanting to validate it even in places where the actual presence of AIDS was kept to a remarkably low level. Their work has become a "classic" in the demography of AIDS.

Of this interpretation, which is moral as well as culturalist, of African sexuality, there exists a biological version that takes on an explicitly racial form in the scientific literature. It is to be found in an article published in an international journal of the social sciences; it caused some reprobation at the time but expressed clearly and cynically a view that was more common than one might think. Two Canadian sociobiologists from the University of Western Ontario, Philippe Rushton and Anthony Bogaert (1989: 1214–1218), presented an interpretation that they guaranteed would make it possible to account for the differences between populations in their "susceptibility to AIDS." To do this, they built an indicator of "sexual restraints" by comparing "racial differences" between "Mongoloids," "Caucasoids," and "Negroids" in terms of "allocation of bodily energy to sexual functioning." According to them, "the same racial pattern occurred with gamete production, intercourse frequencies, developmental precocity, primary sexual characteristics (size of penis, vagina, testis, ovaries), secondary sexual characteristics (salient voice, muscularity, buttocks, breasts) and biologic control of behaviour (periodicity of sexual response, predictability of life history from onset of puberty), as well as in androgen levels and sexual attitudes." These configurations revealed a "sexual restraint" more pronounced first among "Mongoloids," then among "Caucasoids," and last among "Negroids," who appeared to be the least inclined both in biology and behavior to control their sexuality.

Returning to a model borrowed from the theory of evolution, they next examined the reproductive strategies following a curve from r at one end, where "organisms produce a large number of offspring but provide little or no parental care," to K at the other end, where "organisms produce very few offspring but invest a large amount in each." On the r side are the "oysters" and the "fish," and on the K side, the "great apes" and the "humans." Among the latter, the same order of "races" is noted as above, "Negroids" being closest to the primates. Besides, as the authors explain, a correlation exists to other indicators such as "health (infant mortality, illness, longevity), brain size and intelligence (cranial capacity, brain weight, test scores), maturation rate (age to hold head erect, age to walk alone, age of death), social organization (marital stability, mental disorder, law-abidingness) and temperament (activity level, anxiety, sociability)." All these elements are presented in comparative tables that inevitably show the "Blacks" to have the least good results, followed by "Whites" and "Orientals." Going on to the subject of AIDS, the researchers showed how all these factors contribute to explaining the intensity of the pandemic in Africa: "sexual precocity," low "social organizational capacities," but also "lowered levels of intelligence" must be considered as risk factors. Their interpretation was always strictly racial in the sense that their data on "Negroids," for example, might just as well come from surveys on black students on American campuses as from epidemiological studies on the African continent. In conclusion, they admit that "some might find disagreeable our approach to race differences." But they defend themselves by saying that "the ultimate aim of science is causally to explain the world around us, rather than only describe it." They justify themselves by saying that their causality is purely genetic.

The self-evident and unchallenged nature of the sexual explanation to account for the epidemic of "African AIDS" and the alacrity with which many jumped on the theme of "sexual promiscuity" with whatever interpretation (cultural or biological, moral or racial) have had two serious consequences, the first practical, the second political.

From the practical point of view, focusing exclusively on sexuality has caused research and discourse to lose sight of any other possible explanation of the epidemic and thus of any other possibility of fighting it.[32] As Eileen Stillwaggon (2003 : 810) has remarked, "mainstream epidemiology has long acknowledged the role of host factors, including poverty, in promoting disease transmission"; however, "when an explanation was sought for the rapid spread of HIV in sub-Saharan Africa, the standard epidemiological cofactors in disease transmission were generally overlooked" and "the behavioural paradigm" was systematically preferred. As we have seen, the question of poverty (cleverly appropriated by the North American dissidents and adopted by the South African president) is today so intricately embedded in the polemic surrounding the denial of a viral etiology that it has become difficult to even discuss it. But it had barely been brought up before. Next to the interpretation in terms of "co-factors," another aspect has been practically absent from scientific discussions: iatrogenetic transmission, particularly in the material used for injections by health care services and for which David Gisselquist (2003) has collected some important pieces of evidence. Aside from the fact that this thesis is crucial for the comprehension of the genesis of the epidemic, it has been substantially documented and has obvious implications for public health policies, by encouraging the health care system to adopt much more active prevention measures. Whatever the degree of importance attributed to these alternative paradigms (social or iatrogenetic) in respect to the dominant ones (behavioral and cultural), the fact that they are not taken into account in the fight against AIDS has certainly had dire consequences for controlling the epidemic, as many specialists today agree.

From a political point of view, the invention of an *"Homo sexualis africanus"* goes hand in hand with a *"cultura sexualis africana"* (to quote Bibeau 1991) and has produced an image of Africa and its inhabitants mixing an imaginary representation of sexuality and decontextualized data on sexual behavior, a vulgate that has spread to Europe and North America. This interpretation in which common sense competes with scientific argumentation has elicited often-violent reactions on the African continent.[33] Behind the discussion on the African origins of AIDS, on where to draw the line between animals and humans, on the hypothetical idiosyncrasy of a bodily habitus, many have recognized the enduring, sometimes crude, sometimes more sophisticated racism, more or less crossed with solicitude, that European and North American scholars are suspected of harboring against Africans. Rereading these texts written less than twenty years ago, it seems difficult to contradict the critics. The rapidity with which so many researchers in public health or social sciences have followed this lead to the exclusion of all others is quite startling. This seems the most recent episode of a long history that has made of Africa, according to Deborah Posel (2004), "the obscene genitalia of the geographical body of the world," and in these conditions, she adds, it is hardly surprising that "the invocations of this story of sexual humiliation and body vexation, both recent and old, play an important role in Thabo Mbeki's style as orator, thinker, and politician." A good number of his speeches indeed refer to this corpus of ancient and contemporary prejudices.

Mentioning all those who as time went by have construed the stigmatized image of an African population wallowing in hedonism that today, with AIDS, is reaping the logical consequences of their sexual license, President Mbeki exclaimed during his Fort Hare lecture, "Convinced that we are but natural-born, promiscuous carriers of germs, unique in the world, they proclaim that our continent is doomed to an inevitable mortal end because of our unconquerable devotion to the sin of lust." Those who heard him and commented on his words saw in them the near-delirious expression of racist paranoia. But considering what has been written on AIDS during the past twenty years in the light of the analyses produced over the course of the previous two centuries, his speech sounds less strange. During the repatriation ceremony of Saartje Baartmann's remains,[34] Mbeki made a speech in which he evoked this past again to speak of the present: "It was not the lonely African woman in Europe, alienated from her identity and her motherland, who was the barbarian but those who treated her with barbaric brutality. Among the truly monstrous were the leading scientists of the day, who sought to feed a rabid racism, such as the distinguished anatomist, Baron Georges Cuvier, who dissected Saartje's body and said after he had dismembered her: 'These races with depressed and compressed skulls are condemned to a never-ending inferiority. . . . Her moves had something that reminded one of the monkey and her external genitalia recalled those of the orang-utang.'" Recalling the presentation of those organs by the same scientist to the Academy of Medicine, the South African president added, "The story of Saartje Baartmann is the story of the African people of our country. It is a story of the loss of our ancient freedom. It is a story of our dispossession of the land and the means that gave us an independent livelihood. It is a story of our reduction to the status of object that could be owned, used and disposed by others." The first two decades of the history of AIDS show that racial prejudice about African sexuality, though euphemized, has far from disappeared from scientific discourse. As to politicians, the chronicle of the South African epidemic shows they had nothing to envy them for.

Racism as Usual

"If AIDS stops black population growth, it would be like Father Christmas." The scene takes place at the Parliament of the Republic of South Africa on May 18, 1990, and the health minister is quoting a representative, Clive Derby-Lewis. The debate is raging between the two main parties of the white legislative assembly in the tricameral Parliament: the National Party in power, who is in the midst of the negotiation of the democratic transition with the ANC, and the Conservative Party in the opposition after having splintered off from the former, considered too lukewarm in its application of apartheid. The health minister, Rina Venter, has just accused the representative of having publicly and insultingly rejoiced at the fact that AIDS is progressing among Africans. At the same time, she is answering a similar attack leveled by the Conservatives: one of their representatives, F. H. Pauw, has claimed that members of the National Party are campaigning nationwide to reassure their white voters concerning the discussions under way with the opponents in exile by saying that thanks to AIDS the black population will in five years become a minority and that their constituency thus will no longer be a threat to white supremacy: "When one bases one's guarantees and one's hope of solving the problems of our country on AIDS, this is a reflection of the level to which one has sunk."[35] This bitter exchange illustrates the unbridled racial violence that was common among the white parties during the last years of apartheid. It also shows how, within this ambit, AIDS immediately became a deeply polemical political issue. Since the beginning, it was a subject of virulent controversy and systematic disqualification in the public arenas. Never was it a neutral object that it was possible to discuss quietly and for which efficient programs could be planned.

The first two cases of AIDS in South Africa were reported in 1982—the year after the publication of the initial observations in the United States.[36] They concerned white homosexuals whom the deputy director general of the Health Department, Dr. J. Gilliard, labeled "isolated cases," thus indicating what was to become the government's major political argument: the infection was confined to "high-risk groups," and prevention should aim at keeping it from spreading among the "public at large." During the first five years, the government's line was thus both to acknowledge the existence of a "group at risk" (homosexuals)—although, in the words of Coen Slabber, director general of the Health Department, in September 1987, "homosexuality is not accepted by the majority of the population and certainly not by the Afrikaans-speaking population"—and to neglect testing and prevention among the black population, since it was no use to launch a campaign "too early, too heavy," as the Health Department's spokesman, George Watermayer, put it in February 1988: "it is to our advantage that we were able to learn from the international campaign, the explicit nature of which could have resulted in resistance."[37] Given these conditions, the creation in 1985 of the AIDS Advisory Group composed of physicians and researchers who were supposed to advise the government could hardly be expected to have any real implications. Official policy, as expressed by the director general of the Health Department in 1987, rested on the principle that AIDS was the "homosexual community's own affair" and that the state must not interfere.

However, it can be said in the health officials' defense that dominant epidemiological discourse at the time had it that, with the exception of homosexuals, the South African population was exempt from the AIDS virus. "Absence of HIV Infection in Prostitutes" and "Lack of Evidence of HIV Infection in Drug Abusers" are among the reassuring titles of scientific articles presenting South African surveys in 1986 and 1987.[38] Cases only trickled into official statistics: 2 in 1982, 4 in 1983, 8 in 1984, 8 again in 1985, 24 in 1986, 38 in 1987; the curve accelerated as of the following year, with 87 cases in 1988 and 139 in 1989. When one examines the 326 files of South African patients reported through 1990, 71 percent were Whites, 24 percent Africans, 4 percent Coloured, and 1 percent Indians, according to the classifications of the time; as to the hypothetical risk factors, one can note that 66 percent mentioned homosexual practices, 5 percent had been transfused, 4 percent were hemophiliacs, and 3 percent were children, which led one to conclude by default that the remaining 22 percent had been infected through heterosexual relations. There was probably massive underreporting of cases among the inhabitants of the townships and homelands, where health services were much less efficient than those serving the white populations.[39] This is indeed what the results of a serological test regularly carried out in the blood banks seem to indicate. Of the 710,000 donors registered until 1988, 244 were contaminated by HIV, among whom 180 were

Africans (81 men and 99 women) and 56 were whites (55 men and 1 woman). When these figures are extrapolated to the corresponding populations, we obtain rates of seroprevalence that, though still low, already reveal the "Africanization" of the epidemic: respectively, 0.01 and 0.001 percent among white men and women, 0.05 and 0.06 percent among African men and women; it means that rates were five times higher for African men and sixty times for African women than for their white counterparts. What is more, a study done in the South Transvaal during prenatal visits shows that between May 1987 and August 1988, the levels of seroprevalence had risen from 0.04 to 0.34 percent among African women, meaning the rate doubled every six months.[40] All this goes to show that the more closely statistics are scrutinized, taking into account both the problems of access to screening and the dynamics of development of the epidemic, the more obvious it becomes that a serious evolution exists within the African population during the second half of the 1990s. But in reality, until the end of the 1980s rare were those who dared such an observation.

From 1987 on, official discourse nevertheless began to change, and, though trying to avoid worrying the general population, Health Minister Willie van Niekerk recognized the existence of the risk of infection for which he clearly indicated the cause, without explicitly naming the populations involved: white homosexuals but also, for the first time, African heterosexuals. "Promiscuity is the greatest danger," he said, "whether one likes it or not. We have to say that. It is a fact. There is no way one can say: 'I still want to sleep around, but I don't want to get AIDS.'" His successor, Rina Venter, was to take up the same refrain a little later: "The problem of AIDS is that it is not primarily a medical problem. It relates to social behavior." Thereafter, the problem was to modify—that is, to moralize—sexual activity, notably by preaching conjugal fidelity. Free condom distribution hardly fit into such a program, being associated with licentious conduct. An editorial writer for the *Daily Dispatch* wrote on January 21, 1988, "In the threat there is a positive force for the strengthening of the family and monogamous relationships. It should not be an alternative in direction from not using condoms to using them (as some recent advertisements would have us to believe) but to return to a better and saner way of life in constancy and relationships from marriage to grave. There would be greater emphasis on morality and much lesser on the prophylactic." Educating the population was the new creed.

The first all-out prevention campaign orchestrated by the McCann advertising agency was launched in 1988. Differentialism remained well ingrained in people's minds as cross-country rioting submitted the regime to greater pressure and apartheid was day after day coming apart. The campaign was conceived differently according to population.[41] For whites, a considerate version sensitive to people's feelings, using a euphemistic and allusive approach through graffiti, told the story of a young man whose all too liberated sex life had caused him to be infected with HIV. For Africans, a brutal and simplistic set of pictures showing a coffin being lowered into the ground with messages implicitly reproducing the classical stereotypes of sexual promiscuity. In fact, that differentiation was only the ordinary expression of the community-defined view of public health of the times, based on distinctive premises that encounter the racist ideology of the political authorities. "Recognizing cultural relativity," to quote Butchart (1998), was part of the "codes" through which doctors imagine their intervention among the African populations: one must adapt to their specific realities. At the same time, health services deployed a less sophisticated version of racial segregation. Access to serodiagnosis was unequal: African or Coloured patients often found themselves turned away. Treatment by the sole available antiretroviral, AZT, was reserved for whites' hospitals.[42] Basically, nothing in this was really new in a health system organized through a not only separate but also unequal distribution of public property, according to a program of "unification and fragmentation of the state," as Posel (1991) points out: the ideology of the general good (for the whites) underpinning the discourse of apartheid was always intimately connected to the pragmatism of the specific interest (also of the whites) that constitutes the basis of colonial capitalism.

But the main victims of the repressive politics of the South African government were the foreign laborers, especially in the mining industry. Systematic authoritarian screening carried out in 1986 by the Chamber of Mines among 30,000 workers brought to light that 0.02 percent of South Africans were infected with HIV; this figure reached 0.05 percent for those from Swaziland, 0.09 percent for those from Mozambique and Lesotho, 0.34 percent for those from Botswana, and 3.76 percent for those from Malawi (Jochelson 2001). As in the past for tuberculosis, immigrants were accused of harboring the disease. Once again they were the scapegoats in the epidemiological crisis. When the results were published, the response of the health minister was immediate and violent. Beginning in 1988, more than one thousand migrant workers from Malawi, Uganda, Zambia, and Zimbabwe were thrown out of the country.[43] To justify internationally its policy of obligatory screening and forced displacement, the government de-

clared that it was only applying the same rules as the United States, the So-
viet Union, and China, which were then testing foreigners before allowing
them admission and organizing biological discrimination rarely denounced
at the time. In the history of AIDS, stigmatizing immigrants is the ordinary
way of expressing xenophobic demagogy in Africa where "men from Zaïre"
in Congo, "women from Ghana" in Ivory Coast, and many others were
handed over to public revenge and then brutal expulsions,[44] as well as in Europe where foreigners (Africans in particular) were commonly singled out
by the extreme right-wing parties. In South Africa, stigmatization has temporarily displaced racism from the local black populations to the citizens of
neighboring countries, which has left a lasting mark on the interpretation
of the link between AIDS and immigration. More subtly, it made breaking
a work contract of a laborer who was found to be seropositive an acceptable procedure, which in many companies became the ordinary way of
managing the workforce. The life stories I collected in the field testify to the
fact that the threat of infection continues to justify xenophobia and discrimination in the workplace today.

Toward the end of the 1980s, as the epidemic continued to progress more
and more visibly among the native African population and as the internationally boycotted regime was more and more shaken by youth riots in the
townships, AIDS became a political issue used by the protagonists in a violently polemical context. On one side, nationalists and conservatives
lashed out against the African population, their propaganda using the illness to discredit the black opposition and terrorize the white electorate. The
evocation *swart gewaar* (black peril) was revived. Tracts made the rounds of
the country. One of them accused members of the ANC in exile of im-
porting AIDS into South Africa; beneath the drawing of a black guerillero,
this strange caption: "He who dies naturally never cries. He who has AIDS
cries and dies. Socialize with ANC freedom fighters and cry and die from
AIDS." Another document invoked the "twenty-five million who would be
dead or dying by the end of the century," while "up to seven million would
be raving mad before dying." An opuscule titled *AIDS: Countdown to
Doomsday* speaks of "infected terrorists" who "come to live in the townships
and infect the prostitutes." In the months after the ban was lifted on opposition parties, a brochure addressed to the families of returning militants
informed them that they would be submitted to quarantines and compulsory tests.[45] From then on, AIDS was associated with stigma, fear, and suspicion. On the other side, African activists from the antiapartheid struggle
spoke out against the manipulations of the white authorities. Prevention

programs were debunked as "typical of the government's racist propaganda" and the timorous free condom campaign presented as "a plot devised by the government, supported by the employers, and pumped through a restricted press to convince black people to have less sex and therefore fewer babies." The acronym of the illness was ironically rephrased by some as signifying "Afrikaner Invention to Deprive us of Sex." The theory that HIV might have originated in American military laboratories appeared in an article in *Sechaba,* the journal of the ANC in exile.[46] Given such conditions, where AIDS was seen by some as an instrument serving to destabilize the black population and by others as mere racist propaganda, it was practically impossible to implement an authentic policy to combat the illness. Inside the country, only some modest community actions tried to make the public sensitive to the dangers of HIV, but more often than not they were met with disbelief. Outside, the Maputo conference in 1990 brought together militants of the ANC in exile and activists of the Mass Democratic Movement: it was to be the point of departure of mobilization against AIDS in South Africa as of 1994.

It is nevertheless clear that during the last half of the 1980s, AIDS was far from being the number one priority on the political agenda of the government or of its conservative or progressive counterparts. As William Beinart (2001: 254) has written, the period might be summed up in three words: "insurrection, fragmentation, negotiations." In 1985 a state of emergency was proclaimed and the violence of the public police force became general. Tens of thousands of black demonstrators and activists were arrested, hundreds of young people killed by the police and the army during the riots or in prisons. Pressures from international institutions as well as from South African business circles nevertheless obliged the government to begin to reform and negotiate. Between 1987 and 1990 informal contacts were made with Nelson Mandela (who was still in prison) and with Thabo Mbeki (who was in charge of international relations for the ANC in exile), among others. At the same time, the fissures in the system of racial segregation became more and more apparent, with black families moving around and even into the cities becoming more and more common. For a majority of South Africans, the end of apartheid was in sight. In these conditions, the government's margin was very narrow indeed to maneuver against an infection long underestimated, especially in the black population. Either it was accused of not doing enough (it was then attributed to its indifference to the victims of the infection) or, on the contrary, it was reproached for

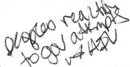

wanting to do too much (it was then suspected of trying to institute birth control by recommending the use of condoms).

It was an impossible situation. As summed up by Ivan Toms, who like many other AIDS activists was also a militant in the fight against apartheid: "There is no possibility that the present government could, even if it has the inclination, run an effective campaign to limit the spread of HIV infection. It has no credibility or legitimacy whatsoever among Blacks."[47] While social unrest shook the apartheid system, segregation exposed its contradictions for the last time as the epidemic revealed the practical consequences of the regime (aside from homosexuals, whites were far less affected by the illness than blacks) and its obvious limits (the authorities were no longer legitimately speaking in the name of the state, except to the nationalist minority, which increased its provocative declarations). In the wake of apartheid, however, the political outline of AIDS had been clearly traced: racialization and xenophobia, suspicion and accusation, dramatization and violence. Yet, at the time, very few South Africans would have imagined that in the darkest recesses of the white establishment whose days of absolute power were numbered, a program of chemical and biological warfare against the black populations was brewing and that HIV was proposed as one of its weapons. That truth was only to come out in the late 1990s.

The Smile of Death

In 2001, at the start of my investigations, as I was asking a young African doctor in the public health sector what she thought of the climate of skepticism surrounding AIDS, her immediate response was to name Wouter Basson. She explained that since 1998, when the Truth and Reconciliation Commission hearings had shed light on the activities carried out within the intelligence services program Project Coast, the white authorities were suspected of being responsible for the spread of the AIDS virus: "people are well aware that that is why it has become a black people's illness," she commented. During the years that followed, I often heard people talk about this. In Limpopo Province, a male AIDS patient with whom I had several conversations told me one day, referring to a long-lasting injected contraceptive, "Most women were infected through this Depropovera on purpose so that they could then infect men. This Wouter Basson was the one who planned that to get rid of black people. He also planted HIV-positive women in Hillbrow to contaminate us, because he knew we were hiding there. In Pedi we call him the Monster." He added, "I heard the same thing in the Northern Province in '95–96. There was this doctor. She was suspected of infecting people. They said she was ill and she didn't want to die alone. She was suspended but was never charged." On another occasion, a young woman suffering from AIDS in Alexandra township was voicing her doubts about the fact that only the black populations appeared to be infected when her cousin interrupted her, exclaiming, "It's like this other doctor who draws blood from black patients and injected oranges whatever whatever whatever . . . so that it must be supplied to black communities and then started spreading like that no knowing that I am HIV-positive because I am eating oranges. And I pass it to my partner, that's how many people got it—Which doctor is it?—It was a doctor from overseas who once confessed he was spreading. I don't know if he did kill himself or was arrested. He said he was enjoying killing people more especially blacks.—Do you know his name?—I can't remember it. It was in the papers and on TV." Reacting later to these repeated examples, a colleague and friend, who lives in Soweto, made the following comment: "In all the funerals I go to I hear people say: it's Basson, it's Basson. In townships HIV and Basson are the same." During the years when AIDS began to loom over the national political scene, the man whom the newspapers called "Dr. Death" was in the center of the most upsetting rumors and the most terrible revelations. But who is he?

Basson is first of all a smile and a wink to the public caught by a photographer. His grinning face made the front page of the papers on April 12, 2002, the day after he was acquitted by the Pretoria High Court. The same ironic expression was on his face when four years earlier he testified disdainfully before the Truth and Reconciliation Commission. It had then been felt that his case was too serious to fit the commission's criteria and that he should be dealt with by the ordinary criminal justice system. That smile and wink is an obvious provocation for all those who suffered under apartheid or fought against it, as well as an attempt to stain the person being addressed through this intimate complicity. In the short story "The Spy Who Loved Me," Maureen Isaacson describes how ill at ease her narrator was to find herself several times in the presence of a secret agent and "hero of the ancient regime" being investigated by the Truth and Reconciliation Commission whose hearings she was covering for the press.[48] She interviewed him and immediately felt uncomfortable under his stare. One day, as she was driving, she discovered him in her rearview mirror. Just a few minutes before she had heard his lawyer explaining to the amnesty committee how sorry the man was for what he had done. Now she was catching him laughing in private with his lawyer at the good trick they had played on the judges. "Inducing paranoia is his business," she writes. Another time she was swimming at her club when she saw him get into the water. She writes, "It formed a stain on the crystal blue." And from then on she changed her working hours to avoid him. Later, her car stalls as it is getting dark, and suddenly appearing, he offers to take her home. Because of the lateness of the hour and the fact that she happens to be far from home, she feels obliged to accept his ambiguous offer in spite of herself. Her comment: "He is the one seeking freedom and pardon, yet I feel guilty." One look, one word, even worse one smile, and she feels complicit in his crimes. To relax in the same place where he is, to speak with him in a neutral manner, even just to exchange a glance must make him think she is on his side. "He has infiltrated my life like a virus," she concludes. The comparison could not be more suggestive. Like Wouter Basson, the man in the short story is caught up in sordid machinations. Like him, he denies everything or says he only obeyed orders. Like him, he laughs at the law that is powerless to prove his crimes. Like him, too, he is bald and wears African-style shirts, ironically of the same kind favored by Nelson Mandela.

The existence of a chemical and biological warfare program was revealed publicly during the last moments of the Truth and Reconciliation Commission's mandate. Until then there had only been vague rumors that no reasonable person would pay attention to. Two elements contributed to the discovery of Project Coast: the arrest of Wouter Basson at the beginning of 1997 for drug dealing, during which a suitcase full of sensitive documents was found; and the confession of Jan Lourens, one of his close collaborators, who in January 1998 explained to the commission about the work that was going on in a secret laboratory. From that point on, "amid allegations of gross misuse of public funds poured into a project so secret that at any given time only a handful of the most senior SADF [South African Defence Forces] officers even knew of its existence, stories began to emerge of cruel animal experiments, plans to breed a super wolf-dog, the search for the ultimate murder weapon impossible to detect during autopsy and sinister research on a contraceptive aimed specifically at South Africa's black population" (Burger and Gould 2002: 7). On June 8, 1998, the Truth and Reconciliation Commission began its Chemical and Biological Warfare Hearings, not without first having rejected a request for adjournment filed by the representative of Nelson Mandela's government who, curiously, feared the revelations that would be made about the program. The public hearings lasted until July 31. The hearings' transcript takes up 668 pages.

Wouter Basson himself refused to be heard. Only in the last days of the commission's mandate was he summoned to appear, but he denied all the charges. Of his presence at the hearings one will later mostly remember his provocations.

On October 4, 1999, the Pretoria High Court thus began his trial, one of the longest and most costly in the history of South African justice. The three hundred days it lasted fill 30,000 pages of transcripts. Pleading not guilty to all 67 charges brought against him, among which 11 were for murder—one affair involved the assassination of two hundred soldiers of Swapo, the Namibian liberation army—he was cleared of one charge after the other by Judge Willie Hartzenberg.[49] The latter, the younger brother of Apartheid Conservative Party leader Ferdi Hartzenberg, did not rest until he had proved, against all evidence to the contrary, Basson's innocence. For the first time in the court annals of South Africa, the attorney general representing the state, Anton Ackerman, demanded that the judge step down because of his bias. His demand was rejected. On April 11, 2002, the former director of the chemical and biological warfare program was acquitted. "The court walls have echoed with chilling tales of hundreds killed under the auspices of apartheid's chief director of death, but the judge says he has difficulty finding a complainant," wrote the journalist Zelda Venter of the *Star* on the eve of the judgment whose outcome seemed inevitable. "Judgment tomorrow will not so much close a door on a murky part of SA's past," she added, "as it will put a plaster on a seeping wound that has shown little sign of healing." The next day, Wouter Basson, who had indeed been acquitted, was on the front page of all the dailies, sending the public a smile of victory and a wink of complicity.

The world discovered the name "anthrax" in the aftermath of the attacks of September 11, 2001. Everyone recalls the wave of panic that followed the sending of letters containing the virulent baccillus. Yet when this happened few remembered the use the South African intelligence services had made of the same microbe.[50] Along with the *vibrio cholerae,* the *clostridium botulinium,* and various salmonellas, it belongs to the bacterial colonies that had been jealously preserved and that the military physicians meant to use to eliminate political enemies (the most famous being the secretary general of the Council of Churches of South Africa, Reverend Frank Chikane, who nearly died in April 1989) or even entire populations (as in the case of refugee camps in Namibia where the water supply was contaminated by cholera toward the end of 1989). But that was only one of the many activities directed by Wouter Basson. The documents of the Truth and Reconciliation Commission and the transcript of the Pretoria High Court trial, plus investigations by journalists and researchers,[51] allow us to reconstitute today the life and work of that military physician.

At the beginning of the 1980s, South African army headquarters developed the concepts of "total war" in order to "ensure the survival of the state." The threat to white hegemony represented by the insurrection of the townships and by the opposition in exile justified that every possible means be employed. The most secret of them all was Project Coast, which was supposed to set up a chemical and biological warfare program. Basson became its director. Testifying before the Truth and Reconciliation Commission, Dr. Daan Goosen, one of his closest collaborators, reported they had the following exchange:[52] "I asked Dr. Basson: Why are you involved in this? And he said: I've got one daughter and one day when black people take over the country and my daughter asks me: Daddy, what did you do to prevent this? my conscience would be clean." It is therefore with the desire to have a clean racist conscience, if one may say so, that Basson launched a series of research experiments in his laboratory. One of the most important consisted in carrying out a "sterilization program" among African women and men; to do so, a "vaccine" was needed that could be administered by mouth unbeknownst to the persons themselves. Other investigations concerned cancerous products, aggressive tear gases, and other toxic substances capable of acting selectively on the black populations. To carry out their research, Basson and his acolytes received considerable financing that they barely had to account for. Generally speaking, the military administration claimed to know nothing of what went on in Project Coast.

"HIV blood was stored for war": the sentence occupied the entire front page of the *Citizen* on May 25, 2000. "I Froze Blood That Had HIV," was the headline of the *Sowetan* the same day. These revelations were made at Basson's trial by Dr. Mike Odendaal, the microbiologist of Project Coast. He described how somebody had brought him a bottle of blood from a person infected with AIDS on behalf of the program's director, specifying that it was meant for "a political opponent." Nothing more happened, and nobody knew if the blood was ever put to use. But it echoed another scandal that took place a few months before, for which there is more information reported in the *Weekly Mail and Guardian* on November 12, 1999, under the title, "Apartheid Forces Spread AIDS."[53] It was not Project Coast that was being challenged this time but the no less daunting Vlakplaas, a group belonging to the Security Forces and its director, Colonel Eugene De Kock, nicknamed "Prime Evil" by his collaborators. According to two former officers of the unit, Willie Nortje and Brood van Herden, who testified abroad about their own involvement in this new affair, their chief had devised a plan to spread AIDS among the black population. Four "askaris"— members of the ANC who had defected to the white authorities—who had AIDS had been brought back to Johannesburg and given employment as security agents in two hotels used by prostitutes in Hillsbrow, the red-light district. Their mission was to infect the prostitutes, who would then infect their clients. The amnesty committee of the Truth and Reconciliation Commission reported the two men's accusations. But as Basson would do after him, in front of the commission, De Kock denied all responsibility for this plan without excluding the possibility that one of his collaborators might have taken the initiative. Less fortunate than his compatriot responsible for the chemical and biological warfare program, he was condemned in his trial to 262 years in prison for the numerous other crimes he had organized or committed.

For some years anthropologists have been intrigued by the production of "conspiracy theories," reviving the political scientist Richard Hofstadter's scientific program inaugurated in 1952 in an attempt to comprehend the "paranoid style" in politics (Marcus 1999). In so doing, they follow a line that parallels sociology, which prefers to look at "rumors," this time following in the footsteps of two psychologists, Gordon Allport and Leo Postman, who in 1947 spoke of "collective fear" (Aldrin 2003). Naturally, everyone can see that conspiracy theories depend on the circulation of "false news," in the words of the historian Marc Bloch ([1921] 1999), whereas "rumors" imply forms that the ethnologist Gérard Althabe (1969) defined as being "oppression in the imaginary." The two fields share the same preoccupation and mirror each other. From the presence of aliens and the existence of flying saucers through the assassination of John F. Kennedy and the death of Lady Diana, conspiracy theories based on rumors share a common structure that connects those who propagate them and those who study them. To the typically paranoid idea of the persecuted, who think that some are in on the secret but are hiding what they know from them, corresponds the nearly symmetrical idea of the researcher, which has it that people believe in fictions but that their beliefs must be respected. That is why these stories may be called "hystories" (Showalter 1997). Originally, anthropology was precisely developed on that basis by refusing to laugh or smile at witchcraft, magic, myths, and even, since Evans-Pritchard, by taking them very seriously indeed. But this did not imply believing in them, precisely because they are beliefs. The balance between actors and observers, between natives and ethnologists is certainly reassuring, both intellectually and ethically. It allows one to unveil the mechanics of an "age of anxiety" (Parish 2001) that has given rise to a multitude of such fables all the while protecting the "other's reasoning" (Stoczkowski 2001) as being real thinking. It does, however, elude one possibility—that the facts reported might just be true.

That is precisely the sort of unusual figure that the history of AIDS in South Africa obliges us to think about. Since on top of everything else it is taking place on the African continent, we have become accustomed to thinking that "an old leftover of persecution interpretations" (Zempléni 1975) exists and that the notion that AIDS has a foreign, often white, origin belongs to the timeless logic of a phantasmagoric relationship to domination and change, as illustrated by the work of the Manchester school on the "meaning of misfortune" (Mitchell [1965] 1987). However, in the present case, we must imagine a situation in which the paranoid beliefs of township inhabitants and cabinet members encounter the verified facts of a genocidal plot. Under apartheid, the imaginary of the extermination of African populations had become standard in policies seeking to eliminate "political adversaries" and eradicate the "black race." Thus it is no longer a question of examining long-lived beliefs but of understanding a certain reality. Of course, rumors render a confused version of history, as we have seen in the interviews. In the former homelands, the "antifertility program" and the "askari project" are rolled into one by asserting that long-lasting contraceptive injections were used to infect women, as if the conjunction between sterilization and contamination paralleled racial eradication. In the townships, freezing the AIDS virus for criminal ends was extrapolated to the actual act of inoculating "oranges," which was probably mixed with the attested use of cholera in orange juice, and the South African physician became a foreign "doctor," in relation to his international network, or, more simply, as if evil actions fatally came from elsewhere. But the framework of representations does reemploy the fragments of a truth that comes out little by little concerning the intentions of the ancient regime.

Let there be no misunderstanding here. I am not suggesting that the spread of the epidemic in South Africa, in spite of the fact that it remains unexplained in the eyes of specialists, is due to an actual plot that has actually been carried through. It is rather a question of thinking out the "conspiracy theory" in South Africa along a dual perspective. The first consists in taking seriously the fact that these "things," however incredible they might be, did exist not only in the collective imagination of African populations but also as part of the secret project of the white authorities. To the usual relativism of social scientists dealing with such cases, we have to oppose the positivism of attested facts. The second supposes one ask oneself what consequences the frequent mention of these worrying and fragmentary "revelations" might bring to bear on a social group. In other words, beyond established evidence of the crimes, we have to consider the sort of general atmosphere of mystery and impunity around the criminals that in the end makes the mere idea of a plot realistic for large segments of the population. The two elements are joined in what one might call the paranoid configuration of postapartheid times, in which delirium belongs to reality and apartheid has outlived itself.

Let us return one last time to Wouter Basson. The acquitted doctor started practicing again as a cardiologist at Pretoria Academic Hospital (formerly Hendrik Verwoerd Hospital, named after the apartheid ideologist) and has been working there without interruption since 1994. In spite of the repeated protests of certain of his colleagues, the man that the newspapers baptized "our country's Dr. Mengele" is on the payroll of the Gauteng Province Health Department and has been kept on in the official organization of physicians of the Health Professions Council.[54] For many of those men and women with whom I talked this over in the neighborhoods of Johannesburg and the provinces of South Africa, particularly after the conclusion of his trial, the fact that he is so protected raises painful doubts about the permanence of shady connections between the regime of yesterday and the powers of today.

PROPOSITION 4: THE HISTORY OF THE VANQUISHED

History is written according to two patterns, that of the victors, linear, coherent, completely bent toward its end, and that of the vanquished, fragmentary, uneven, full of trial and error, dispair, and expectation.[55] "It is a principle based on experience which is always verified that history is always made in the short term by the winners who, though they may prolong their victory over the medium term, can in no case dominate over the long term," writes the German historian Reinhart Koselleck (1997: 238). Such an interpretation may appear optimistic or even demagogic when held up against the facts. Yet it contains a profound truth that transcends the question of knowing whether yesterday's vanquished may hope to be tomorrow's victors. Whereas on the side of the victors "the historian is easily inclined to interpret a success won in the short term by an *ex post* teleology of the long term," as Koselleck explains, on the side of the vanquished, on the contrary, "the primary experience is that it all happened differently from what they expected or hoped." In other words, the confidence of the former makes them discover a direction to history, whereas the astonishment of the second deeply imprints a historical meaning. This is not to say that history "from below" is necessarily truer than history "from above." It is rather a matter of considering that the ordeals lived through in one's flesh and blood say more about the social world than the developments reshaped by the mind, because they connect the present to the experience of the past in order to build the future rather than connect the present to the project of the future in order to erase the past. There are things one does not forget.

Beginning his speech upon the return of the Saartje Baartmann's remains on August 9, 2002, Thabo Mbeki warned his audience: "We cannot undo the damage that was done to her. But at least we can summon the courage to speak the naked but healing truth that must comfort her wherever she may be. I speak of courage because there are many in our country who urge constantly that we should not speak of the past. They pour scorn on those who speak about who we are, where we come from and why we are what we are today. They make bold to say the past is no longer, and all what remains is a future that will be." The phrase "at least" in the second sentence must be given its full weight: when history has not been on one's side, at least its telling should be. The South African president is regularly accused of using collective memory to justify the position of his party and back up his own authority. It is true that the rhetoric of the president is constantly delving into the past to recall the violence that the African peoples were the victims of, first through European colonization and then through white domination. But he is also speaking of what really existed. As John Comaroff and Jean Comaroff (1997: 411) have written, "Nonetheless, the happenings with which we are concerned had a palpable logic: structures of inequality and exploitation were established, racialized distinctions were inscribed on the landscape, hegemonies emerged that turned hybrid realities into discriminating dualisms, elites and underclasses became implicated in each other's lives and identities." That past is not so far off; adults still remember it.[56] To grasp what is being played out today one therefore must look for what was being played out yesterday. Not for the sake of nostalgia or memories but because the mark is still deeply engraved. Walter Benjamin (1968: 258) wrote of the classic historians (epitomized, according to him, by Fustel de Coulanges), "they blot out everything they know about the later course of history," and "their empathy with the victor invariably benefits the rulers." To this version, he opposed a different reading in which the present throws light on the past, the only way to seize the stakes of the moment in which we are living on the rebound. He called this "to brush history against the grain." That is what I have been attempting to do.

To the strictly contemporaneous approaches that would have the history of the AIDS pandemic begin in the 1990s, when its progression started to gain momentum, and who therefore lock its interpretation into an impossible dialogue between the government and its opponents, I have tried to substitute a genealogy of the epidemic. This approach first means revisiting the long experience of public health used as an instrument to legitimate racial segregation, contributing to the exploitation of the workforce and building up subjectivity through domination: the fact that health policies and medical practices were also ways of treating patients and preventing illnesses obviously changes nothing. It also means considering, within the shorter period of the presence of AIDS in history, the continental and national contexts in which the representations of the origin of the virus and the mechanisms of its propagation, the racially differentiated programs to combat the illness and care for the sick, the operations of destabilization and elimination of the African majority of the country developed throughout the first decade of the epidemic: again the fact that other types of discourse, more prudent, could also be heard and that other actions, more respectful, were undertaken does not diminish their impact. The stigmatization represented by the categorization of a so-called African sexuality in the language of nature and promiscuity, the denial contained in the fact that only sexual behavior was questioned to the detriment of socioeconomic determinants, and finally the violence symbolized by the conception of plans of total race wars have made their mark throughout the twentieth century and plunge their roots into the beyond. "History weighs more than reality," complained Susann Coosen, a political scientist at the University of Port Elizabeth, in an opinion piece on the 2004 election campaign.[57] Perhaps we should say rather that history, too, is reality.

In view of this genealogy, the structures of the official response to AIDS can be understood as being something else than the denial that common sense has reduced them to. They fall into place around two sets of moral economies that are also two sorts of relationships to time. The first is the economy of resentment. This is a relationship to the past. We know that for Nietzsche, feeling resentment is what typifies the painful relationship that dominated people have to their history. It is an "invasion of conscience by memory traces," as Gilles Deleuze (1962: 131) has put it. That is why it paralyzes action. In Nietzsche's vision, dominated people, absorbed in the discovery of the imprints left by time and the denunciation of their authors, are caught up in a powerlessness that they justify by their history. For many in South Africa and particularly for those who underwent and sometimes combated apartheid, AIDS is an experience in the strong sense of the word. They relive and feel anew the past of violence, humiliation, and loss of dignity that they either experienced themselves or experienced through the accounts of parents and relatives. Tuberculosis and syphilis, medical discourses and moral lessons, the image of sexuality and the exploration of bodies spring to life once again as people experience the epidemic. The second is an economy of suspicion. It is a relationship to the present. Its source can be found in the analysis of ideology proposed by Marx, a prelude to the generalization of the idea that those who dominate hide the workings of their domination from the people they dominate. The notion that something essential is being kept from us about the truth of the world and that it is in the interest of those who hold the reins of power to hide it from us is a common belief. The theory has received official approval from a contemporary school of thought in the social sciences, which Jacques Rancière (1998: 99) sees as "a nihilist interpretation of suspicion theories." AIDS in South Africa, as in many other places on the continent, has bred doubt and mistrust: doubt concerning its reality, mistrust of its specialists. The expression of culturalist and racist prejudices in the years that followed its discovery, the attacks on the sexual behavior and local traditions, imposing solutions emanating from both a minimalist and an oversimplified view of what Africans needed or what they were willing to accept, confirmed them in their skepticism and suspicion. Finally, South African medicine and science, compromised by their active or passive collaboration with the apartheid regime and its crimes, sometimes with the complicity of the intelligence services of the Western states, have discredited anything that might be forthcoming from the white world or even from the West.

Let us make no mistake. It is because the vision of the vanquished is articulated around these two sets of moral economies that it manages to express a truth that the history of the victors refuses to name: for resentment concerns authenticated facts of the past, just as suspicion implies documented realities of the present. These two moral economies can thus not only be rationally analyzed, they also correspond to an essential moment of truth for South African society. If one does not want to recognize them for what they are, one runs the risk of doing nothing more than recriminate and complain, two reactions that have been especially common in South Africa over the past ten years every time the subject of AIDS is broached.

Yet these two perspectives do not obliterate the future, for two reasons. First, other dynamics exist in South African society, and it is obviously impossible to limit the answers to AIDS and more broadly to social problems solely to the above-mentioned duality of resentment and suspicion. Aside from resentment (and to stay within a Nietzschean typology), there are active forces in those who strive for social change. Concerning suspicion (and to stay within a Marxian approach), many social actors do implement praxis rather than ideology. It is therefore impossible to reduce South African politics to a single interpretation, even if it allows us to somewhat apprehend the incomprehensible. Second, the present government and the popular support it receives can no longer be explained by a clearly defined situation of domination. At least on the political level, the vanquished of yesterday are the victors of today. This novel situation has as its consequence that the parties in power and their elites cannot with impunity keep the South African nation that they now rule in the sole logics of resentment and suspicion. They have already been subjected to critiques from people who want acts rather than words and who are beginning to see them as the new dominators.

"What might it be to tell a 'free' story in South Africa, about memory and democracy, and about the intricate relations between individual and collective memory?" Sarah Nuttall (1998: 75) asked in a book on how memory operates in politics, art, and literature. The answer probably lies in the plural experiences of history cautiously rewritten by the Truth and Reconciliation Commission and violently mobilized around the AIDS epidemic. Probably, too, in giving the past the time it needs to be written.

FIVE

The Embodiment of the World

The past is all the fact I have
Memory my only fiction
Below the silent sanction of the stars.

PATRICK CULLINAN
"My Predawn Owl"

ON MARCH 30, 2004, a meeting of the AIDS Consortium was held in Johannesburg at the headquarters of COSATU, the Congress of South African Trade Unions. This organization, which united most of the NGOs that have been combating AIDS in South Africa for more than twelve years, is dominated by the two heavyweights in the field, the National Association of People Living with AIDS and the Treatment Action Campaign. Members of both organizations whom I saw in the days preceding the meeting had warned me it would probably be stormy. It was. In an e-mail to his fellow members, TAC treasurer Mark Heywood reported as follows:

Today I attended the AIDS Consortium meeting that was the subject of attack by NAPWA members. Apart from their general unruly and threatening conduct it is necessary to report and condemn the racism that is being fomented and encouraged by NAPWA's leadership. The very first comment by a NAPWA member included a racist attack on a white member of the AIDS Consortium Executive, Chloe Hardy, who was told that "we are sick of white people sitting at the front of the meeting; it causes us pain," to applause from the NAPWA leaders. At the end of the meeting, Thandoxolo Doro, the national organiser of NAPWA, confronted me aggressively and shouted "We are sick of you fucking white racists taking advantage of black people with HIV/AIDS." As he and other NAPWA members advanced on me I was removed for my safety by an employee of

COSATU and others. After the meeting had ended, the NAPWA members toyi-toyied in the meeting room and outside led by NAPWA Director Nkululeko Nxesi, singing "Mark Heywood the white racist has succeeded in dividing black people—that was his agenda all the time." An intervention to stop this by Mazibuko Jara, the Chairperson of the AIDS Consortium, led to a new chant that Jara was the new "black bourgeoisie."

Although it may appear strange to the foreign reader, this scene will hardly surprise observers of the South African situation. Competition between the two organizations goes back a long way, even though at the beginning they were allies and even though they often work together in the field. Their rivalry arises from the usual competition for more or less scarce resources (not only for financial means but also for the symbolic capital and the political influence it represents). But it also reflects sociological differences: TAC is more urban and international and has a relatively small number of Africans in its most visible avant-garde (though its officials are always careful to make sure the diversity of its members is represented in public events), whereas NAPWA is more representative of the country overall, including rural areas, and is firmly anchored nationally, with a large majority of African patients (contrary to TAC, its policies have been less and less welcoming to other groups). But beyond those differences, there is their choice of allies—NAPWA sides with the ANC; TAC, with COSATU— 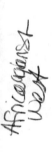 and their strategies—in 2003 TAC organized a campaign for civil disobedience against the government whereas NAPWA sponsored the Black Easter campaign against the pharmaceutical industry. All these differences account for the bitterness of the dispute during the AIDS Consortium. The rhetoric employed points to what is at stake, something far more general than AIDS and specifically written into South Africa's history. As it happens, behind the conflict lay the suspicion that NAPWA was guilty of misappropriating funds and favoring nepotism, as a result of which TAC had pressured for an audit.[1] That audit had been assigned to a British woman, and to avoid the taint of collusion and racism, it was decided that she should be not only a foreigner but also black. The audit confirmed the lack of financial transparency and revealed serious fraud. But, in spite of efforts to avoid racializing the conflict, the color line was once again summoned to interpret the facts. The day after the spectacular quarrel, NAPWA and several other organizations announced that a forum of black associations against AIDS would soon be held. An anecdotal but significant sign of the social efficacy of this racial interpretation is that just before the meeting, a young home-based care volunteer in Alexandra explained her version of the conflict to us in the most impartial manner possible. There had been, she said, an audit done by a "white man" (as we saw, the auditor was a black woman) who "obviously" concluded that this "African association" had problems. The link between the two facts—the color of the skin of the expert and the negative result—seemed logical. This young volunteer had lived in the Free State, at the experimental heart of the apartheid machine, until the age of twenty. For her, the affair was much more trivial than when, as a child, she had seen an Afrikaner shoot an African's dog for the mere reason that it had copulated with a white man's female dog. For her, a racialized worldview went without saying.

The body is not only the immediate physical presence of an individual in the world; it is also where the past has made its mark. Or rather the body is a presence unto oneself and unto the world, embedded in a history that is both individual and collective: the trajectory of a life and the experience of a group. The mark of time is engraved so deeply as to be imperceptible: when perceiving ordinary objects and when going about one's daily business, in the wear and tear of the physical organism and the exposure to the risk of illness. In other words, it is beyond the separation of culture and nature. Often, however, history is obscured and the body, existing in the here and now, seems to the observer—or to oneself—like a presence without a past. That is the case when ways of being or doing are treated strictly in terms of rationality or intentionality: the actor who calculates, deliberates, and decides seems to escape determinism and even temporality. That is also the case when sex or color differences are naturalized or on the contrary, but that comes to more or less the same thing, when they are denied: the questions of gender and race then become impossible to think, because they are taken out of social time. The history of AIDS, especially on the African continent, confirms how efficient such a blotting out has been: in practice, population surveys and prevention programs essentially based on the standard comprehension of knowledge, attitudes, and practices, elude the temporal inscription of individuals and the groups to which they belong; more subtly, the sexual and racial dimensions of the epidemic have often, at least in official speeches and policies, been treated ahistorically, throwing the former back on facts of pure sexual violence and concealing the latter officially in order to avoid stigmatization.

But bodies resist the obliteration of the mark left by history. They resist both in the subject's perception and in the objects perceived. Let us reconsider two scenes already described. When the health minister said to the public health doctor during a discussion on AIDS policies, "You cannot understand because you are white," she was speaking both of herself perceiving and of the other being perceived through racial categories that at the moment appeared to supersede all the others she could have mustered.[2] When, speaking about the difficulties of implementing programs for AIDS testing and prevention in her area, the subdistrict director declared, "I've got an objective view of these things because I'm in a favourable situation, but if you were traumatized since you were a child, you would be quite emotional about it," she was expressing her own conception of the two ways one can see the world—according to whether you are white and privileged or black and oppressed.[3] Whether it is a question (as in the first case) of an apparently immediate perception of the intersubjective relation or (as in the second) of a reflection on that perception by the different interlocutors, racial characterization amounts to what Everett Hughes (1945) has called the "main status" (as opposed to the "subordinate status"), the one that comes before the others and pushes them into second place.[4] Differences in speech (subjectivity vs. objectivity) and asymmetries in positions (involvement vs. detachment) only confirm this as an intrinsic feature of the construction of identity and otherness, since not only does it enter into people's weltanschauung, it functions differently depending on one's historical situation. Both women shared a certain experience on the apartheid battlefield. Yet the health minister allowed her "African" origin to take precedence the instant she put down the public health specialist as "white" in racial and even racist terms. Conversely, the director was counting on her "Afrikaner" resources to keep the conflicts she was describing at a distance, significantly avoiding the reference to color and preferring the less essentialist word *traumatized*.[5] But let us not be misled by what such examples might signify. Racial ascription is still today the most effective factor in the construction of representations and the elaboration of expectations concerning the others in South Africa. It does not, however, preclude other attributes, in particular, status, class, gender, and region of origin.

The idea here is thus very general. It aims at ascertaining how what Alfred Schutz (1962: 7) calls "the common-sense constructs used by men in everyday life" is built. He continues: "Let us try to characterize the way in which the wide-awake grown-up man looks at the intersubjective world of daily life with which and upon which he acts as a man amidst his fellow men. This world existed before our birth, experienced and interpreted by others, our predecessors, as an organized world. Now it is given to our experience and interpretation." The world in which we act and interact seems to be a given, he writes, and when we do or think something we are usually convinced we are acting or reflecting in a private, individual manner and making spontaneous choices. In fact, we are always delving into a "stock of previous experiences, our own or those handed down to us by our parents or our teachers." It is through them that the past is embodied in our present but also, more materialistically, that individual and collective history is embodied in what we are. This phenomenological approach, which is a radical rejection of behaviorism, allows us to restore their width and breadth to actions and interactions by taking into account both their inscription in the world and their meaning for the individuals. For this reason the Austrian sociologist prefers to speak of "conducts" rather than "behaviors." The studies of risk practices as they have been carried out for AIDS and in Africa particularly would have much to gain from that analytic displacement.[6] To understand why and how social agents act and interact as they do and, for example, why violence has crept into the very heart of gender relations in the townships or how sexuality is negotiated between desire and commerce, we must explore the everyday life-world and the history by which it is informed.

From that point of view, the author who has never stopped questioning our bodily inscription in the world and who—borrowing among all available disciplines, from psychology to neurology, from psychoanalysis to biology, from physiology to pathology—has taken the risk of creating a "phenomenology of perception," placing it at the inception of all science, including sociology, is Maurice Merleau-Ponty (1945). As he writes, "The whole universe of science is constructed on the lived world and if we want to think out science itself rigorously, to appreciate its meaning and scope exactly, we must first awake this experience of the world of which it is the secondary expression. To comprehend thus essentially means to describe what we know of the world and how we know it. And we know not through our intellect but through our experience" (ii). Better yet: "The world is not what I think but what I live" (xii). For children born in South Africa under apartheid, knowing the world in black and white is initially the consequence of their daily experience, which naturally depends on their own perception of the color spectrum; only in a secondary intellectual move can they develop an analytic approach to justify or criticize racial inequality. The same goes for all social experience. The true mark of history is inscribed in the materiality of the physical and psychic being: "The specific past which is our body can only be seized by an individual life because it has never transcended it, because it secretly nurtures it and partly uses its strengths—because it remains its present" (101). The body is therefore a past embodied in a present. It is the tangible trace of time, the mark that brings it up to date. To grasp the world, to act oneself and interact with others, it is all we own—but we own it all.

In the sociological tradition, the "habitus"—a concept proposed by Marcel Mauss (1980) and pursued by Pierre Bourdieu (1980: 88)—elaborates the phenomenological interpretation (without always explicitly referring to it): "The conditionings associated with a particular class of conditions of existence produce habitus, systems of sustainable and transposable dispositions, structured structures predisposed to function as structuring structures, i.e., as principles generating and organizing practices and representations which can be objectively adapted to their goal without supposing the conscious aim of the ends and the explicit mastering of the operations which are necessary to attain them." The analysts of the South African political situation who interpret the racial rhetoric of public debates as being merely the cynical manipulation of an efficient resource (in other words, corresponding to strategic calculations) are consciously or unconsciously circumventing the fact that it is above all a reference shared by most of the social agents (i.e., it is embodied). Certainly, the health minister, the organization leader, or the simple citizen uses race as a tactic to discredit their adversaries. Doubtless, too, this act is effective precisely because it is stating the socially most plausible truth in this context. A language—the language of race, as it happens—is useful only if it is meaningful—as it is here with respect to a specific history. Incidentally, it would be erroneous to consider that the racial or racist vocabulary only exists on one side of the color line, that is, among African people, as it is often claimed by those who criticize the government's racialization of issues. In fact, it may even exist more brutally where it is denied. A public health professor who had lectured on the unequal distribution of AIDS in South Africa told me that at the end of her class the only students who had expressed interest and asked questions were black, whereas the only aggressive reaction came from a white student who asserted furiously that racial differences no longer existed and that even in Sandton (the wealthiest neighborhood in Johannesburg) the biggest cars nowadays belonged to Africans (suffice to go there on a Saturday morning and wander through the luxurious mall to realize how little truth the assertion contains, but this comment shows how, even in small numbers, rich blacks are always the most visible to many whites).

In fact, one can follow Bernard Lahire (1998: 53) and distinguish "two trends among the theories of action and of the actor" according to the way 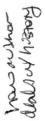 they deal with history. "There are, on the one hand, models that confer a definite and decisive role to the actor's past and more particularly to his/her very first experiences (the various psychological theories, the psychoanalytic theory and the theory of the habitus) and, on the other hand, models that describe and analyze moments of action or interaction or the given state of a system of action without bothering about the actors' past (the theory of rational choice, methodological individualism, symbolic interactionism, ethnomethodology)." Most work on AIDS, large statistical surveys as well as many ethnographic studies, leans on the second approach. Needless to say that my perspective is of the first sort. Not as a postulate but as a theoretically founded fact—how can one separate, even analytically, an individual or a group from its history?—and an empirically verified reality— how can the spread of AIDS, its interpretations and the controversies surrounding it, be understood otherwise? Linking past and present in biographies and narratives as well as in situations and interactions is what I attempt in this chapter, first by seeking to grasp the social configurations that underpin the AIDS scene, then by trying to demonstrate how they are incorporated into people's itineraries and lives.

BEHIND THE LANDSCAPES

> *that province in their blood*
> *whites cannot understand*
> *around us the city hums*
> *with the quarrel of machines*
> *a culture of barbed wire*
> *and speaking wallets*
> *of which we are the heirs*
>
> KELWYN SOLE
> *"Invention of Tradition"*

"Blood pours from the wounds of a dead body, staining the ground below. Steel rods rise from the ground, encircling the body like a cage. Sheets of newspapers, swept up by a gust of wind, flutter in the air, some fixing on the body, others floating to another part of this desolate landscape. A red chalk outline draws itself around the body, directly onto the barren land. Shrouded in papers, the corpse is absorbed by and transformed into the grim terrain itself. Ultimately, rocks, mountains of dirt, steel pylons, car tracks, weeds, and craterlike pools of blue water are all that remain." William Kentridge's graphic artwork is remarkable in that it can be read like a documentary in which drawings come to life to create a world where oneiric poetry and social criticism mix. The film *Felix in exile* in charcoal and pastel on paper was created in 1994 and lasts a little over eight minutes. One of the first sequences, described by Staci Boris in the excerpt above, shows the disappearance of a corpse, swallowed up by the gold mines of Johannesburg's East Rand. As the associate curator of the Chicago Museum of Contemporary Art puts it, this vision "vividly illustrates one of the major themes running through Kentridge's work—the hidden histories of the landscapes—and poses questions of how a landscape is constructed and represented and whose stories it ultimately tells, if those stories are remembered and told at all." For the artist himself, his images are not intended as "illustrations of apartheid"; rather they "are certainly spawned by, and feed off, the brutalized society left in its wake." What one can name postapartheid is contained entirely in this observation and that intention. AIDS and more generally the political and social landscape since 1994 have been interpreted as a tabula rasa, or, at the very least, the aim has been to build a new society so radically different that the old one would disappear from memory. Some have wanted to believe in the future; others have sought to bury the past. But it is becoming more and more evident that present-day landscapes contain hidden histories that cannot be gotten rid of by applying a politics of forgetting. To fully grasp the human tragedy of AIDS, it is impossible to overlook the work of unearthing the historically constituted structures that lie beneath the surface, since most of them persist ten years after the first democratic elections and are present today in the debates that rage across the public sphere. However, this is not a question of mere determinism. Inequality, violence, and human displacements, in their relation to the epidemic, are not simply the causes of the propagation of the illness and the reasons it did so in such an uneven manner. They are also a description of the conditions and ordeals that the patients experience concretely.

The Redemption of the Mine

"The Miners' Revenge." In Gold Reef City's amusement park, between Johannesburg and Soweto, dedicated to the memory of the Rand gold mines, one of the best liked and most feared sites bears that curious name. I never understood what it meant, except to imagine that the terror that grips middle-class children as they hang over the gaping pit in the large mining chariot is a form of revenge for the suffering experienced in the past—and still today—to allow the mining industry to develop and the South African economy to flourish, both to the sole advantage of white capitalism built on racial segregation. Although it is doubtful that the miners are effectively getting their revenge, one could consider that the mine is being redeemed symbolically through AIDS. Toward the end of the 1990s public authorities and private firms finally decided to take the epidemiological situation of the mining industry seriously: "Indications show that forty-five percent of South African mine workers are HIV positive," Susan Shabangu, minister of mines and industry, announced in November 1999, as demographic studies revealed that the epidemic threatened to kill 10 percent of the labor force each year.[7] In the face of that reality, the large companies first tried to solve the problem as they had done in the past for tuberculosis (Packard 1989), that is, through selecting workers by making serological tests mandatory prior to hiring (similar to the clinical tests of yesteryear that eliminated the physically inapt candidates) and especially by not renewing an infected person's contract (as in the case of the bacillus in the past). In August 2000, as insistent rumors about this unethical practice were circulating, Labor Minister Membathisi Mdladlana publicly intervened to say that "if it is true employers in the mining sector sever contracts of workers because they are HIV-positive, undoubtedly these actions are illegal," and to declare that he was "prepared to raise the question with the mining sector for it to be addressed as a matter of urgency."[8] The rumors proved not unfounded, and the practices reminded everybody of the policy of systematic testing during apartheid and the wave of expulsions of foreign workers that followed in 1988.

A complete turnabout in policy on the part of the mining industry thus took place in 2001 when Anglo Platinum and De Beers, the two largest South African platinum and diamond companies, respectively, in a competition of generosity, declared almost simultaneously that they had decided to implement a prevention, testing, and care program using a "global" approach careful to respect "anonymity" and to fight against "discrimination." At the beginning of the following year, they were joined by several other global firms such as Sony, Daimler Chrysler, and BMW under the auspices of the South African Business Coalition in a venture with relatively broad but vague objectives.[9] Finally, in August 2002, in the context then dominated by the decision taken by the Constitutional Court against the government in the case of the prevention of mother-to-child transmission and by TAC's renewed attacks on the health minister over gaining ac-

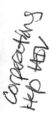

cess to drugs, Anglo American, the giant of the mining industry, federating Anglo Gold, Anglo Platinum, and Anglo Coal and controlling nearly 50 percent of De Beers' stocks, shortcut the public authorities by announcing they were going to initiate antiretroviral therapy for their 134,000 workers who suffered from AIDS.[10] The huge mining conglomerate, which at the time of apartheid had unscrupulously exploited workers and discharged them when they were sick, was now held up both nationally and internationally as a model of humanitarianism.

During the breakfast offered in the luxurious rooms of a hotel in the residential section of Rosebank at the beginning of April 2003, Anglo Gold announced the preliminary results of the treatment given to its sick miners. Journalists and representatives of the various departments were invited. The lecturer—the physician in charge of the program—first gave an overview of the company's health services that included two hospitals, six dispensaries, and 10,000 employees and reminded the audience of the many activities initiated by the firm for the benefit of their 40,000 workers, from voluntary counseling and testing to home-based care, through awareness campaigns and peer education; orphans, too, had become a recent preoccupation and, as she explained, "Anglo Gold had made an important donation to develop programs in favor of AIDS orphans." She then presented her data: of the 138 HIV-positive workers known to require treatment, 121 had accepted it and 8 had interrupted it, so that in the end 113 patients were receiving antiretroviral multitherapy, among whom half suffered from more or less serious side effects; the overall cost was estimated at 25.8 million rands for 2003 (about U.S. $3 million), of which 13.7 million rands were spent for the patients undergoing treatment, amounting to 669 rands per employee and per year, that is, 55 rands over the monthly payment of the insurance premiums (note that the annual gold production of South Africa comes to 12 billion rands). The lecturer added, anticipating the questions of those who would find the cost of this act too high in the context of international competition on the gold market: "The reality is you need to do something and it is going to cost you something." But so as not to leave her audience with a dry list of figures and costs, she ended her PowerPoint presentation by projecting two photographs: the first showed a little white boy; the second, little black children, accompanied by this moving comment: "The reason, I ask myself, why we are doing all this? [first slide, she smiles proudly] There we go, this is the light of my life. . . . [second slide, she keeps smiling but in a compassionate way] and these are the lights of the other people's lives that are no more, they are the orphans in our Carletonville home-based care projects. . . . Thank you for your attention." Applause burst forth.

Obviously, I was interested by her presentation, but I was intrigued, too: the South African program that all the newspapers, including the foreign press, were praising for being so generous only concerned a little over one hundred patients. Somebody indeed asked the lecturer about this. She answered that out of 40,000 employees, they estimated that "25 to 30 percent," that is, 13,000 persons, were HIV-positive, of whom 3,000 required treatment. But she did not comment on the fact that barely one out of thirty was actually receiving multitherapy. The reasons for this mediocre outcome were probably many and complex, but whatever the case may be, the final result made the company's medical director, who took the floor next, seem quite presumptuous when, after having scathingly spoken about the government's policies regarding antiretroviral therapy and proudly presented the actions of his company's health service, he exclaimed, "What we have here is a National Health Service that works!"[11] The leap from the 121 patients his service had placed under treatment to the 5 million HIV-positive persons whom the public authorities had to care for was presented as a mere difference in degree.

Yet it is he who, when he spoke after his younger colleague, gave us the key to the entire performance. Like a juggler accustomed to this sort of act, he began by a joke in which American lawyers were compared to rats before continuing in a solemn tone: "Of course, apartheid is the deep wound in the soul and psyche of South Africa. And healing that wound is the work of generations and is an agenda for 42 million South Africans. The only question is how much assistance we need from Mr. Fagan and New York City lawyers in order to come to terms with our own past and whether we have remedies right at home in a sober environment with a good court system and a vibrant dialogue between social partners." Everyone understood he was referring to a case that the Khulumani Support Group and the Apartheid Claims Task Force had just brought against Anglo American, De Beers, and other multinationals in the United States for the damages done during the apartheid regime. The lawyer, Ed Fagan, was a precursor in this sort of reparations claim, since he had won from the German firms and government a U.S. $5 billion fund to compensate Jews for having had to do forced labor under the Nazi regime.[12] President Thabo Mbeki was not in favor of the South African groups' legal action, but he was talking with the mining sector in order to obtain a contribution to the reparations fund for apartheid victims certified by the Truth and Reconciliation Commission.

Archbishop Desmond Tutu, who had presided over the commission, had also intervened to push the mining sector to participate in that patriotic effort and thus outstrip the legal action taken against the multinationals.

Therefore, the generosity toward AIDS patients and the publicity it afforded the mining industry pointed to a double strategy. On the one hand, the firms negotiated partnerships with the unions, which had the authority to approve agreements on health care costs, while attempting to keep the government benevolently neutral, since it had reacted with hostility to their discriminatory policy. On the other hand, they tried to use those programs as moral guarantees in the eyes of the international community at a time when the fact that they had been profoundly compromised under the apartheid regime threatened to put them in a bad position, including to their stockholders, especially the Americans, who are often vulnerable to arguments involving "ethical capitalism."[13] In other words, they were buying their good name, and, compared to their U.S. $25 billion turnover and nearly $2 billion profit in 2003, the $2 million given to the program for HIV-positive patients was not too steep—in any case, much less than the amounts that had been calculated for reparations.

The lecturer's compassion and her director's sarcasm thus swept under the carpet the mining industry's historical responsibility for the system of apartheid (for which it was accused in the courts) and also for the development of the AIDS epidemic (as is less well known). The survey done in Carletonville (Williams et al. 2000), the largest gold mining complex in the world, situated in the Rand near Johannesburg, is one of the most incriminating pieces of evidence. It revealed that 28.5 percent of the miners are infected with the AIDS virus. The authors sketch the following description of the mine's social environment:

> The population of Carletonville town is about 20,000 while that of Khutsong is estimated to be 150,000. The mines house an additional 60,000 to 80,000 migrant workers. Most mine workers live in ten single sex hostels close to the mine shafts. Living conditions are basic and between four and fifteen workers share a room where each man has a bed and a locker or cupboard space. Close to the mine hostels there are shebeens (informal bars) and hotspots (where commercial sex workers meet clients). Some hotspots are informal settlements; others are simply open areas in the veld. From early morning the first customers, miners returning from the night shift, come and go, buying alcohol and sex. The shacks are generally owned by older women, often former sex workers, who sell liquor and pro-

vide accommodation to three or four sex workers in order to attract men to the premises. The sex workers who work permanently in the hotspots are joined on weekends by women from Khutsong or from other places such as Soweto. Miners who see their wives and families between once a month and once a year are ready clients, and often form casual relationships with sex workers.

In these "hotspots," 68.6 percent of women were infected by HIV; however, even among those residing in Khutsong township, the rate of infection reached 37.4 percent.

Given that description and those figures, the slides and jokes of the Anglo Gold lecturer were out of place, as were her humorous understatements and the audience's mirth as she talked about the prevention implemented by the firm—precisely at the Carletonville site, whereas we had come to luxurious Rosebank to listen to her: "Of course, there is abstinence and monogamy. It is essential. People need to have their choice, but it is not the front line of our approach [murmurs and laughter]. We have programs including condoms that are free from the state. Well, we try to count how many condoms are distributed, but obviously we can't monitor how many of them are used [murmurs and laughter]. In the next slide we are going to show you how many are distributed. I must be honest I don't know why we are providing these statistics. It always raises a bit of alarm to tell that, companywide, per month, our employees use 1.31 condoms [at this, the public burst out laughing]." In the Carletonville survey, 61 percent of the men and 66 percent of the women had never used a condom in their lives. Even with occasional partners, only 21 percent of the men and 34 percent of the women said they used one regularly. And we have seen that over a quarter of the men and nearly half the women were HIV-positive. It gives one an idea of how great the danger of infection is for all those concerned, even when the number of partners is small. Far from being contingent, simply contextual as it were, the high prevalence of the infection and the high risk level are the outcome of the way mining is organized, especially among migrant workers: "There is no other country in the world whose urban industries, whether mining or manufacturing, have employed such a large proportion of oscillating migrants for so long a period of time," writes Francis Wilson (2001: 105). This policy has had an equally unmatched human cost.

As noted by Jeeves and Crush (1995: 2), "the herding of South African black mine workers into communal single-sex barracks away from their families has a long history." In the second half of the nineteenth century, when gold and diamonds were discovered, it was necessary to attract a labor force into the mines that were developing at full speed. As the white workforce was insufficient, Africans from the national territories or from neighboring countries were increasingly brought in in large numbers. For practical reasons, the thousands of African workers were put near the mines in vast "compounds" of collective and rudimentary housing. This system dominated as of the 1890s. A few attempts were made at the beginning of the twentieth century to stabilize the families on "labor farms" or "tin towns" near the mine pits, but, faced with the risk of uncontrolled expansion of such a residential system not far from the white cities, segregationist logic finally prevailed and the so-called Natives Urban Area Act of 1923 gave the towns the power to regulate the Africans' living conditions. At the same time, the need for workers increased, but the government was opposed (essentially to protect the domestic labor market) to calling on foreign workers as had been the case for Chinese in the 1900s and Mozambicans in the 1910s.

The first important segregation law, the Natives Land Act of 1913, had reduced the space Africans were authorized to occupy to "reserves" that covered only 13 percent of the nation's territory, which naturally proved insufficient to ensure the survival of these populations and forced the men in particular to look for jobs abroad. With the agricultural depression of the 1930s, this workforce turned to the mines, which employed 160,000 workers at the end of the decade. According to the industry, united in the powerful Chamber of Mines, they should, in pure entrepreneurial logic, always be considered a migrant workforce: precarious employment was thus built through temporary contracts that made it possible to renew the workforce especially when illness or exhaustion made laborers incapable of continuing in the mines; it also prevented workers from organizing in unions, since their contracts were temporary and there was always the threat of being terminated; above all, it ensured the externalization of the reproduction of the workforce, because the families subsisting on their plots of land guaranteed its continuity and renewal (Wolpe [1972] 1995). It is thus easy to understand how the system of crowding workers into permanently transitory and rudimentary "compounds" first, "hostels" later, was an intrinsic part of life in the mine and the situation that allowed for the greatest profits. In 1992 almost six hundred of these collective and temporary lodgings officially numbered 530,000 beds of which 313,000 were in the Rand region alone (Minnaar 1995). Though family housing was announced a few years ago in order to humanize life in the mines, it has been implemented only marginally.

Thus conceived and upheld, the mining economy—and most industries, for that matter—favors the conditions for the AIDS epidemic to develop not only around the mines themselves but also throughout the country. In the mines, separating the working men from their families and especially from their wives, who remain in their villages, induces the development of leisure places combining drink and prostitution, promoted or simply tolerated by the companies because they keep workers in the workplace, as Mamphela Ramphele (1993) has described in her book on the "hostels" of Cape Town. In fact, every form of sexual economy exists, from the prostitutes who live at the edge of the mine and take part in activities more or less controlled by their older sisters to girlfriends with whom conjugal-type relations give rise to a second homestead with children, through occasional relations with women living in the neighboring townships. Besides, these various modalities are not mutually exclusive in the miners' individual life stories, for, though they have built up a preferential relationship with one woman, they may still have sexual relations with prostitutes. Nevertheless, "the economy of desire," to use a phrase coined by Dunbar Moodie (2001) in the biographies of miners of the Pondoland region in the former Transkei, is not limited to the alternative of "country women" (wives remaining in the villages) or "town women" (more or less ephemeral girlfriends around the hostels or in the township); they also include the "mine wives," young men working under the protection of older men whom they service sexually in a relatively stable and long-term fashion.

This local configuration of sexuality in the mines nevertheless becomes meaningful, on the one hand, in the larger context of the construction of social identities, masculine identities in particular, and, on the other hand, in the context of the conditions of existence and especially of working conditions, masculinity and work being closely connected. This is what Catherine Campbell (1997) has shown in her study of the Rand. The notion of risk, as she explains, is not only part of the miner's daily experience of being exposed to accidents or to witnessing the accidents of others but also part of the omnipresent ideology of virility, consisting in having to face danger and never show fear: "You show your manhood by going underground, working in difficult conditions—this shows that you are man enough to accept that if you die you are just dead," says one of her interviewees.[14] Henceforth, the less visible and more remote risk of being infected by AIDS is considered a mundane sort of danger. All the more as the ordinary circumstances of sexuality in the specific places of the shebeens and at those particular times when one is drunk are not the ones covered by the prevention campaigns, which address rational beings in controlled situations.

The psychoanalyst Christophe Dejours (1993: 33–34) has suggested an analysis of these "defensive ideologies" that are specific to dangerous occupations and that aim to "mask, contain and hide a particularly serious form of fear" related to the objective conditions of the activity. These ideologies lead to risk taking but also facilitate the development of alcoholism or violence. The mine and its environment thus reenact, in a near-experimental fashion, the conditions of production and reproduction of the AIDS epidemic. In the random sample of the Carletonville survey (Williams et al. 2000), 53.8 percent of the women ages 20 to 24 and 58.1 percent of those ages 25 to 29 in Khutsong were HIV-positive. When the women residing in this township of 150,000 were questioned on their personal history, 22 percent of those who declared they had a single partner in all their lives were contaminated by HIV; this proportion rose to 34.5 percent when they had two partners and 49.7 percent when they had three. Put otherwise, in this high-risk environment of the mine and its surroundings, the very question of multiple partners corresponding to the various forms of occasional relations and often stigmatized as "sexual promiscuity" is no longer relevant for a large proportion of the population, in particular, women: any love affair exposes one to a very high risk of infection, especially as the use of condoms is not well accepted. Of course, when they go home to their villages, the infected miners may in turn transmit the virus to their wives and through them to their children.

In the imagination of African populations the mine has often been figured as cannibalistic. There is a trace of that in the songs collected by David Coplan (2001) among the Lesotho migrants. That picture has long been supported by the number of deaths caused by accidents, tuberculosis, silicosis, and the diverse illnesses that are the result of bad working, living, eating, and hygienic conditions.[15] For the 500,000 workers employed in mining today, as well as for their wives, girlfriends, and children, the mine as cannibalistic now makes sense for AIDS as well—if not an occupational illness, AIDS is at least a pathology closely related to the ways this workforce is employed. In view of this century-long political economy of the epidemic, one can thus wonder about the moral economy of the AIDS policy recently announced by the mining industry.

Of Inequality as Obscene

"The truth is that poverty causes illness and death. The truth is also that ill health causes poverty. As we work during Health Month to address issues of health, including AIDS, we must understand these fundamental truths as a necessary condition for the success of the sustained campaign we must wage to ensure the continuous improvement of the health of our people." With this credo published on April 5, 2002, in the newsletter of the party in power, *ANC Today*,[16] Thabo Mbeki inaugurated "Health Month," dedicated to promoting action in that field. Like every other time the words *poverty* and *AIDS* were linked in one of his speeches, interviews, or texts, activists and editorial writers were quick to react, seeing in the president's declaration the evidence that several months after having officially announced he would no longer interfere in the AIDS debate, he was still prey to the virus of dissidence. Since the beginning of the pandemic, the focus of discourse and policies throughout the world solely on the medical aspects of the illness, and since the beginning of the South African controversy, solely on the availability of drugs, has made the social issues (both carried and revealed by AIDS) practically inexpressible. Of course, a number of opposition critics have conceded that poverty is certainly a serious problem, that if one were taking antiretroviral drugs, one should also be able to eat— it was hardly possible to do otherwise than admit it—but rare indeed were those who were willing to draw the conclusion, both about what happened yesterday and about what is happening today. As we have seen, the case of the mining companies is paradigmatic: one can set up care programs (for reasons that are not only humanitarian) provided one does not bring up the past or question the present (there can be neither recognition nor reparation, no more than change in the working and living conditions that facilitate the spread of the infection).

As Lock (1997: 210) has written about North America (but her remark applies more generally), "Efforts to reduce suffering have habitually focused on control and repair of individual bodies. The social origins of suffering and distress, including poverty, and discrimination, even if fleetingly recognized, are set aside, while effort is expended in controlling disease and adverting death through biomedical manipulations. Disputes with respect to biomedical technologies usually revolve around the question of individual rights, autonomy, and justice." No more in South Africa than elsewhere has it been possible to treat the question of inequalities when dealing with

AIDS. Elisabeth Costello, in the eponymous novel by the South African writer J. M. Coetzee, tries, as she prepares a lecture, to explain to herself why the book of one of her colleagues, Paul West, deeply troubled and upset her.[17] After thinking for a long time she suddenly realizes: "*Obscene.* That is the word, a word of contested etymology, that she must hold on to as a talisman. She chooses to believe that obscene means off-stage. To save our humanity, certain things that we may want to see (may want to see because we are human!) must remain off-stage." Talking about poverty *and* AIDS in South Africa has similarly become obscene.

Yet it is hard to avoid that question when considering the figures or carrying out fieldwork. Statistics and ethnography converge to assert the existence of considerable inequalities in the distribution of the illness but also in its consequences. The indicator usually employed in international comparisons to evaluate the distribution of wealth is the Gini index, which measures the proximity to or distance from the real curve of the way resources are distributed among the population: of the 105 countries for which this information is available in 2000, South Africa was 101st, the 20 percent poorest disposing of 2.9 percent of the resources while 20 percent of the wealthiest disposed of 64.8 percent.[18] These inequalities largely correspond to the color line: 60.7 percent of Africans, 38.2 percent of Coloured, 5.4 percent of Indians and 1 percent of Whites are poor. Considered from the point of view of employment, the disparities are just as obvious: 38.3 percent of Africans, 20.8 percent of Coloured, 11.3 percent of Indians, and 4.3 percent Whites are unemployed. In the poorest African quintile, the proportion of persons declaring they were unemployed reaches 54.3 percent; given the actual distribution of the population, it is significantly impossible to calculate such a rate for Whites in the two poorest quintiles—because they are practically absent of them. The differentiation in occupational categories also reveals spectacular disparities: Africans account for 29.1 percent of management, 36.8 percent of professionals, 51.9 percent of technicians, 78.5 percent of unskilled workers, and 87.2 percent of domestic employees; Whites, for 54.8 percent of management, 51.1 percent of professionals, 33.1 percent of technicians, 3.2 percent of unskilled workers, and 0.3 percent of domestic employees.[19] During the first decade after the end of apartheid, these inequalities had not diminished.

Though an African middle class and even leisure class have grown up over the past ten years, notably within the framework of the affirmative action policy known as "Black empowerment," they remain an extremely small minority of the African population, contrary to what the common rhetoric aiming to deny socioracial inequalities would have us believe.[20] Though it is true that Mbeki's famous speech about the "two nations"— one "white, relatively prosperous," the other "black and poor"—errs by seemingly ignoring the segment of the population that is both black and prosperous, he nevertheless is stating a profound truth about the gap between "the theoretical right to equal opportunity" and the empirical fact "that it is equally incapable of realisation." These socioeconomic and socioracial inequalities have a considerable human cost.[21] Between 1996 and 2001—during the period preceding the heavy impact of AIDS on mortality—Africans had a life expectancy of 54.8 years; Coloured, 59.6 years; Indians, 70.2 years; and Whites, 73.7 years. Given the distribution of the epidemic and the inequality of access to treatment, the trend can only be a widening of the gap. Infant mortality is 54.3 per thousand live births for Africans, 36.3 for Coloured, 9.9 for Indians, and 7.3 for Whites; these disparities have been constant throughout the twentieth century. Thus, in Johannesburg, the differences between the mortality rates for White and African children were 1 to 10 at the end of the 1930s and 1 to 5 at the start of the 1960s. The epidemiology of AIDS prolongs and sometimes redesigns the contours of these social and racial inequalities.

According to the so-called Nelson Mandela National Survey, the rate of seroprevalence among adults ages 15 to 49 is 15.6 percent, but it reaches 28.4 percent in areas known as "urban informal" (townships for the main part) against 12.4 percent in so-called tribal areas (especially the former homelands). It is 18.8 percent for Africans, 6.7 percent for Coloured, 2.3 percent for Indians, and 5.7 percent for Whites. When one considers economic capital, poor households, that is, those that declared they did not have enough resources to satisfy their basic needs, have the highest rates. But in terms of cultural capital, educated households, corresponding to a high school education, are the most affected.[22] These results suggest a complex relationship between place of residence, socioracial group, income, and education. Leigh Johnson and Debbie Budlender propose the following characterization to account of this relationship. The populations with the highest risk of infection correspond to the townships and the rural areas where there are many migrant workers, especially among people with an intermediate education and employed in unskilled jobs and, to a lesser extent, in families with very little schooling and either unemployed or precariously employed. At both ends of the spectrum, the wealthiest and best-educated categories, on the one hand, and the most rural and the poorest, on the other hand, present the lowest risk levels.[23] The statistical relationship between AIDS and poverty is thus not linear.

In a given milieu, however, the statistical association between HIV prevalence, socioracial belonging, and socioeconomic conditions is much more constant, as demonstrated by the surveys carried out in the industrial sector. Prevalence there is twice as high among unskilled workers as among management and eight times higher among Africans than whites. Among Africans, if one considers their position in the company, taking 1 as the reference point for unskilled workers, the proportion of infection is only 0.67 for skilled workers and 0.3 for middle management. In each of these categories, whites are five times less often infected than are Africans. Finally, socioracial and socioeconomic inequalities come together to create a risk ten times greater for the African unskilled worker compared to the white manager. But to obtain a realistic view of the epidemiological landscape, it is necessary to add that, of course, there are many more Africans than whites among unskilled workers, the ratio being reversed for management, a fact that in absolute terms creates even greater disparities. Thus one can see how unequally AIDS is striking South African society. In this respect, rather than insist on the relationship between poverty and AIDS, as is usually done, it is probably more relevant to analyze the situation in terms of social inequalities understood as being economic, racial, and also gender-defined. Even if it is not the most appropriate tool to grasp inequality, ethnography confirms and refines these remarks. In particular, it allows one to apprehend the diversity and complexity of the mechanisms through which social factors insinuate themselves into the body and, more precisely, how history inscribes it with AIDS. This means renouncing simplistic determinisms and statistical reasoning.

Let us take the case of Sophia, a young woman from Alexandra. She was born in Soweto in a poor family comprising her mother, her stepfather, and her brother. She grew up in Natal, raised for a couple of years by one of her grandmothers. She then spent three years in a boarding school in Pretoria. When she interrupted her schooling at age fourteen to live with her boyfriend, who was only one year older, her mother was pleased because the boyfriend kept her and treated her well. Despite his young age, the boy was involved in several illicit activities, namely, theft in Hillbrow, a neighborhood of Johannesburg that had a reputation for being shady. His father, who belonged to a Soweto gang, had been shot by the police, and he had been raised by his mother, a household employee. The young couple settled down in a small apartment. But their relationship was less idyllic than it appeared. He often stayed away for several days, and she suspected he was seeing other girls. He was jealous and beat her when he thought she was being unfaithful or even when she showed too much consideration for their friends. One day, she fell ill, took a serological test, and discovered her infection: she was not even fifteen. At first, she did not dare tell him. When she finally did, he refused to believe her. Later, they had a baby, who was not infected. Shortly after, they separated. Today, she survives thanks to her disability grant and the child grant she receives for her son, which together amount to 860 rands a month. She is not getting any antiretroviral drugs, and she has been ill for approximately ten years.

Let us now consider Justine, an older woman from Limpopo Province. She is forty-eight. She was born on a farm near Tzaneen. Her parents worked there, and it is where she spent her childhood and adolescence. The school was on the farm, and when she was fourteen she, too, began to work for the farmer. The salaries were extremely low, but the family had a vegetable garden and their employer gave them a bag of corn and some salt every month. When Justine married an automobile mechanic from Ticky-line, she went to live with him, and they had a child. Then, since he could not manage to finish paying the dowry *(lobola),* her parents took advantage of a visit to keep the child as a hostage. When Justine's husband discovered this, he beat her, and she went back to her parents to hide. She lived on the farm for eleven years, then got tired of it. Leaving her son with her parents, she went to work as a domestic first in Pretoria for three years and then in Johannesburg for eight years. She had a boyfriend in Pretoria, a Ndebele plumber who had migrated from Lebowa homeland. When they became aware of the relationship, her employers took her to the doctor one day and forced her to get an intrauterine device. Later she left her job and moved to Johannesburg. Therefore she had to separate from her boyfriend and became involved with another man from Lesotho. With the first as well as the second, the material arrangements were the following: since she occupied lodgings in her employers' courtyard reserved for the salaried workers, she put her boyfriend up in her room; the boyfriend would give her money, food, and sometimes gifts. Both men were very kind to her, as she recalls. She does not know when she became infected. What she does know is that when she fell sick, her employers sent her to a doctor, and when they learned about her condition, they fired her and gave her compensation. She then had to go back to the North. Too feeble today to work, she can no longer stay with her parents, who are retired. She lives on her sister's property in a tiny shack under the glaring sun. Since nobody ever explained to her what she was entitled to, she receives no social grants. She goes to the hospital once a month to fetch her treatment, which obviously includes no antiretroviral drugs but vitamins and antibiotics. Her dream is to have enough money so as not to have to depend on her family and to be able to live with her son, unemployed today and also supported by a relative.

For Sophia as well as for Justine, it is far more by taking the social context and its reproduction into account than by studying the relations of cause and effect in a deterministic way that one can see how illness has been engraved in their histories. The young woman from Alexandra had a fragmented childhood and adolescence—several places of residence and ways of life—before meeting a barely grown-up boy who was socialized in delinquency and violence (following in his father's footsteps). To a certain extent, her mother gave her to this boy as she had previously to the grandmother and the boarding school, conscious that she herself was unable to raise her and happy to have her cared for by another. The urban setting of prostitution, drug dealing, and illicit activities that became the couple's surroundings is much more than a spatial framework; it is a real actor on the AIDS scene. Taking off from there, the infection discovered at age fourteen is little more than a by-product of circumstances, the outcome of both structure and environment. The woman from Tickyline followed a quite different itinerary. First, her story is one of ordinary exploitation on a farm repeated from generation to generation, with a marriage that appears to offer a way out of this no-future universe but that turns out to be a failure, at least in part for economic reasons. Later, it becomes the classic itinerary of working migration and discovery of domestic life among the urban bourgeoisie, including new forms of domination that go as far as regulating sexuality and procreation and new forms of constraint that include destabilizing the couple's relationship. Illness here means losing one's job. The dialectics of AIDS and poverty are manifest in this biography in which the latter makes the former possible and in which the former in turn exacerbates the latter, in a vicious circle.

Disability grants, when they are available, can reverse the dynamics, and though it cannot treat the infection, it can at least alleviate poverty. AIDS then is not only a calamity; it can also become a resource. This cruel reality underlines what is at stake in welfare policies, as imperfect as they may be. In the end, saying that poverty causes AIDS is inexact, especially if such a statement serves to exclude its viral etiology. Yet there is a profound truth behind the factual error: the stories reported here provide an interpretive

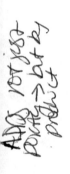

AIDS not just poverty → but by product

grid of the risk of infection that it is difficult to imagine could apply to the conditions and ways of life of the middle class or the well-off bourgeoisie. Ethnography cannot elucidate all the social mechanisms by which an illness is transmitted. It can, however, describe the worlds in which certain facts are not only possible but likely (for instance, leaving home at age fourteen to live with a delinquent in a dangerous place) while they would be unthinkable in another world (what is common in Alexandra township is simply inconceivable in the suburb of Sandton, only a few kilometers away). This comment seems so obvious that it is difficult to believe people have torn each other to pieces over it.

From One Violence to the Next

"A Society of Rapists." This is the title of Charlene Smith's article on statistics on sexual violence in South Africa that appeared in *Weekly Mail and Guardian* on April 7, 2000. Her statistics were impressive: "The danger of being raped is five times higher in South Africa than in the US."[24] She herself had been the victim of rape in her home a year before and had made it publicly known in the press, telling her story with a courage everyone had admired. Her attacker, a young African, was identified some time later and had just been sentenced to thirty-two years in prison by an Afrikaner judge. From her own experience, she drew broader conclusions: "Confronting rape is to acknowledge that HIV is rampant in South Africa not just through sexual promiscuity. AIDS is storming across the continent because of despicable attitudes and practices toward women and children—and rape leads the field." Again mixing her personal story and general considerations, she criticized the government for not having implemented in public health services the antiretroviral prophylaxis after rape that she herself had had access to in the private sector: "The government has been offered AZT at the lowest price in the world," she wrote, "300 rands or around 50 US dollars for the necessary 28-day supply. It has been rejected." The article caused a stir in South Africa.

Indeed, if Charlene Smith's intention was to provoke shock, she must have been gratified to see that her words had become the subject of polemics at the highest levels. Soon after, in his letter of July 1, 2000, addressed to opposition leader Tony Leon with whom he was having an apparently courteous but definitely incisive debate over AIDS and particularly over the effectiveness of and need for antiretroviral prophylaxis after rape, Thabo Mbeki expressed his indignation that her article had been published in an influential national newspaper and, even worse, that an interview with her had been published in the *Washington Post,* thus opening the polemic to an international audience: "Reflecting a view about rape in our country, Charlene Smith was sufficiently brave, or blinded with racist rage, publicly to make the deeply offensive statement that rape is an endemic feature of African society."[25] The president went on, quoting the journalist, who had written: " 'We won't end this epidemic until we understand the role of tradition and religion—and of a culture in which rape is endemic and has become a prime means of transmitting the disease to young women as well as children.'" And he associated those words with the "hysterical estimates of the incidence of HIV in our country and in sub-Saharan Africa made by some international organizations," seeing in them the expression of deeply ingrained prejudices against Africans.

AIDS, rape, culture, racism: the discursive network of a new polemic was in the making. The primary motive of the debate with Tony Leon over HIV prophylaxis after rape, to which Mbeki had brought facts taken from international scientific literature, once again giving his adversary a lesson in medicine, slipped into the background. The insistence with which he argued and the virulence of his tone betrayed that something else lurked behind an apparently technical discussion. Beyond the question of how to deal with rape, the history of race relations surfaced once again. In his answer on July 28, Leon defended the journalist: "Nowhere in this quote does Charlene Smith make a racial distinction between black, coloured, Indian or white South Africans." *Stricto sensu,* the opposition leader was right. For those who read the articles, however, the allusions were perfectly transparent. The portrait the journalist painted of the rapists—up to the references to "tradition," "culture," "sexual promiscuity," "sugar daddies," and "virgin-cleansing"—included all the commonplaces about "African sexuality": never has one of these themes been associated with the white world. And not only was it of Africans that she implicitly spoke, she also associated rape and AIDS, establishing a causal relation between the two. In his letter dated August 15, Mbeki returned to the subject, and after having expressed again his sympathy for the journalist's traumatic experience and recalled that he had personally intervened to accelerate the search for the rapist, he concluded: "All rape is reprehensible. I was as distressed when I heard about Ms. Smith's rape as happens whenever I hear of any incident of rape. I have not sought to vilify Ms. Smith. But neither do I accept that her terrible and unacceptable ordeal gives her licence to propagate racism, as I am convinced her published comments do." This exchange is only one of many episodes in which rape and racism have been linked.

In this polemical context, the very real association between sexual violence and the incidence of AIDS is a delicate matter, especially in view of the history of prejudice concerning African sexuality, but also of the sociology of facts that involve sexual violence. The difficulty is even greater as sexual violence has been publicized through dramatic stories that have obscured rather than clarified the problem. The affair that stirred up the most intense public feeling was the rape of a nine-month-old coloured child in a township of the Northern Cape. "Suffer, Little Children," read the headline of the *Weekly Mail and Guardian* on November 9, 2001. Beneath the headline, taking up two-thirds of the newspaper's front page, was a photograph of the child's mother sitting between another woman and a child, the mother covering her face with one hand, probably as much to hide her sorrow as to avoid the camera's inquisitive gaze. The caption read: "A relative of the nine-month-old Louisvale baby who was raped comforts Gertruida Rens and her granddaughter Valencia. It was to Rens' home that the baby's grandmother brought the child the night she was assaulted. In the weak light of Rens' lounge the women discovered a bleeding, gaping wound as they parted the infant's legs." Six men were arrested in the neighborhood, two as rape suspects and the others as accomplices. All were drunk. The two suspects were a family friend and the child's great-grandfather. The event received considerable publicity, seeming to confirm the idea of the bestiality and inhumanity of South African men even more than the reality of the rape. It combined two main taboos: child abuse and incest. However, it overshadowed both the ordinariness of violence and the complex nature of its causes. Not that such dramas are exceptional.

The story told by Astrid, a young woman whom I met in Alexandra, is revealing in this respect. To the mundane question I asked practically at the beginning of her interview, "So you were raised by your mom and dad?" she replied unexpectedly: "Ya, my mom and dad. So unfortunately, when I contracted this HIV, I've been raped by my father. He was a caring and loving father at home. He used to buy us gifts, food and so on. But the problem is on that day maybe he didn't know what he was doing [she interrupts herself, overwhelmed by emotion]." The rape happened during a wedding that was attended by the whole family. Astrid was then sixteen. She had left the party before the others to finish her homework. A little later she heard her father enter the house. He was drunk. He forced her to open her door. He raped her twice. She told her mother, who ordered her to keep quiet: "Because he's the only one who is working, let's not put him to jail, because we are going to suffer." But shortly after, Astrid developed "sores" on her genitals. She went to a doctor and had to tell him what had happened. That is when her serological status was revealed. Her family got together, and her parents said she was going to die. From that day on, they ignored her. However, with the help of a social worker, the young woman handed her father over to the police. He was sentenced to eight years. She ran away from her family to escape retaliation. Such testimony, or Magda's, which I recount below, attests to the reality of sexual violence within families. But it must not cover up the ordinary occurrence of rape.

In their review of available data in South Africa, after having reiterated the difficulty of obtaining information on such a sensitive subject, Rachel Jewkes and Naeema Abrahams (2002) report several series of statistics. According to the declarations recorded by the police, the annual number of rapes actually committed is 210 per 100,000 women, compared to 80 per 100,000 in the United States (data covering the general South African population show in addition that only 15 percent of women who reported having been forced to have sexual relations filed an official complaint). According to a Health Department national survey, 7 percent of women say they have experienced sexual violence (that is, forced or persuaded to have sex against their will) in the course of their lives, and this figure, paradoxically, is higher the younger the woman. In research carried out at a medical-legal clinic in Hillbrow that centralizes the cases of persons living north of Johannesburg, 12 percent of rape victims were less than sixteen years old and 75 percent were between seventeen and thirty-five (one-third of these cases had been victims of gang rape). In another study, this time in the southern district of Johannesburg, it was found, contrary to what one often hears, that 55 percent of the women said their aggressor was a total stranger and 22 percent said that they knew their attacker on sight (however, the younger the victim, the more often the rape was committed by an acquaintance). Overall, the data reveal that the most common scenario is an attack that occurs on the way to work and with the threat of a weapon. In addition, most of the rapes are committed within the same so-called racial groups, again countering the common representations. Moreover, white women report sexual violence twice as often as African women. As to sexual abuse before the age of fifteen, the results of two studies converge: the frequency of rape during that period was found to be 1.2 percent and 1.6 percent respectively, almost always after age ten. Finally, concerning the supposed but rarely proven relationship between sexual violence and AIDS, a study done at four health centers in Soweto has established that HIV infection is statistically associated with the violent character or the dominant nature of the usual partner rather than to sexual abuse during adolescence or rape committed by a stranger. These figures, besides contradicting newspaper sensationalism, invite us to reflect beyond the question of rape to that of violence in gender relations.

In many of the stories I collected told by women and sometimes also by men, violence could be read between the lines, in a sort of counterpoint to the statement I so often heard: "He was nice to me." The meaning of this expression is always the same: it implies giving money and presents, buying clothes and drinks, or when the woman has children, treating them well. The fact that the man is jealous and sometimes brutal is often considered the counterpart of the attention and gifts the woman receives from him. Some of the reported facts, obviously, are less benign, but the most common situation is ordinary violence that takes place in a negotiated context. In his study in the KwaZulu-Natal, Mark Hunter (2002: 101, 112) describes two sorts of ordinary sexual transactions in which sex is part of an exchange between young men and women and which differ from prostitution, on the one hand, and from conjugality, on the other: he categorizes them as "sex linked to subsistence" and "sex linked to consumption." The first type, most often observed among migrant women living in "informal settlements," corresponds to economically and socially very vulnerable situations in which the woman, in a highly dominated position, exchanges sex for basic necessities: food, a roof over her head, clothing, protection for the children. The second, frequent among women who are more stably settled in the townships, is a more balanced situation between young women and their "sugar daddies," with a seemingly satisfactory relationship for both. In reality, the boundary between the two types is relatively permeable, as the following exchange (reported by the same author) illustrates: "How many boyfriends do you have?—Three.—Why do you have three boyfriends?—Because I have many needs.—What needs?—To dress, I don't work, a cell phone . . . doing my hair so that I am beautiful for my boyfriends, they won't love an ugly person.—What do they give you?—One money . . . another groceries . . . another buys me clothes.—And your mother knows where the groceries come from?—She knows, she doesn't say anything because of the situation of hunger at home." From food to cell phone, from clothing to hairdresser, from necessity to appearance, the expectations are many and the dividing line somewhat confused between sex for subsistence and sex for consumption.

Olga's story illustrates this confusion. She is a young woman I met in the rural township of Lenyenye. She is thirty-eight and not working. She lives in a small two-room house. She has had two children, now eighteen and twelve, with the same man, to whom she was married. They have separated but remain friends, and he continues to give her money every month. One year after their separation, she began having boyfriends. "I was suffering at that time, she explains. I didn't like to do it, but the father was not supportive, so I had to." Yet she protests she is not like those women who "go around" or who "go to shebeens": on the contrary, she "stays at home." She finds lovers when she goes downtown. "When I have to buy things for my children, that's when I meet guys, they talk to me at the bus stop in Tzaneen." Most of these men are not from the region. "They come from far, so why spend their money in a hotel?" So she takes them to her place. Their relationship lasts some time, and they see each other on weekends until the love affair ends, that is, until the man's money runs out. Each time she has a new boyfriend, she makes sure he knows her situation immediately: "When I meet a man, I would tell him, 'If you want to come with me, you should know five things: I have children; you have to respect them; you must buy them clothes; you must bring them food; you must support them.' Some say no." She often changes boyfriends (she says: "every month"), but she avoids having several at the same time, for fear of retaliation (she explains: "if a man would come a week later and find another man here, he might want his money back and even shoot me"). In her neat little parlor, she tries to stay pretty, in spite of the gauntness brought on by the illness. Coquette in a brightly colored dress, carefully made up, she concludes: "We need men because of the support they give to our children and to ourselves—because of their money." Olga claims her boyfriends have never been violent with her. In fact, for her, violence is above all that which is attached to her social condition, the impossibility of finding a job, the need to look for protectors to be able to live with her children: "Money was the only reason why I started to have boyfriends." As she speaks of that period of her life when she began having one affair after the other, she uses the words I most often heard in similar circumstances: "I was suffering." These women's suffering is a social suffering indeed, in the sense that it is socially produced. This violence is structural violence, because it is related to the unequal structures of society. For Paul Farmer (1997: 280), "The world's poor are the chief victims of structural violence—a violence which has thus far defied the analysis of many seeking to understand the nature and distribution of extreme suffering. Why might this be so? One answer is that the poor are not only more likely to suffer, they are also more likely to have their suffering silenced." The undeniable violence of the physical domination that many South African women experience on the part of their companions must not obliterate the equally undeniable violence of their material existence, which leads them to expose themselves to those economic and sexual exchanges. This is precisely what they call suffering.

WITHIN THE NARRATIVES

because of you
this country no longer lies
between us but within

ANTJIE KROG

"For All Voices, for All Victims"

"What I didn't want to write was just another township or protest novel shrilly pronouncing the execration of apartheid. I wanted the critique of the accursed doctrine to emerge automatically out of the objective social relationships between two individuals. . . . In fact I have an aversion for the township novels and their predictable plots. I know of no township novel which is able to reflect on its own method, on what it is doing while telling its story." In the preface to his internationally famous novel *Mating Birds,* Lewis Nkosi departs from the militant literature that he considers too demonstrative, too explicit, too conventional, and which in the end reveals little of the complexity and the truth of social relations under apartheid.[26] On the contrary, literature must render the very stuff things are made of, their blatant evidence at the same time as their subtle uncertainty for those who live them. The same goes for anthropology. The way it analyzes the structures and processes of domination, exploitation, and segregation tends to function by generalizations and simplifications that no longer reflect individual and collective experiences.[27] As noted by Peter Delius (1996: 3) in his history of a rural society in the province of North Transvaal (today Limpopo), analysis of change has long been satisfied with "catch-all and external categories such as 'tribesman,' 'peasant' or 'proletarian,'" which of course "were not without some explanatory power" but which "could not capture the identities within, or the content of, struggles and transformations in the countryside." Historiography and ethnography put the flesh back in the society being investigated. Thus I would like to add to the landscapes, whose underpinnings I attempted to analyze, a few narratives to show how their realities are inscribed in the itineraries of the men and women who, at a given time in their lives, we just see as AIDS patients. My aim is to allow the social configurations to come alive in individual histories, or yet again, using a classical distinction, to reveal the constraints of structure and the freedom of agency. But perhaps we must go further—not beyond but within the narratives. As we all know, interviews render more or less linear and coherent stories that sketch a life or fragments thereof, thus representing a privileged medium to attain people's experiences. Nevertheless, they are not the whole story. Not only do observations and archives come to complete and elucidate them, but their very materiality must be explored from the point of view of the speech forms and the interactive situation. That is the approach I would now like to apply to three biographies (the first of which is in fact the biography of a couple): first, by questioning the place of the anthropologist on the ethnographic scene and particularly the moral dimension that frequently operates unconsciously; next, by examining the conditions of the production of narratives bearing on the most private sort of violence; finally, by returning to the question of the limited space in which the possible is deployed. Naturally, in addition to its theoretical perspective, each story speaks simply about people and their lives.

An Investigation of Morality

Anthropologists have long portrayed themselves as scientists who describe, analyze, and interpret the social universe, in particular, the social universe of others, a proposition that seemed all the more natural as the dominant position in which they themselves were caught up as members of colonial society facilitated the task of carrying out fieldwork. More recently, however, as a result of the transformations in the global order but also of their changed relationship to the others (which, as is well known, largely results from the resistance encountered in their fieldwork), anthropologists have become witnesses who report, retell, and attest to what they hear and see. I would like here to introduce another figure, less discussed than the first two and far less studied: next to the scientist and the witness, the anthropologist also appears as a moral actor. Plenty of criticism has been leveled against anthropology over the past quarter of a century—often from within the discipline itself. Its epistemology has been reevaluated: ethnographies have been called "fictions," and the truths pronounced about the other have been judged "inherently partial—committed and incomplete" (Clifford and Marcus 1986: 7). Its politics too have been discussed, this time from its geographic and cultural borders, in the name of a "subaltern" position or a "post-colonial" theory (Bhabha 1994; Mignolo 2000). Part of what constitutes the anthropological experience nevertheless seems to me to have remained in the dark: a form of moral commitment to the world.

By this expression, I mean the analytic separation between good and evil and the choice of the former against the latter: it is therefore a question of both delimitation and implication. It is probable that such a moral commitment has never been clearer than today, as crusades for the human rights and the rights of peoples in which anthropologists imagine themselves to possess a natural authority become more and more common and as ethical charters of the discipline are written that attempt to guarantee acceptable conditions for the practice of anthropology in contexts that have become unfavorable (Pels 1999). It would, however, be a mistake to turn a blind eye to the fact that, in the same way as Durkheim's sociology and to a certain extent Weber's, the anthropology of Boas and from a different angle Mauss has always been a moral discipline—a discipline that contains in its intellectual project a more or less explicit definition of good and evil and whose involvement in the social world emanated from a more or less elaborate ethical code (Wax 2003). That dimension went unnoticed for a long time, hidden, as it were, by the utilitarianism of applied anthropology or by the protests of critical anthropologists—in other words, by what in the first case was called practical and in the second political. Yet that dimension is somehow genetically constitutive of the relation to the others as established by the discipline, since that relation is necessarily imagined from a moral point of view of the self, which academic texts and official accounts try to erase but which field notes and autobiographical narratives reveal much more surely.

To illustrate this assertion, I will keep to my own investigations. The question certainly deserves to be thought out more carefully at the present time when, especially in France where in the name of an "anthropology in the *polis*," some of its most qualified representatives have turned into censors and prescribers, trespassing on science to tell society what is good for it and to denounce agents who are doing wrong. But instead of discussing them, I want to present a personal anecdote that I hope makes my proposal and its critical implications acceptable, for, in spite of its locally limited character, I believe it expresses broader truths about what drives social scientists in the field and about what they feel in situations that often trigger implicit evaluations, about the judgments they bear on the actors and actions they observe. I therefore elaborate on it for what it teaches us about the anthropologist as subject—and more specifically about the rarely explicit moral dimension of the anthropologist's relation to the people being studied—but also of course for what it teaches us about anthropological objects—in the present case about the conditions of possibility of loving in the time of AIDS.

We are in Limpopo Province, in one of those inhabited areas too large to be qualified as a village, too little structured to be called a town, as it often happens in the former homelands—in this case, the Lebowa. It is a sort of township in the country. The interview is drawing to a close. What we have just been told has stirred me. Or should I say, angered me. And upset me. Night has fallen. I think over the story and what it can mean. The young woman we have just heard tell her story is well known to me. We met a year earlier, when we first came to work in the region. I also know her husband and have known him even longer; I met him in Soweto, quite a while before coming here. I shall call them Phindile and Mesias. Both are HIV-positive, and both have publicly revealed their serological status. Mesias spent years in the township where he first lived with a prostitute, then married a woman with whom he had a child who died early from AIDS, and finally decided to retire to his parents' village where he became an AIDS activist. He has become a local figure because he divulged his illness over the radio and now is an educational volunteer. Phindile is a young country woman who has never left the region. Before she met Mesias, she lived with her mother and her divorced older sister and took care of the latter's handicapped child. The contrast in the couple is striking both in their physical appearance and their ways of doing things, his elegant urbanity versus her somewhat awkward restraint. For a long time, conflicts between the two families prevented them from living together. A few months ago, they managed to find a small house to rent, and that is where they now live, with the little handicapped boy they fostered. I share with them the intimacy of daily meals and conversations about all sorts of things, of the kind that make for friendship but not indiscretion. That is often the way it is with fieldwork companions. This evening, with the consent of both, I have conducted a real interview with Phindile; tomorrow it will be Mesias's turn. The situation is much more delicate than I had imagined or, to be honest, than I had wanted to admit. What I find out cannot help but change my impression of them both. They know it, and the fact they agree to speak to me at such a cost is proof of their trust. At the same time, I suppose that Phindile needs to tell her story to somebody and that only I, an outsider, was able to hear it without it having any serious consequences for the couple. I also guess that Mesias, a religious man, wants to relieve his conscience.

Phindile barely waits for the tape recorder to be plugged in to start revealing her secret: "When I first met Mesias, in 2001, I did not know much about AIDS. At the time, I did not know my status. He has infected me, because he never used to discuss his status with me as well. I had no idea he was HIV-positive. At the time, I didn't even know my own situation. We met, it was on Good Friday and from then on we were courting together." Their love affair began then. A few days later, Mesias's sister-in-law, with whom he is not on good terms, told Phindile that her lover had AIDS and that due to it he had lost a child. The young woman was terribly upset by the revelation: "I felt very scared and bad, because I had heard that there is a pandemic . . . That night I couldn't sleep. I still recall when I was afraid to ask him if he had some such epidemic." After a few weeks during which they continued seeing each other, she took the risk of asking him about it: he adamantly denied being infected. A little later, she found a printed sheet among his papers that contained the result of a serological test that said he was HIV-positive. She asked him again: somewhat embarrassed, he explained it was simply a document distributed to all the prevention volunteers. "It took nine to ten months before he told me the truth, and all that time we had sex without using condoms." I now realize that the man whom I know as one of the local promoter of AIDS prevention has not applied to himself the principle he teaches others. A few weeks after he had revealed his serological status to her, Phindile took a test that turned out positive, but she says she is not angry with him. From then on they have had "protected sex" since they have decided not to have children. A few moments later I learn that before knowing Mesias she had had a baby with a man whom she left because he was an alcoholic and violent. She had never mentioned this part of her life before. The child died shortly after birth, from pneumonia according to the doctors, from a hereditary disease according to her family. The father also died a few months later. She remained alone until she met Mesias.

Today they are both ill but do not want to take antiretroviral drugs because they fear the side effects. At any rate, to know if they need this treatment, a CD4 count would be necessary, but it is too expensive. They have more confidence in the natural remedies promoted by the health minister, in particular, beets and garlic, for they are too poor to buy olive oil, which is also recommended, and above all the concoctions made with tea, coffee, and fish oil prepared at the Zion Christian Church that they both attend. Phindile also declares she takes the cotrimoxazole given out at the health center as a prophylaxis for several opportunistic infections, unbeknownst to her priest "so as not to disappoint him." Henceforth, the illness has become not only a form of daily ordeal, with its symptoms and worries, but also a resource thanks to which they have been able to make their place in their local society. Mesias just began working with a prevention organization, and Phindile has responsibilities in the local branch of the national patients' organization, NAPWA. They have also received some financial benefits and a certain degree of social recognition through their involvement in community activities.

Later that day, I write in my notebook: "We come out of the room fairly shaken by the narrative. Outside, in front of the house, where we are having dinner with a group already there, a page from a newspaper, half torn, lies on the humid earth. Without thinking I pick it up and read the title of an article: 'SA Men Must Learn to Respect Their Women.' A strange coincidence that gives a sort of general meaning to the story we heard." In fact, I am disturbed in a complex and ambiguous manner. My feeling is linked to my reprobation of Mesias's attitude, who by not saying anything to Phindile and not using condoms has probably infected her, but it is also related to my disappointment at having been deceived by this man who is dedicated to fighting the epidemic. At that moment, it is clear that I have less sympathy for my research companion. I realize it, and it bothers me, since it means that in spite of myself I am beginning to judge rather than analyze his behavior. Reprobation is stronger than understanding. A few minutes later, when we are again alone, I confide my doubts to our South African research assistant. "Phindile was already HIV-positive when she met Mesias," he remarks with quiet assurance. "She was infected by her other boyfriend and their child died of AIDS." He does not seem particularly shocked by her story. Perhaps as a South African man he is in fact siding with another South African man, by making his unscrupulous behavior appear mundane. Or perhaps, having been raised in the midst of cynical gender relations, he has a different view on the young woman's life. Whatever the case may be, he does not seem the least given to moral evaluation. For him, these are things that simply happen. Besides, I must admit that his interpretation is plausible—at least as plausible as mine.

The next day, Mesias gives us a long interview as he had agreed. He probably suspects that Phindile has talked to us about their secret. It is even possible that she told him about it. The fact is, he begins on the same theme. "Maybe I must start from the beginning," he declares somewhat formally. "The time of diagnosis, the life in between, and until now. So I was diagnosed in 1993, and I have had a very big problem because, you know, I was trapped in a situation where I had a child with a lady and after that she passed away because of the very same pandemic. After all that, when I stand up on my feet saying no more again, I started having a problem of the previous years. Going back to the denial stage with my new wife. And then breaking those promises that I will not infect or whatever other people. We had unprotected sex. Sometimes when you need a person it's very hard to say, 'Hey, I'm just like this,' because you must have heard that most of the people, when they hear that you are HIV-positive or you have AIDS, they won't agree maybe to stay with you or to make friends with you. It's the most difficult thing that a person can ever experience. Because if you check, most of the guys in this kind of business you find they end up having children. So you might ask yourself, 'Why do they say to people they need to protect themselves, but at the end of the day you find this couple has got a baby. So this is where questions are posed to us as role models in the community." For more than fifteen minutes, he speaks in a muddled manner about the painful situation of being such a different man in private from what he preaches in public, about having built his new life without having given up the old one, about having betrayed the trust of the woman he wanted to marry. He continues: "And then until someone disclosed my status to her and she came back to me and said, 'Mesias, why are you hiding something like this?' I said, 'No I'm not hiding.' And she said, 'Why are you having a lot of material about AIDS?' I said, 'No I'm just a volunteer.' Until she came to realize that I was lying to her, and then she confronted me and I had no way out and I had to be open with her and I said, 'No I'm HIV-positive.' And she said, 'There is no problem. Even if you are like that you are still Mesias, you are still my lover, and I'm still going to be your wife.'" He seems moved.

Rereading the transcription of the interview, I realize that through my questions I unconsciously returned twice to the story, making him tell it again, implicitly checking his version against his wife's, questioning him about how he felt about lying to her, asking him to be precise about the time it took him to finally admit the truth. But we not only scrutinize the facts, we also judge. The anthropological study tends to resemble a morality investigation. Indeed, as is well known, an interview often takes on the form of a confession. Here, it completes the process: it pinpoints a fault and absolves its author. An act of contrition concludes it: "It might happen and it might not that maybe she came being positive or maybe she came not being positive and then she got this thing from me. That is two possibilities. But I don't take that one that she came being positive. I take the blame as Mesias. I take the blame." Truth-telling has brought redemption. Through our interview, the penitent is looking for reconciliation with himself but also with us. The ethnographic encounter reveals its ambiguity.

From the beginning of the epidemic, research on AIDS has concentrated on the problem of transmission to which, as Gerald Oppenheimer (1988) has shown, epidemiology brought elements of objectification and interpretation. The first observations in the United States in the early 1980s were followed by the meticulous reconstitution of "sexual networks" and to the obsessive search for the "first case." In France, questions in the compulsory declaration forms and classifications in the health information system were built around "transmission groups," a supposedly less stigmatizing label than "risk groups"; let it be said in passing that to be African became almost automatically synonymous with "heterosexual transmission," as if Africans could not be homosexuals or drug users. In Africa itself, focusing on this issue led to the desperate quest for the origin of the virus and to dangerous hypotheses concerning the forms of transmission between man and animal but also between human beings. Thinking about transmission, which was obviously logical and legitimate given the natural history of the illness and the possibilities of preventive measures, had as its corollary the production of the representation of a danger against which one must protect oneself, for example, by organizing tests at the borders as many countries did (United States, China, Russia, Belgium) and, more discreetly, through some of its consulates in Africa (France). In many countries the question of legally penalizing those persons who could be proven to have knowingly infected their partners arose again and again. Aloïs Hahn, Willy Eirmbter, and Jacob Rüdiger (1994) have shown in a questionnaire survey in Germany that representing AIDS as a "permanent danger of contamination," as the "consequence of and the punishment for a fault," or promoting "avoidance and exclusion attitudes in the private life" and wishing to see "obligatory anti-AIDS measures, including generalizing the test," are statistically linked. Thus there exists a close relationship between the images of the illness as being "very infectious" and a repressive constellation simultaneously moral, social, and political.

A decade later, even if this configuration is still operative, it is now in competition with another one, liberal this time. Under the combined effect of the actions of patients' organizations but more profoundly of the transformation of the contemporary ethos, an ideology has developed that exonerates the sick, preaches tolerance toward them, and claims respect of their rights. In the new liberal constellation—largely dominant in international circles and the only one considered legitimate today in public discourse—the moral dimension—though it has distanced itself from the logics of sin and punishment—reappears in the form of what Michel Foucault (1994: 139) called a "pastoral technology." One must no longer punish, exclude, or oblige but protect. Protect yourself so as to protect others: we know that this has been the preventive message to counteract the supposed selfishness of those who, once infected, would no longer be interested in the fate of others or, even more, would be happy to drag their spouse or partners down in their misfortune. The care of the self supposedly guarantees the care of others.

At an international conference in Heidelberg, where I had given a lecture explaining that in South Africa the levels of prevalence were so high that it was no longer necessary to point to any particular sexual behavior to account for the spread of the illness, a Harvard biologist approached me and asked in great anguish, "But how can they be protected then?" The question clearly troubled her deeply, and though she had never set foot in Africa, she felt personally concerned by the sick people I had spoken about but also by the healthy ones living near them. The manner in which she expressed doubts about my answer, which she considered unsatisfactory because in her view it was impossible to let things go on this way, revealed her concern beyond what one expects in similar scientific circumstances. Very often, in South Africa or Europe, that question is asked, generally with a hint of reproach for the anthropologist who studies but does so little to make people change their behavior.

This pastoral altruism, which is probably legitimate and even a good thing as an abstract principle, is nevertheless problematic in concrete situations. In fact, if the others do not conform to one's expectations, then disappointment and frustration set in proportionately, and, in certain cases, the violence of the reaction is in proportion of the emotion initially invested in that gratifying moral sentiment. I have frequently witnessed that ambiguous ethical involvement among health professionals and social workers facing the sick or the needy whom they tried to assist and whose lack of will to extract themselves from their situations finally infuriates to the point that they end up stigmatizing even more dramatically those they originally wanted to help. It seems to me that anthropologists, especially when they are concerned with serious problems, do not escape such a moral undertaking and its emotional consequences. Thinking of my own colleagues, I have come across this tendency many times—in informal exchanges more than in scientific writings, however.

The debate between Roy D'Andrade (1995) and Nancy Scheper-Hughes

(1995) has the merit of having begun the much-needed discussion about the existence of "moral models in anthropology." It has especially shed light on the ethical questions raised by engagement in the social sciences. Perhaps it tells us more, however, about the important decisions confronting anthropologists, between objectivism and involvement, than about the small stakes they face in the field. More about the epistemological and political dimensions than about the morals of the profession. In my professional experience, that dimension crosses the line of demarcation between those who believe in a positivist model and those who prefer a militant one: no one can avoid it. And perhaps it cannot be otherwise.

To return to Mesias and Phindile, the former was right in saying that hiding the fact of being HIV-positive happens all the time, and the latter may have been less deceived than it seemed at first. Moreover, comparing their two narratives refutes the commonplace so often heard according to which a person (usually a man) willfully infects his partner to take her down with him into illness and death. As it happens, the cruel paradox is that, one the contrary, it is because he loved her that Mesias did not tell Phindile he was HIV-positive. He explains that he saw her as the woman who would remain steadfast when the illness had cut him off from the rest of the world, reliable enough so as not to wrong him with other men and devoted enough so as to stay with him in his last moments. He fought with his family to force them to accept her as his wife and acquired a piece of land on which he is building a house to leave her after his death. The lack of courage manifested by not telling her he was sick resulted from his fear of estranging her if he confessed at the beginning of their relationship. This fear is not unfounded.

A young woman from Tickyline explained to me what happened when she decided to "disclose her status" to the men who courted her: "Each time I told them, they left and never came back." Conversely, another young woman in Lenyenye declared to me that she never told her boyfriend but asked him to use condoms, which he did: "If I'd tell him, maybe he'd leave me and my children and I would remain with nothing." Not to say anything, and therefore to endanger the other's life, is an attitude I frequently heard my interviewees admit, especially at the beginning of their illness. Much more than an intention to harm, as it is often said, it is the profound contradiction between the desire for the other and the fear of losing him or her that makes them choose the ambiguous solution that mixes a life project and a deadly risk. Men more often than women play that dangerous game in the love—and sex—transaction. Some women prefer on the contrary to reveal their status to their partners or to negotiate the use of condoms ("I tell him it's because I don't know what he does on his side," cleverly explained a young woman from Alexandra who was HIV-positive). This apparent sexual division of responsibility for the transmission of the infection—in which men dissimulate and women tell—is far from being the general rule, however. Many women admitted they prefer to say nothing to their partners for fear of raising his suspicion if they mentioned condoms. Sometimes the couple thus bases its relationship on a mutual lie. For instance, an immigrant woman living precariously in Soweto had a test at the hospital and discovered she was HIV-positive. After having hesitated for a long time, dreading her boyfriend would throw her out, she finally decided to talk to him. She then realized, when cleaning up their bedroom, that he was taking the same drugs she did. Actually both were sick and had hidden the truth from each other.

In the Heart of the Country

Each township possesses its official storyteller and symbolic novel.[28] For Alexandra, it is Wally Mongane Serote, author of *To Every Birth Its Blood*. The large neighborhood is Johannesburg's oldest township since the destruction of Sophiatown in 1955. The 500,000 inhabitants crowd onto a small territory in rows of shacks on pieces of land ever more populated. The area is delimited by tiny, narrow streets, huge and multistory immigrant hostels where in the 1990s the murderous confrontations between the Inkatha and the ANC took place, and a few low-rent apartment buildings. When leaving Alexandra one progressively penetrates into the suburb of Sandton, with its sumptuous villas, whose walls are topped by barbed wire and protected by armed guards, and its luxurious shopping centers where an essentially white bourgeoisie comes to stroll. In all of South Africa, there is hardly another place where the urban contrast is harsher or where social and racial inequalities are more shockingly obvious. Different from Soweto and its neatly drawn neighborhoods end on end, Alexandra is a township both imprisoned in the insurmountable confines of its segregation past and intimately present at the very heart of the great metropolis. The precarious housing piling up, swallowing up the courtyards and filling every nook and cranny, gives the impression of sediment in which the different temporal strata of the city can be read, up to the most ephemeral constructions where, arriving from the countryside or from abroad, the last waves of immigrants have come to live.

From all the interviews we did there emerge two narrative lines reconstructing this recent past. On one side, violence—that of the police, of course, but perhaps even more that of the gangs and the *tsotsis* (delinquents) and, later, that of the civil war under the state of emergency. On the other side, resistance—the memory of the comrades demonstrating and feverishly *toyi-toying* but also the forcible enrollment of the inhabitants in the fight against white power and the chastisement of those accused of collaboration by "necklacing" (fire put to a tire around the victim's neck). "Now we have light in the streets, but before it was dark at night, a woman remembers. Everybody was hiding for fear of *tsotsis*. White police were hard on us too. They came down at night looking for those guys or checking our permit. If we didn't have it, we were sent to jail for two days. During the day, we had the street committees. If you don't go with the comrades, they come and fetch you at your place. If you miss rallies, they would call you informer. And punishment could be from being beaten to being burnt alive. It was difficult at the beginning, but then I enjoyed it. That time, it was nice. They forced me and scared me, but then I did enjoy it. I even got a bullet from the police once." Relatively pacified compared to those years of fire and brimstone, the township today remains unsure and precarious.

Magda lives in Alexandra.[29] I have known her for a long time and we have agreed to start her story again from the beginning because I only know it in the fragments she revealed each time we met. She begins all of a sudden, and after a few rushed sentences, all at once releases the violence of her life.

> Okay. Myself when I was here I was staying with my granny in Lesotho. And then my uncle was raping us every time, you see. And my mother come and say to my granny, "I want to take my child and go with her to Natal." And then my granny say, "Okay you can take her because there is a problem." And then my mother and my stepfather took me from Lesotho and came with me in Natal. And when we were there my mother go back to her mother's place [to work]. And then that man [the stepfather] again sleep with us [my sister and me], sleep with me every day. Myself I say, "What can I do now?" And then there is nothing I can do because that man promised us he can kill us and then because he is doing that gun, we don't know, he know how to make it, self-made gun, I don't know what. And then he said he wanted to do the child with me and then myself I say, "So, how?" And he said my mother is not making the baby, so he wants to make the baby with me. And I said, "Hey, nothing I can do." My stepsister told me, "Magda, we are going." I said, "Where?" She said, "Joburg." I

said, "Okay, it's fine, I can go." And then I never tell anybody, because my mother at the time when we leave Lesotho, you see, she said, "If my husband can sleep with my child, I can kill the child." Because she know, my mother, she know her husband used to sleep with her friends and everybody. Okay, when I'm there, I never tell my mother because from the first time she told me that if I can tell her that story, she is going to kill me. Okay, my sister took me to Joburg. She was staying at Elisabeth Hotel down here. And then when I am there my sister told me, "Okay, this is Joburg, you are going to get nothing if you don't have a boyfriend." "Hey," I said, "what can I do?" She said, "There are a lot of people. You can get a boyfriend, you see." Okay, she takes me to a bar and she say, "There are guys there, they are working, choose which one you want." And I said, "I don't want a boyfriend." She said, "Choose, you're going to get nothing if you don't have a boyfriend, I must choose the best boyfriend for you." So I take one and then after that my sister told me, "Hey! you choose the wrong person. Where is the money now? You can't sleep with somebody who don't give money." And then come when I would get the job and I was working domestic worker. And then after that I'm not staying with her now, I stay by the kitchen in the employer's house. And then I get another boyfriend staying with me.

For over half an hour the flow of short sentences continues, uninterrupted and confused, jerky and panting, telling her stories of love, of suffering, then of her illness and treatments.

Let us reconstruct Magda's biography through her narrative but also the fragments of discussion collected through the years I have known her. She is thirty. She was born in a village in the Lesotho. She was raised there by her grandmother, with a sister four years older and from a different father. Her parents were separated, and her mother reproached her father for not sending them money: he had disappeared, and she had gone to Natal where she worked and married. One of her mother's younger brothers also lived with the two girls at the family property: he is the one who abused her regularly. He had been married but had left his wife when she gave birth to twins: one of them had died, and he wanted to sell the other because twins were considered to have evil powers; his wife had opposed him, he had threatened her, and she had run back to her mother's. She had thus grown up with her older sister in that poor and violent environment, among an affectionate grandmother who hardly wielded any authority, an incestuous uncle who terrified her, and two cousins her age. She remembers that her uncle raped her for the first time when she was seven or eight. Then it became a habit, especially each time he drank too much. She liked school but was hardly able to attend: she was locked in the domestic chores of their rural existence, fetching wood and taking care of the animals.

When she was fifteen, her mother came to get her and her sister. She had been told by the grandmother about the incestuous relations with the uncle. When she took Magda away to the small town in Natal where she lived with her husband, her mother threatened to kill her if she slept with him. It was clear that she thought her daughter was partly responsible for the rapes she had been victim of, on the one hand, and that she knew her husband had affairs with other women, on the other. Shortly after having settled down with her mother and stepfather, Magda was regularly forced to have sexual relations with him. He was a violent man who manufactured arms during that period when, stirred up by the white authorities, the conflicts between the Zulu of the Inkatha and the Sotho of the ANC were often murderous. He had told her he would not hesitate to get rid of her if she revealed anything. Her mother pretended not to see what was going on. Each time she left for a few hours, the stepfather abused Magda. During the three years spent with them, she had also had a love affair with a boy her age. When she turned eighteen she managed to escape from the family prison and went to Johannesburg.

In the city, she now must provide for her needs. Her cousin (whom she calls "sister" in her narrative) puts her up in the room she shares with her boyfriend but tells her bluntly that it will not last long. She explains what Magda must do to survive: find a man who can support her. She takes her to a bar known for that type of encounter near the hotel where she lives: "We went to that club Kiss Kiss and then we seat and the guys from Elizabeth Hotel they were wearing nice. She say, 'You can choose one.' Me I say, 'I want that one,' and then he buy beer. Dry we drink. We enjoyed that day and then after that we go and sleep." The man she just met also works in this hotel. He spends his nights in the employee's dorms where the beds are separated simply by a curtain. That is where she sleeps for the first six months of her stay in the city. Every evening she must arrive late and every morning leave early because "they don't want any girls down there." At least she has a roof over her head. But her boyfriend, who has a wife and a little girl back in their village, has no intention of paying for her food. During the day, Magda therefore must find something to eat: "There were many girls in the room. We were staying the whole night, but early we must go outside the hotel all the ladies. Myself I must go and check the other guys or to look for the job. To eat you can get another boyfriend so that you can eat because my sister she can tell me, 'If you're hungry to get food you must get boyfriends so that you can eat.'—And where do you find them?—The guys? By the street! But sometimes if you find them by the street they can say, 'Let's go to the room and you go to the room and you get the food there.'—Did they give you food or money?—Sometimes they give you eat first, sometimes no money, sometimes they can give you money, but it's no money because ten rands is not money, or five rands, just for cold drinks. And you eat and you do sex and you go." This life lasts six months.

She eventually finds employment as domestic worker for a Coloured family. She has room and board there, sleeping on a mattress in the living room. She earns 150 rands a month, but she receives less if she does her work badly and especially if she ruins the laundry while ironing. In her rare spare time she goes out with her boyfriend of the moment who offers her gifts and shows her the city. A girlfriend takes her one day to a hotel in Hillbrow, in the northern quarter of Johannesburg. She meets women there who work as prostitutes for 100 rands per client. One of them tells her laughingly that she has a regular client so big and strong that he makes her bleed every time: "She said, 'Every day you see, I'm bleeding. I can sleep with the others first before I can sleep with that one. Because while you're bleeding, the customer is still waiting.'" But Magda explains that this sort of life makes her feel uncomfortable. At that time she herself had a regular boyfriend. He drinks a lot, and when he is drunk he beats her. She has changed jobs and now works in a small Indian textile factory where she makes buttons for 150 rands a week. A few months later, she becomes pregnant, but her little girl dies shortly after birth. She is told the infant died of AIDS. She and her boyfriend take the serological tests and discover they are both infected. They part a few months later.

Until recently, historical, anthropological, and sociological work in South Africa hardly dealt with the question of sexuality, in particular, sexual violence.[30] The silence on this topic, in contrast to the recent impressive corpus produced by the social sciences, the epidemiological statistics, the administrative data, and the organizations' studies on these two themes, tends to make people believe that sexual violence is a new reality, thus contributing to make it a particularly delicate object to deal with, since this would relate sexual violence to postapartheid. Of course, it is not sexual violence that is new but its public acknowledgment. Zazah Khuzwayo's book *Never Been at Home* is a landmark in this respect, since, halfway between an ethnographic testimonial and an autobiographical novel, it recounts a childhood and adolescence in the province of the Natal spent with a violent policeman father who sexually abuses his daughters and a loving mother who herself is a victim of her brutal husband.[31] The white world is practically absent; everything takes place in the domestic sphere, the village, and the township. The same is true in Magda's story: in Lesotho as in Natal, and even in Johannesburg, apartheid is all the more powerful given that it is invisible and that the little girl's and later the young woman's life is placed in a framework of experience from which whites are totally excluded so that all the violence appears as a purely African problem. However, staying at this level of interpretation would mean losing sight of the conditions that make that violence possible (though not of its mechanical determinism, of course): the mother's migration for work, which caused her to be separated from her daughters; the absence of state regulation in the so-called African territories that are therefore left to corrupt local authorities; the pauperization of rural society and the exodus to the city in a context of precariousness and vulnerability that affects women especially; and finally the anomie of the last decade of apartheid during which the cruelty of social relations was the rule in a country that had become impossible to govern.

If one reads Magda's discourse literally, considering even the detached way in which she reports the most terrible facts, her life seems a catalog of all the violence that could possibly be exerted on women's bodies: forced incest with a maternal uncle; routine rape by the stepfather; transactional sex for a bed to sleep in, a meal to eat, sometimes only a drink; the brutality of physical power relations with successive boyfriends; AIDS as the result of this long history of violence (of course, nobody knows how she became infected, and making her stepfather responsible for it in front of her mother expresses her desire for revenge for having been abandoned to all the men who abused her one after the other). In the face of this masculine violence, not only have other women been useless to her, but they have even facilitated it by their silence, their threats, their orders, or their advice: a grandmother who sees everything but says nothing for years; a mother who swears she will kill her if she sleeps with her husband; a cousin who tells her to look for men if she wants to survive; a girlfriend who invites her to a place of prostitution (she herself sets the limit when bargaining over sex). We have thus delineated all the forms of what Janet Maia Wojcicki (2002) calls "survival sex," which belongs to a history of sexual domination (rape during childhood and adolescence) and has its place in a continuum between the simple guarantee of the minimal conditions of existence and the satisfaction of a few modest desires. The negotiated order of sex one often refers to is here quite secondary compared to its constrained order.

But Magda's story could also be interpreted in another way—not only as the itinerary of a victim of male violence and the hardships of the times but also as the itinerary of a reconquest, of autonomy and identity. After her little girl died, she left the father with whom she was always fighting and who beat her. She found a protector who did not demand sexual payment from her and allowed her to train as a dressmaker and acquire a sewing machine. She joined a local organization in her neighborhood where she is employed for 700 rands a month doing home-based care for AIDS patients. She has been able to register with social services, and though she works, she gets a disability grant in the same amount. She has been called on to participate in various actions of the Treatment Action Campaign, becoming a well-known activist whose story has been told in several newspaper articles. She gave birth to another child, who, thanks to her network, benefited from the prevention of mother-to-child transmission program by nevirapine. And last, for the same reasons, she has been placed under antiretroviral multitherapy as part of the protocol of clinical trial before the government authorized its use in the public services. All this demonstrates that, far from being crushed by the ordeals she has been through all her life, she has been able to build an autonomous space: she is physically strong since she has started receiving treatment, financially independent from the men she continues to see, active in the collective struggle against the epidemic—thanks to her strength and generous personality she shows what resisting misfortune means. But not everyone has that strength.

A World Apart

Globalization has not reached Tickyline. At least that is what I often thought during my stay there in April 2003. The second war in Iraq had just begun, and the American troops had launched their land attack on Baghdad. The entire world was watching the valley of the Tigris and the Euphrates, following the progress of the invasion on CNN. But never, in Tickyline or in the nearby township of Lenyenye where I went several times, was I able to find national papers to get fresh news of the war. Never, during my visits, did I hear a radio or see a television set. Never did the question of these events that occupied the attention of the entire planet arise in our conversations. Tickyline and its surroundings still seemed to be "a world apart,"[32] as if its history under apartheid had continued. This large village in the province of the Limpopo belongs to the former homeland of the Lebowa, a dismembered territory where the segregationist regime had placed the members of what was known as the Pedi ethnic group by displacing entire families (thus freeing land for Afrikaner farmers). Apartheid's capacity for invention in this matter was nevertheless relative. The forced displacements had begun well before the regime was installed; it goes back to the military conquest of the Pedi kingdom by the British troops, when "reserves" were stipulated in the Native Land Act of 1913.

Tickyline still figures under its original name, Ramalema, in the records of the health subdistrict. The white authorities ordered the expropriation of the territory when ore was discovered, and the inhabitants were relocated a few miles from there. However, the industrial plan was dropped and the mine project abandoned. But the huge properties of the ancestors were lost for good, replaced by "rurbanized" plots, and the traditional chieftaincies were dismantled, replaced by legal but illegitimate bantustan authorities.[33] In everyday life, this usually meant impoverishment. "The only change I saw," explains one of the displaced women, today seventy-five years old, "was that women were forced to work and that men had to leave for jobs in Johannesburg, because of lack of resources." The new location is inhabited today by nearly 8,000 people. In reality, it has no discontinuity from the surrounding villages, for instance with Sunnyside. This semiurban ensemble thus counts almost 15,000 people on the edges of Lenyenye township, the main regional center inhabited by 12,000 people. During my various stays, I never met a single white person in or around Tickyline. To see one, I had to leave the precincts of the former homeland and visit the immense farms or the nearby town of Tzaneen—which is what the men and women of the region in fact did, essentially to find a way of making a living. The men would work on the fruit plantations or in small businesses, when they were not obliged to look even farther away, in Gauteng in particular. The women would sometimes be employed in domestic work or the commercial sector, but some of them also would have to depend on the men they encountered, who gave them a little money in exchange for sex. Living in Tickyline today is hardly any different from what it was before 1994. The borders of the former homeland still hem in a world outside this world,[34] where nobody talks about the war in Iraq, where the African populations still live cut off from white society, except for the economic sphere where they are exploited.

This is where Joseph has spent his entire life. He is forty-four but looks twenty years older. His face and body are marked by the wear of work and the devastation of illness. He was born on one of the nearby farms. His parents lived there in huts with eleven other families, also employed by the white owner, Mr. Jansen. Joseph's father worked the land, his mother helped in the kitchen. They also grew vegetables on a small plot of land and raised a few animals. There were five children in the family. Besides the small salary, the farmer gave them corn every month. The children helped their parents on the farm very early on. At fourteen, Joseph was also working and paid 150 rands a month. He recalls how severe Mr. Jansen was and the harshness of the punishments. Several times, he was beaten for having disobeyed, always following the same scenario. He would get caught (while fishing in the river, for instance), brought by the owner to the center of the farm to be whipped in front of the small community (so that humiliation was added to pain), stretched out on a bench with his pants down and hit on the buttocks (this procedure is a quasi-paradigm of the physical punishments imposed on Africans by their white masters all over the continent). On one day when he had been beaten that way (he was then twenty) he ran away and filed a complaint at the first police station he came to. It was the last time he was punished thus by the farmer.

This is also when he decided to leave for the small town of Mujaji, where he obtained a job as a gardener in the public service sector of the bantustan government. He married a woman who worked as a servant for an African family. After three years, Mr. Jansen, who was short of cheap labor, came to take him back. But as Joseph did not want to return to the farm where the salary was much lower compared to the one he received in his new job, the farmer went to see the director of the Lebowa administration, who asked his gardener to return to his former employer (a significant example of the way powerful white owners made arrangements with local African authorities). Joseph worked at the farm until the mid-1990s, when Mr. Jansen, whose business began to decline because of competition from international fruit producers, decided to sell out and retire. In spite of the meager salaries and severe punishments, Joseph says his former boss "treated them well," referring to the fact that he gave them monthly fifty kilos of "mealie meal," the Africans' staple diet. This authoritarian and protective model was the usual form of paternalism in the Afrikaner rural world.

After two years spent in the service of another small farmer who also had to give up his land, Joseph was hired on a large property. Thirty-four people worked and lived there. Discipline was strict; the workers were often insulted and sometimes hit. Labor was organized factory-style, and as in the mining sector, the workforce was housed in hostels where most of the men lived alone even if they were married. At first, Joseph shared a small room with his wife, both of them working for a salary of 150 rands a month, he gathering, she sorting out bananas and avocados. But soon, after a quarrel, Joseph's wife went back to her family in Mujaji and he started living like a bachelor again. The workers' existence on the farm was organized like clockwork. During the week they worked hard from 5:30 A.M. to 4:30 P.M. They had Saturdays and Sundays off. There was music in the shebeen (a bar improvised in the midst of the farm's shacks) that served beer and especially *nxomboti*, the locally produced fermented drink; it was sold for 2 rands a pot, so they drank large quantities of it.[35] Women from around came to visit: officially, they were there to buy bananas that they would sell at the local markets, but they had their routine with the men and often became their official companions.

Joseph protests that he did not "sleep with those women" but says he had several "girlfriends" to whom he offered drinks in exchange for sex. Of one of them he says, "I think I got my illness from one of these women. Maria was her name. She used to cook for me. She was my girlfriend. And then I heard that she was ill. The farm owner had chased her because she was ill and had infected men." Sometime later he too fell sick. He had vomiting, diarrhea, and a rash. He went to see a private doctor who only treated his symptoms. At that time he had another girlfriend who worked at a nearby farm and came to see him on weekends. He had met her at the shebeen where he had offered her a beer. Thereafter they saw each other on a steady basis. When she discovered he was sick, she stopped coming. In January 2003 his clinical condition worsened. He was taken by ambulance to the Shiluvane health center and admitted. He stayed there for five days. Before he left the farm, his employer had told him not to worry, that he would get his work back when he returned. When he reappeared one week later, carrying the medical certificate that listed the name of his illness, the boss fired him outright. No explanation, no indemnity, not even a document that would allow him to collect unemployment. When he insisted on his rights, the boss took out his gun and threatened to shoot him if ever he saw him again. Joseph left. Considerably weakened, he never found work again.

Joseph felt it was now impossible for him to return to his wife and their two children, ages fourteen and seventeen. They were on good terms, he says, but she was now living with another man. Impossible too to go to stay with his parents, who got a small pension but would not be able to support him. So he asked his sister and brother who live in Tickyline with their respective families to put him up. When he came out of the hospital and confided to them that he had AIDS, their relationship deteriorated rapidly. "When I started to get ill they distanced themselves. They would not give me food. They left me apart from the family." On the large family property, he was confined in a small room in the rear courtyard. He was not allowed to use the toilet, and when they went out, the sister and brother locked the door. He ate alone, provided he paid for his own food; if not, he got nothing. He constantly had to put up with vexations, and they never missed an opportunity to make him feel how unwelcome he was. He attended the local support group for AIDS patients every week. There, with half a dozen other HIV-positive persons like himself and a few NGO monitors, they talked about their problems and tried to develop a vegetable garden project. The morning session ended with a copious meal that was his only substantial intake of the week. Sometimes he got a food package. Antiretroviral drugs were not available at the public health care services, but he was treated for an opportunistic infection that greatly improved his general condition. And the hospital's social worker filed for a disability grant for him; a few months after losing his job, Joseph once again started to get money—700 rands a month. His life really changed after that. Thanks to the grant, he could leave the family home and rent a shack in the village. It is built of sheet metal and wooden planks, and when it rains, it is flooded. But at least he is independent. Since his brother and sister found out he gets good money, he has become *persona grata* again.

When I last saw him, a year after we had first met, Joseph was a different man. I had known him thin, introverted, taciturn, in rags. Now I found him good-looking, smiling, talkative, almost elegant in a cotton shirt and linen trousers. He now rents a room in a small compound, sort of a collective residence. He earns some money by helping a mason make bricks. He tells me he is even considering getting remarried.

An ordinary story, taken from among several collected in the same region and all describing the same hard life on the farms, the same cold-blooded racism of the white owners, the same precariousness of employment and resources, the same instability of man-woman relationships, the same violent ostracism of the sick.[36] Joseph has never left Tickyline and its surroundings. He moves from one place to another, always as a result of decisions made by others or forced by circumstance and always remaining within the same small perimeter. Unlike Poppie Nongena, the heroine of Elsa Joubert's eponymous novel who, from exile to exile, crosses the entire country, Joseph is an immobile displaced person.[37] He has never been to Johannesburg; his parents had told him life was too violent there. He has only known the margins of the homelands, those farms where the workers' families reside in a situation of economic dependence transmitted from generation to generation. He has lived the transformation from the farming economy of small family properties to the industrialization of import-export firms. But the main difference from his point of view between the farm where he started at age fourteen and the farm from which he was driven away at age forty-four lies in whether his employers were a little "nicer" or a little less "nice" to their workers, whether or not they whipped them, whether or not they gave them "mealie meal." After thirty years of work, he cannot do better than rent a small room where he lives alone in one of the village compounds.

It is in the historical context that one can grasp the objective conditions of the production and reproduction of AIDS. First, there is the manner in which human lives are controlled by the employer who decides to take his worker back against his will by going to fetch him in his new job or, conversely, to get rid of a sick man or woman regardless of the existing labor laws. The African worker's body is not his own. The farmer can get hold of it and exploit it and discipline it, then get rid of it when it has become useless and thus discardable. Joseph had to leave his wife in Mujaji to return to the farm. Breaking couples apart for the benefit of the economy is typical of colonial capitalism in its different shapes and forms. Second, there is the way the workers' daily life is organized: the hours and salaries that do not allow them to live elsewhere than in shacks or in hostels; the organization of their leisure time essentially based on alcohol and women. One must call attention here to the effects of the shifts in the organization of labor, from a family-based form, in which the domestic economy is made to serve the paternalistic company, to an individual form, in which men and women are usually separated in conformity with the industrial model. Sexual transactions based on the man buying drinks, clothes, and gifts are not exclusive of the fact that real couples form, often for short periods, establishing relations of mutual assistance (the woman makes the meals), protection (the man defends his girlfriend), and, of course, affection. Given such historical, economic, and social realities—where everything seems to favor the development of the epidemic—it is not difficult understand the extent to which the rational actor paradigm and the behavioral-cultural interpretation that usually are taken to account for the transmission of AIDS prove unsatisfactory. It may be added also that in the industrial model of a plantation, under the pressure of health institutions, a nurse goes once a month to the hostels to care for the sick and hand out condoms—a noble effort but totally out of step with reality if one considers the conditions of existence of the men and women living on these farms.

My first impression was that the small world of Tickyline lay outside the big world where the Gulf War was taking place. The truth is, of course, at least partly different. With the pressure of major national as well as international transformations, things change even in the former homelands and the surrounding farms. The small landowners like Joseph's first two employers either sold out to large firms as part of the growing industrialization of the fruit and vegetable sector or to African farmers within the framework of the Restitution of Land Rights Act implemented by the Ministry of Agriculture.[38] The manager of a thousand-hectare farm employing one hundred fifty workers not far from Lenyenye explained to me this double shift. On one side, he said, immense properties develop through a series of acquisitions among the multinational fruit exporters. The one where he works has businesses across the country and shareholders the world over, the main one being French. Health and labor regulations are strictly supervised in the firm, which also signed a European charter for "quality control and ethics," and it must respect the norms in matters of remuneration, social security, and medical care: the minimum wage is 700 rands, unemployment insurance is mandatory, a doctor is available free of charge for employees for an accident in the workplace or withheld from salaries in the case of illness. Of course, compared to the number of people looking for work in the region, the number of people employed by this type of company is limited but nevertheless significant as a form of normalization of agriculture in general. On the other side, he continues, agrarian reform leads to splitting up the properties. His father, for instance, owned three hundred hectares and employed about fifty people. Claims for restitution by families who were entitled to the land before expropriation during the twentieth century arrived at a time when he was having trouble making the farm pay. He was thus extremely satisfied with the compensations offered. Today on his former land there are thirteen small farms belonging to African peasants.

Between the two extremes—which can be considered beneficial for most of the local population, whether its members become employees with better salaries or owners in the name of agrarian reform—it is likely that a majority of the farms are continuing to function according to one or the other of the two old models, the traditional paternalistic model and the closed industrial model, which, as we have seen, considerably restrict individuals' movements. If, as Anthony Giddens (1984: 169–170) has written, "constraint cannot be taken as a uniquely defining quality of structure" and "structure is always both enabling and constraining," there are still social configurations in which agency remains extremely limited. South African society under apartheid and even during postapartheid is of that kind. In Joseph's story, a window opened on new possibilities: obtaining a disability grant from the government. It has allowed him to recover some of his autonomy in relation to his family and some dignity in relation to himself. Often criticized, social policies on AIDS do have this capacity.

PROPOSITION 5 : THE FORMS OF EXPERIENCE

Writing about the experience of violence and inequality involves the symmetrical risk of giving in to either the pathos of denunciation or the exaltation of rebellion—a trap that Nancy Scheper-Hughes (1992: 533) describes in the conclusion of her own work on disease and death in Brazil: "In writing against cultures and institutions of fear and domination, the critical thinker falls into a classic double bind. Either one attributes great explanatory power to the fact of oppression (but in doing so one can reduce the subjectivity and agency of subjects to a discourse on victimization) or one can try to locate the everyday form of resistance in the mundane tactics and practices of the oppressed, the weapons of the weak (here one run the risk of romanticizing human suffering or trivializing its effects on the human spirit, consciousness, and will)." Her words echo the historian Belinda Bozzoli's reconstituting of the itineraries of South African women (1991: 239): "This study has attempted to question two extremes of approach: the 'victimology' that caricatures black South Africans as the somewhat pathetic objects of colonialism, racism, oppression, poverty, patriarchy, and capitalism; and the converse of this, the 'rah rah' approach which makes romantic, celebratory, and teleological assumptions about Black South African consciousness and struggle." I hope that the sort of misery I have described here escapes miserabilism and that my discourse on the victims of structural violence has not become victimology. I have no doubt, however, that these life stories leave little room for romanticism and that their recounting has avoided the pitfall of demagogic enthusiasm.

As a matter of fact, in the tension thus created that also more generally opposes structure and agency, South African history, especially the part of that history that concerns the African or black population, makes the analysis point toward constraint rather than freedom. How could three hundred years of oppression and exploitation, more than a century of discrimination and segregation ending up in the project of apartheid that affects every facet of life and creeps into every pore of the body, leave people with real decision-making power as to their own destiny in the townships and above all in the homelands? This is not to deny the fact that every agent is called upon to make choices—though completely overdetermined by the socio-economic and political-juridical structures—or to say that these periods did not witness any resistance or rebellion, personal strategies and collective actions—but there again, actors' autonomy was severely hampered by the systems of domination.

For Magda, moving between her Lesotho, Natal, and Alexandra, and for Joseph, enclosed in his Lebowa and the neighboring farms of the Transvaal, however different their lives and the forms of violence and inequality they experienced may have been, agency was restricted; and their biographies often resemble a repertoire of events inscribed in situations of poverty and relations of power. The illness itself, which is neither a biological fatality nor a cultural curiosity but the result of those inequalities and that violence, in the end comes to inhibit the field of the possible even more, if only by the physical weakness it causes. Of course, the closer one comes to individual experiences, the more the breadth of each story; the singularity of each trajectory and the personality of each agent bring with them unexpected coherences and bifurcations, unforeseen rationalities and desires that cannot be compressed in the unrelenting game of structures. Magda recuperates her autonomy by joining a home-based care association, participating in activists' demonstrations, obtaining before anyone else antiretroviral treatment during pregnancy and after delivery, or simply by learning to negotiate her relationship with men better. Joseph, in spite of the stronger economic and social constraints that weigh on the rural world than on urban society, recaptures a space in which to move, modest but one he never possessed before, independently from the arrogant authority of his white employers and the deleterious malevolence of hostile relatives, and he even considers marrying again and becoming a landowner. In both cases, it is not without significance that AIDS is paradoxically what allows them to withdraw from the spiral of misfortune and domination, directly for Magda through her involvement in militancy and indirectly for Joseph thanks to his disability grant. Illness is also a social resource.

To account for the epidemic of AIDS in South Africa, for its unprecedented progression and its unequal distribution, for the profusion of controversies and the difficulties to act, for the past that encumbers it and the present with which it forces one to live, we need a theory of the embodi-

ment of the social world, that is, of the way in which history has surreptitiously and decisively infiltrated every interstice of life, words and acts, representations and praxis. Borrowing from the phenomenological interpretation adopted by sociology after Bourdieu (1979) and reformulated in
anthropology by Thomas Csordas (2002), we may attempt to articulate
what I have proposed to name condition (life embedded in the economic
and social reality), on the one hand, and experience (life lived both individually and collectively), on the other.[39] This is what I have tried to do here
by associating landscapes and narratives, structural effects and agents'
strategies, the world of mines and farms and the trajectories of men and
women. It is in this way that the "experience of the body" that Merleau-
Ponty (1945) has spoken about can become what he calls "being an experience," in other words, a presence unto oneself, unto others, and unto the
world that necessarily preserves the mark of the past, the past one lived oneself as well as the past experienced by the group to which one belongs. But
that experience is not homogeneous and does not follow a straight line.
Here, another philosophical tradition must be called upon: hermeneutics.
For Wilhelm Dilthey (1976), the universe of experience is not uniform. On
the one hand, there is the daily experience passively lived through and
recorded. On the other hand, there are experiences that form and transform
those who have lived them. These facts or moments that emerge from the
temporal flow are what structure the meaning of life. As Victor Turner
wrote (1986: 35–36), "These experiences that erupt from or disrupt rou-
tinized, repetitive behavior begin with shocks of pain or pleasure. Such
shocks are evocative: they summon up precedents and likenesses from the
conscious and the unconscious past—for the unusual has its traditions as
well as the usual. Then the emotions of past experiences color the images
and outlines revived by present shock." Both as the individual reality of the
sick person and as the collective reality of a social group, AIDS has that effect of making the past color the present.

Achmat Dangor's novel *Bitter Fruit,* considered one of the emblematic
works of postapartheid literature, recounts such an experience.[40] It begins
abruptly: "It was inevitable. One day Silas would run into someone of the
past, someone who had been in a position of power and had abused it.
Someone who had affected his life, not in the vague, rather grand way in
which everybody had been affected, as people say, but directly and brutally." Far more than writing up the report of the Truth and Reconciliation
Commission (which is what the main character of the book is doing) whose

contents are precisely the stuff of the history that must be reconstituted, it is thus a banal yet extraordinary event—an unexpected encounter—that unleashes the true resurrection of the period of oppression and upsets the delicate balance of his existence. More than any other experience, AIDS thus unleashes the meaning of things.

SIX

Living with Death

life—
life is worth living
can be lived and must be lived
in their grace
in their search of life
in their search of those simple things which make it life
which make it be lived

MONGANE WALLY SEROTE

Third World Express

"SUCH A LONG TIME SINCE I last saw you. Next time you come I will be dead." In the small living room of the house in Alexandra where she resides, the young AIDS sufferer whom I am visiting after having been away from South Africa for several months greets me with this terrible statement. I would like to be able to express the serene manner she has of being seriously ironic, to describe the sad smile that accompanies her welcome, to communicate the resigned sweetness of the comforting yet desperate words she has for her unexpected visitor. The consequences of her infection are certainly no mystery to her. A few years earlier she lost her boyfriend to the same illness; he was also the father of her only child. Also, she belongs to a support group for HIV-positive persons and has therefore seen her companions in misfortune disappear one after the other. The last time I saw her she spoke at length about a friend's funeral that had greatly impressed her: "I've thought about it all day and all night. I was thinking when it would be my turn." So she knows what awaits her, all the more as the media are full of news about the antiretroviral drugs—the implementation of the national rollout of treatment having just been announced—but she guesses it will have arrived too late for her. Extremely thin and weak, she suffers from bouts of fever and diarrhea. Every time I see her since we first met two years ago, her body seems more evanescent. She does not have much longer to live, and she knows it. Besides, she has done what she has to do before her death. She has made the "memory box" she will leave for her son: a tape on which she has recorded her story in a few dense sentences, a diary containing autobiographical paragraphs, a picture of herself, some clothes, a shoe, and a plaster impression of her palms. She has gone to see the priest to tell him what she would like him to say at her funeral and has chosen the music she wants played on that occasion. Nothing must be left to chance; for she is well aware that, when death comes, relatives tear each other apart, old and new accounts get settled, wounds are engraved for future generations. She knows about the stories of witchcraft that her family-in-law tells about her, making her responsible for the death of the father of her child: "I don't want people to fight for my body." Everything is thus ready for her scheduled end. Or almost everything: she must still go to her father's grave outside Johannesburg to pay her respects for the last time, talk to him about her illness and her child, carry out a ritual of separation that will accomplish what must be accomplished. Behind the apparent calmness of her preparations, the surface sometimes cracks and anguish shows through. "When I'm alone," she says, "I start thinking about those who passed away and I am scared for myself too." Over the two years we have known each other, morbid evocations have thus been the mainstay of our conversations. Yet on this April day in 2004, she expresses something else aside from death. She says she has met a man from her neighborhood: "He came to me and told me he loves me. I told him it's not possible. He said what's the problem. I said I'm positive." In spite of that revelation, he has stayed with her. They do not live together, but he comes daily to see her: "Everything that's happening in my body and in my life, I explain to him." Henceforth she tries to fully enjoy each moment they spend together. He is what now attaches her to the happiness of still being on earth. "I don't want this virus to destroy my life," she explains, though she realizes that all they actually talk about is her illness, her symptoms, her medicines, her anxieties, and, finally, the impossibility of having a normal love life. Suddenly, just a few minutes after having greeted me with her words about death, she exclaims, "I know I will survive, I have faith in this Methodist church." She had announced her death; now she is talking about her rage to live. And it is religion that gives her the hope to which she clings. Just as we are about to part, she tells me of a dream she had the night before. She was sleeping with her friend. Upon awakening, she sees a serpent entering the house. She screams. Her friend tells her to be quiet. The snake circles around her bed, then leaves. "It's the virus coming and going out of your body," comments a girlfriend who was present during the interview. The young woman died a few months later without my having seen her again. Like so many others. Investigating AIDS is like working on sand. Each time I return, I am informed about those whom I know and who are no more. That is the premonition she had when she greeted me the way she did.

Living with death. Living in death. This is what AIDS in South Africa is about. The intimate contradiction of life that one must still live though death is everywhere and though one knows that dying is imminent and inescapable. So people say and ignore. They assert and deny. As a young patient put it, caught between hope one day and renunciation the next: "You know how it is: you want to die and you don't want to die." The contradiction is individual, but it is also collective. Those who have decided once and for all that denial is the simple key to easily understand specific individual and collective practices in South Africa and elsewhere cannot apprehend it. Sick people try to enjoy life that is left to them, they fall in love and make love, they forget to use a condom or to take their medicine—and they are blamed for denying reality. The president challenges mortality statistics, speaks of fighting poverty rather than mastering sexual behavior patterns, brings up the toxicity of the antiretroviral drugs—and once again, the explanation is denial. Things are often more complex and ambivalent: the AIDS patient who says he does not believe he is infected may nevertheless organize his daily life around the illness, and, conversely, the AIDS activist who strives to obtain access to antiretroviral drugs for all may refuse to take them himself for fear of side effects; similarly, the health officer may argue against the figures released about the epidemic all the while implementing prevention programs, and the government may consider finding a vaccine a national priority while casting doubt on the pathogenic nature of the virus. What we must grasp then is the copresence of all these contradictory positions in what we call "denial." Each patient and the nation as a whole are caught up in the "I know, but still" attitude that Freud analyzed as being the very expression of simultaneously acknowledging and refusing reality.[1] With one essential difference, however. Psychoanalysis tries to unveil the contradiction in the belief, but here anthropology has to account for the contradiction that resides in the experience itself.

The ethnographic example chosen by the psychoanalyst Octave Mannoni (1969) is taken from *Sun Chief: The Autobiography of a Hopi Indian*, by Don Talayesva and Leo Simmons. During the kiva ceremony, the young initiated Hopi discover that the Katsina masks that had frightened them so much in their childhood are not evil spirits but their disguised fathers and uncles. However, rather than give up their belief, they make it the foundation of their religion: " 'I know the Katsina are not spirits, they are my fathers and my uncles, but still the Katsina are there when my fathers and uncles dance with their masks on.' Something has somehow gone over to the other side (which is the definition of initiation)." It seems we are hitting upon the hard core of the belief itself: not the illusion of a child, which could be done away with by revealing it is only a fairy tale, but the persuasion of the adults who resist the evidence that the thing does not exist, even when they themselves provide the proof. That tension is probably what allows us to account for the contradictory cognitive positions concerning AIDS: believing in the virus and suspicious that it even exists; promoting antiretroviral drugs for others but being wary of them for oneself.

But there is another tension, this time in the experience itself, which does not derive from representations of reality but from reality as it is lived effectively. How can one live an imminent death? How can one govern a country in the midst of a scheduled catastrophe? We are no longer operating here in the order of the unbelievable but in the order of the intolerable, both individual and collective. I have discussed elsewhere (Fassin 2005) that the only "universal intolerable" might be the perspective of the group disappearing, genocide being the outermost limit. The fact that the reference to "genocide" has been so explicit and so frequent in the recent history of AIDS in South Africa is not a coincidence. In the face of the unbearable, bodies resist. At times to accept the deadline and prepare for it. At other times to reject the imposed reality and invent a new one. To die or be reborn. Truth thus lies at the heart of denial.

DYING

How many more must die
Before things get right?
MZWAKHE MBULI
"It's Too Long"

"The mortality rate in the City of Johannesburg is increasing at such a rate that it is running out of space to bury its dead and is considering using old mineshafts as underground cemeteries. With this in mind, the City Parks is talking to the Chamber of Mines about taking over disused mineshafts to be used as catacombs—underground galleries with recesses for tombs as were common in ancient Roman times. The city is currently burying

20,000 people a year and this figure is expected to rise to 70,000 by 2010. Department of Health statistics show that five years ago, there was a birthrate of 14 per 1,000 and a death rate of 14 per 1,000. This year the birthrate rose to 19.5 per 1,000 while the death rate dropped to 10 per 1,000. 'Johannesburg has a population of 3 million people who eventually will have to be accommodated in a final resting place,' said Alan Buff of City Parks, who is in charge of the cemeteries. 'We need 1,500 ha to take us to 2050.' The city is making provision for the acquisition of an additional 1,000 ha of new land and is investigating alternative methods to cope with the huge demand and expected increase in AIDS deaths. These include freeze-drying by means of liquid nitrogen, mausoleums, i.e., above-ground cemeteries, mass graves and multiple burials. The upright burial or trench system was also being looked at." This article from the *Saturday Star* of November 29, 2002, is one of the many testimonies regularly echoed by the press attesting to the dire situation of mortuary economics in South Africa. And the cemeteries overflowing with corpses are only one of the manifestations of the omnipresence of death. The city walls in the townships of Johannesburg as in the former homelands of Limpopo are placarded with posters advertising tombstones and funeral homes. In Alexandra, traffic is made difficult every Saturday because tents multiply in the streets where people gather in front of the home of the deceased before the funeral. In Lenyenye, people's meager savings are sunk almost entirely into burial societies, which, when the moment comes, guarantee subscribers the necessary sum for their own funerals. Henceforth, South African society is living with death. A sort of normalization has taken place, to the point that nobody is shocked when, during an interview with a patient he has not seen for a while, an anthropologist asks (as if inquiring after a traveling relative), "And is your boyfriend still alive?" The normalization of death, which is something else than simply a mundane reality, is what I would like to apprehend, both as government policy and as people's private experience.

Governing under Uncertainty

When the figures from the annual survey on HIV prevalence among pregnant women came out in 1999, they were interpreted in two opposite ways, as the titles of articles published a few months apart in the *South African Medical Journal* by a team of epidemiologists from the Cape and by functionaries from the Ministry of Health illustrate: "HIV Surveillance Results: Little Grounds for Optimism Yet," for the former; "1999 HIV Surveillance

Results: Little Grounds for Pessimism," for the latter.[2] In fact, when it initially publicized those statistics the government thought it possible to rejoice: for the first time in ten years the deadly trend of AIDS was beginning to reverse. Compared to the previous year, there was a slight change, from 22.8 to 22.4 percent. Above all, the rates for the youngest women clearly were down, from 21 to 16.5 percent for those under the age of twenty and, less dramatic, from 26.1 to 25.6 percent for the twenty to twenty-four age group, which hinted that new infections in the most vulnerable group were decreasing. The good news was relayed by the National Association of People Living with Aids and by the Centre for the Study of Aids at Pretoria University. But according to the director of the Centre for Actuarial Research of the University of Cape Town and his colleagues from the Medical Research Council, such conclusions were unwarranted. In reality, the variations observed were not statistically significant given the size of the sample, as also confirmed by the confidence intervals. Their projections suggested on the contrary that the infection was continuing to spread. While "conceding that it is very difficult to know the truth of the epidemic and that models are limited by the assumptions required," the authors suggested that state authorities should reconsider their optimistic analysis. Responding to this attack, the directors of the Epidemiology Unit of the National Anti-AIDS Programme and the Surveillance System at the Health Department, as well as the statistician from the Medical Research Council, called for caution in handling demographic models, stressing that "they are but models, not reality." They underlined the efforts accomplished over the past years—it was only logical that there should finally be a few positive results—and urged the critics to look at the African situation for once through rosier glasses.

In this context, the 2002 figures were awaited impatiently. The Health Department delayed publishing them for a long time and finally only did so under pressure from the Treatment Action Campaign. The rate was 26.5 percent. It was released with the following comment: "Although we see a slight increase, statistically this increase is not significant and we can confidently say that the prevalence rate has been stabilized."[3] A statistical argument ad hoc that was thus considered relevant now to relativize the apparent worsening of the situation but had not been used to moderate the favorable impression of the trend of the preceding year. Yet, if we look at the past five years, the trend announced by the Health Ministry seems partially accurate: after an exponential progression between 1990 and 1998, the curve had reached a much lower rate of increase, with prevalence of 22.8 percent in 1998, 22.4 percent in 1999, 24.5 percent in 2000, 24.8 percent in 2001, and 26.5 percent in 2002. In other words, stabilization seemed on its way.

Introducing statistics into human reasoning and even into the government of men has been analyzed by Ian Hacking (1990) as a way of "taming chance." Where the action of invisible, supernatural, or even natural powers seemed to triumph over human will, figures, means, and rates were reassuringly rational. Things are not so simple, however. In the case of AIDS in South Africa, statistics have on the contrary brought intellectual and political insecurity. Instead of controlling the facts through established data and demonstrated regularities, one has been confronted by new uncertainties. Thus it was first asserted that 50 percent of the personnel in the health sector were infected; three years later it turned out that only 16 percent were. For the mine workers, it was publicly announced that 50 percent were infected, but the estimate today is about 14 percent. As to the army, not long ago a prevalence as high as 70 percent was announced, whereas the presently accepted figure is 23 percent.[4] The promised order has turned into new disorder. And that disorder concerns what lies at the heart of all public policy: the life and death of the nation's subjects. In her inquiry into the post-Chernobyl era, Adriana Petryna (2002) has shown that catastrophes are not followed by neutral evaluations. They are traversed by politics from beginning to end. Yet statistics—etymologically, the science of the state—are crucial: counting the dead and the living, defining who are the legitimate victims and their eligible heirs. Let us look at a few examples.

In 2001 the Centre for Actuarial Research of the University of Cape Town (the most respected South African demographic laboratory for AIDS statistics) published a series of projections that were to become the main reference for the entire scientific community in the years following. The most dramatic information concerned the loss of twenty years of life expectancy in two decades—a drop from 60 to 40 years between 1990 and 2010. In certain provinces the drop was even more spectacular: 36 years would be lost in KwaZulu-Natal. Almost inconceivable figures, unmatched in modern history, that is, since a statistical science capable of producing mortality tables and modeling its evolution was invented. In 2003, however, the same specialists started to revise their analyses somewhat, using new information and especially refining them by introducing elements of racial differentiation. Most affected were the Africans, with a life expectancy reduced to 40 years, whereas the Coloureds managed to limit their loss to age 55. It was pointed out, incidentally, that no figures were calculated for Whites. In 2004, remarkably, the researcher in charge of the program announced new results. This time, the curve of life expectancy did not go below age 50. Though still confident in his demographic model, Rob Dorrington nevertheless admitted, "There is always some degree of uncertainty about predicting the future. Data on the epidemic in South Africa are scarce so we need to use the imperfect information that we have to forecast the future."[5] The degree of uncertainty here is from twenty to ten years of life expectancy lost over a three-year period of research or even a single year, if one takes into consideration the 2003 update that remained particularly pessimistic for Africans. We are well beyond the variation by a few decimals of prevalence in the antenatal surveys, which was the object of harsh discussions with the Health Department only two years before.

In fact, concerning these annual surveys, the public authorities as well as doctors, researchers, and activists have become accustomed since 1998 to referring to their rates, which range from 22 to 26 percent. They are the basis on which all calculations are made, from the trend in the number of patients or orphans to the projected budgets for medicines or grants. However, in 2002, the first national survey to be carried out on a random sample of people visited and questioned at home, in other words, supposedly representative of the general population, gave results totally different from the previous estimation through sampling pregnant women consulted in the public sector. The prevalence rate was 11.4 percent when considering all ages and 15.6 percent for adults ages 15 to 49. If only the women in that age group were considered, the rate was 17.7 percent, reaching 18.4 percent for African women.[6] Of course, it is easy to understand that by focusing here on African women ages 15 to 49, one tends to find more or less the same population as the one tested during the antenatal visits in public facilities (where over the same period the rate was 26.5 percent). Nonetheless, considering that the figure taken from antenatal clinics (generally used in all the estimates and projections for the entire adult population) is twice as high as the figure obtained in the household survey one sees the degree of uncertainty that the South African government has had to work with for ten years.

Other countries face similar difficulties. In January 2004 the South African investigative journalist Rian Malan granted a spectacular interview to the British magazine the *Spectator*, with the title, "Africa Isn't Dying of AIDS."[7] To denounce figures that were "deliberately exaggerated" by the international community and by NGOs and to criticize the "computerized models" used to predict future patterns, he relied on the statistics that had undergone a revision in several countries. A few weeks earlier, the Demographic and Health Survey of Kenya undertaken by the U.S. Centers for

Disease Control had established the prevalence rate for the population of that country at 6.7 percent, considerably lower than the 9.4 percent that UNAIDS had officially validated until then. These results were also challenged because, as was noted, 14 percent of the women and 13 percent of the men had refused to be tested and may have done so precisely because they thought they were infected. In South Africa, the chair of the Treatment Action Campaign accused the journalist of playing the dissidents' game. However, a few weeks later, as we saw, the director of the Centre for Actuarial Research cut by half the loss of life expectancy by 2010. He thus implicitly admitted that those who asked for a little less pessimism and a little more caution were not necessarily wrong.

Contemporary societies, as Ulrich Beck (1992) has demonstrated, are risk societies in the sense that they produce both the danger that threatens them and the awareness of that peril. Few countries are as directly faced with danger as South Africa, with its devastating AIDS epidemic. However, the idea of risk covers two distinct notions present in common sense as well as in scholarly interpretations. Mary Douglas (1992) calls them "chance" and "danger." There is a risk that an unfortunate event will occur, that is, a probability, and that event itself constitutes a risk, that is, a threat. The first meaning is the epidemiologist's, who calculates "relative risk" and "absolute risk," who looks for "risk factors" and delineates "risk groups." The second meaning is the ecologist's, who questions the security of "nuclear energy" and denounces the dangers of "global warming," promoting instead the benefits of "sustainable development." To govern is to measure the "risk" in the second sense by using the resources of "risk" according to the first sense.

In South Africa, while the specter of a million dead in the near future seems confirmed, the instruments to deal with it remain uncertain. Yet the more uncertain they are, the more adamant the certainties asserted on either side. Similarly, state agencies lack clarity in their communication, and information is treated by the media with the greatest incoherence. In 2002 the South African government ordered a study on mortality from Statistics South Africa, the national demographic institution. "It will give a picture as to what it is that kills people in the country. That is why it is important to have those figures. We must know," declared Thabo Mbeki. On November 19, 2002, the results were supposed to be announced at a press conference in one of the capital's luxurious hotels, but the event was canceled one hour before because the government said it had not been informed. The study was released two days later. In an interval of twenty-four hours, one could thus learn from the press that according to the Medical Research

Council AIDS is "the biggest killer" in South Africa, while according to Statistics SA, "South Africa is dying from non-natural causes," that is, homicides, suicides, and accidents. Obscurity (not knowing) and opacity (not saying) combine to characterize a government of uncertainty.

However, even when the polemic was at its peak, policies continued. By focusing attention on the controversies alone, emphasizing the fights between the Health Department and the Treatment Action Campaign, or reducing Thabo Mbeki's positions exclusively to his association with the dissidents from California and Australia, many observers have missed the everyday work being done in the provincial and national administrations, in hospital wards and health care facilities.[8] These activities were also conducted in a context of uncertainty but with a high level of pragmatism. Rather than a single, clearly defined strategy, diverse tactics are thus implemented. Support groups and home-based care, prophylaxis of opportunistic infections and distribution of food parcels, condom promotion and disability grants. To put it more bluntly, activities stemming from the hypothesis that the virus is sexually transmitted and tasks aiming to correct poverty do not seem opposed. People do things without really being informed and act without being sure of what justifies their actions. A foreign doctor I met in Limpopo implemented the prevention of mother-to-child transmission with nevirapine all the while thinking that dissidents may be right. A South African nurse interviewed in the same province was in charge of counseling and testing but admitted that she feared doing it for herself. The organizer of a support group in a rural dispensary acknowledged that she herself would never use the antiretroviral drugs if she were HIV-positive, a hypothesis that she never even checked out in any case. So one might say that things get done on a day-to-day basis far from the turmoil of the high spheres of the state. The hottest national debates barely scratch the surface of actual practices. The history of the health system, the differentiated logics of the professionals, the restrictions on resources and the limits of competence, the individual projects of agents and the personal experience they have of the illness are just so many factors that, far more than the decisions coming from above, make up the daily routine of AIDS management in this context of uncertainty, where the only thing one can be sure of is that more and more people will get sick and die.

The Materiality of Illness

Questioned about what is the most distressing in her work on behalf of AIDS patients, a young volunteer from one of Alexandra's home-based care organizations responded, "The hardest in this work is when you find maggots in the bed sores, it happened to me last week with a man who died since. Also it is when you have these strange skin lesions like this woman I visited, she looked like a snake." Instead of compassion about the fate of her fellow humans—as I had expected, given the dramatic situations we had just witnessed together—she expresses repulsion at their stricken bodies. No feelings, just sensations. She thus reminds me of the basic truth that in AIDS as in other serious diseases suffering is inscribed in the body, in its material substance, in the most immediate and most elementary way. Illness is a matter of pain and smell, of bodies not washed and festering wounds, of no longer being able to swallow food and of relieving oneself in one's bed. Anthropologists may sometimes forget this fact when they are interested in cultural representations, narrative constructions, and symbolic meanings. Following Arthur Kleinman (1988) and Byron Good (1994), in particular, social scientists working on sickness reacted against purely biomedical analyses to show quite relevantly the importance of narratives and meanings. Against the positivism of a clinical approach that reduces illness to being only an object, with a diagnosis and a prognosis, in short, that reduces it to pathology, their interpretation was attentive to the patient's perspective and restored its rights to the processes of subjectivization that in the end turn the illness into an experience. But of this experience, one too often forgets the physical dimension: it is pain, limited autonomy, a rotting body that mediate the relationship to the social world, as Michael Kelly and David Field (1996) have noted. Put otherwise, the material side of illness—less noble certainly but nevertheless its flesh and blood—has been neglected. Consider the two following paragraphs quoted from my field notes in Alexandra.

> Visit to a patient's home. The concrete house, vast and filthy, deserted (except for children who from time to time run around playing) and ransacked (by the bailiffs who came to do their work for a creditor, probably a shopkeeper). Maria lives alone with five children, the eldest a girl being approximately fifteen. She is almost a skeleton, moaning in the middle of a sunken bed. In her room and the rooms around floats the acrid smell of urine. Two home-based care volunteers are talking to her. Maria is begging them to take her to the hospital. She no longer eats, can no longer swallow her medicine, cannot even get up to relieve herself. She suffers from tuberculosis, but judging from the pile of tablets on her night table, she has not taken her treatment for a while. Her children keep her company because it is vacation, but when school starts again next week she will be alone all

day. This solitude is an isolation that weighs heavily on her. During the day, anxious, she keeps calling her children. At night, her screams wake the family and the neighbors. Given her situation, there is nothing much the volunteers can do except wash her, help her take her medicines and keep her company for a few minutes. Today, however, it may be necessary to do more. We talk it over to see if we can try to find a bed in the hospital. We know it will be difficult, but if we give up it means we condemn her to lie dying in this room, with only her immense anguish for company. We spend half an hour on the phone trying to get an ambulance. To convince the company to budge, we have to state my professional identity with a foreign accent, for it would never work if only the volunteers call for it. Finally, our correspondent sends a car. We let the two volunteers take Maria to the hospital with a letter of recommendation that I write to the doctor. A few hours later I see one of the two young women at the headquarters of the home-based care association. She looks sad, does not join in with her colleagues who are having fun laughing and dancing for one of their birthdays. Maria was examined in the emergency ward. They put a drip on her and told her she would go home afterward. She would not be hospitalized. Her treatment would not be resumed. Actually they considered her lost. The volunteer, ill herself, tells me she thinks of what her own end will be. Like a painful reflection in a mirror, Maria is showing the young woman her own future.

Visit to a patient's home. Ben lives in a single room four by four meters made of cement blocks and divided into four more or less equal parts by wood and cardboard so as to make three tiny rooms and a kitchen. The place has been lent to him by the owner of the house, and he himself puts up friends there. It is dark, smelly, and messy; since there is no furniture, clothing and kitchen utensils pile up on the floor and the occasional chair. Ben is in his corner of the room, lying on his bed. His face is emaciated, his body fleshless. His strength has left him. Four volunteers, all men, have been sent by the association. After having greeted the patient, I retire to the entrance, somewhat embarrassed by all those people around the dying man. Through the thin partition, I hear two of the volunteers washing him. I speak with them a little later. They never had any training in home-based care and so keep to that mere activity of bathing the patients. They tell me that there is a retired nurse who works in the association, but she never accompanies the volunteers because her feet hurt. They do not know Ben. This is the first time they visit him. They have found out that people in the neighborhood feed him because he does not seem to have any family. When I return to the headquarters of the association a few days later, I am told he died the day after our visit. He was twenty-five.

These last moments of truth of the disease are preceded by a series of steps that mark its progressive embodiment. They are the ordeals that the patients must face before their tragic ends. Discovering the infection, sometimes in denial at first, often in despair. Exploring the past, searching for the partner who may have been at the origin of their contamination. Telling their close ones, eventually organizing a family meeting for a disclosure. The rumors that one overhears or guesses, the children kept at a distance at school or in the neighborhood. The attention one starts to pay to what is said about the causes and treatments on the radio or in the street. The medicines one takes, hidden from view, and that one usually ignores since they were only prescribed to avert opportunistic infections and not to treat the disease. With the first symptoms comes the first hospitalization, often the pretext for being fired from the workplace, generally without compensation. With the decline of the body, it becomes harder to preserve one's physical independence, to take care of the children, the house.

Most patients anticipate the end by subscribing to a burial society to make sure that when the end comes, the funeral will be honorable and will not have to be paid for by the family, to make sure that it will be sufficiently dignified too. Some gather souvenirs, beloved objects, flattering photographs, recordings of last wishes in a memory box to leave the children as the last trace of themselves. For those who belong to a support group, a new form of sociability develops as a result of sharing the same illness, often comforting, sometimes difficult because of rivalry and gossip. For those who have the good luck to come across devoted and competent social workers, the application for and access to a disability grant, usually after several months of waiting, brings relative financial independence but is also sometimes lusted after by greedy families. Those who encounter certain humanitarian organizations or participate in clinical trials will have access to an antiretroviral treatment, opening them to the possibility of a longer life, sometimes exposing them to the bad fortune of side effects from which some may even die. Finally, for many of those who do not know or do not want to know, who prefer to hide their serological status or have nobody to confide in—that is, for those whom neither anthropologist nor doctor nor even priest reach—the end means silence and solitude, a silence filled with noise, a solitude filled with malevolence. If one compares the numbers of members of support groups and of patients seen in health facilities to the expected numbers given the statistics of the epidemic, one may assume that this category of the "invisible" is by far the most numerous.

"My life now?" sighed a young woman during one of our last encounters. And she gave the answer herself: "My relatives make it hard." She mentioned the suspicion of witchcraft that her family-in-law held over her, threatening to take away her son even before she died, and all those stories of debts she had because of her own mother's funeral. She did get a disability grant, she said, but "money goes so fast." Each month she received 700 rands (about U.S. $100 at this time) out of which she took 200 to pay for the furniture that her mother had bought on credit before her death. The rest went for medicine (200 rands), food (200 rands), and her younger brother (100 rands). That was her daily life with AIDS: fear of her in-laws, anxiety at the idea of losing her little boy, careful budgeting of her slim grant. Weakened by her infection, wanting to care for herself more efficiently, she could not even imagine paying 650 rands for antiretroviral multitherapy. At that time, the government had not yet applied its roll-out of drugs in the public health-care system and treatments were available only in the private sector. This was October 2003.

A few weeks later, I read two articles in the *New England Journal of Medicine*.[9] The first presented a new antiretroviral drug particularly effective in association with other already known products. The only difficulty was its price, which could come to U.S. $30,000 a year. The writer commented, "Thus at least for the moment the annual cost of medications for HIV may vary by a factor of about 100 depending on which drugs are used, where the patient lives and whether or not the price is discounted." The second article reported the case of a thirty-nine-year-old AIDS patient living on the East Coast in the United States who had received a heart transplant at an advanced stage of his illness because of a serious cardiopathy. Aside from the operation itself, the financial evaluation of the operation included reanimation, immunodepressants to prevent rejection, treatment of complications such as opportunist infections and iatrogenic accidents that might occur in the wake of the intervention or because of the medication, and, of course, antiretroviral multitherapy. The cost, however, was not indicated. "Ethical issues need to be considered, including the appropriateness of expanding the pool of eligible recipients by including patients with an indication for which transplantation has unproven success, at a time when there are inadequate numbers of organs available," the authors wrote. Remembering the young woman in Alexandra and her tight budget that did not allow her to treat her disease, it seemed to me that the inequality of lives in their very material existence, that is, in the amount of money it takes to simply save them, could hardly be more starkly expressed. A few months later, as the government had just announced the roll-out, she told us she was soon going to start the drugs. So she did. But, probably too weak to tolerate them, she died shortly after.

Those Who Remain

A desolate place. The vast concession in Tickyline gives me the same impression each time I come. Not that its actual space is devastated, but it is the feeling that overcomes me when listening to the fragments of history emerging from the interviews and seeing the tired sadness on the faces of my interlocutors. I met them through a volunteer from NAPWA who asked me if I wanted "to meet a family with orphans." The question put me ill at ease: did he think I could in any way be helpful to them, or more probably (considering the discussions we had previously had) that the situation could "interest me"? In fact, the ambivalence of his offer revealed the ambiguity of anthropological expectations. It was dusk when I arrived at the family's place.

It is composed of five small one- to three-room houses. One is used as a collective kitchen. The other four houses are inhabited by three brothers and sisters, their children and grandchildren. A small, parched vegetable garden surrounds it. Rosa, the eldest, is the one who speaks during our first meeting. She is fifty-three and divorced. She has ten children ages twelve to thirty-three. A few months ago she lost her second daughter, twenty-nine, who died of AIDS and left two little girls (from a first father, deceased) and a boy nineteen months old (from a second father, who had left). This little boy is also HIV-positive, and his sickness is already showing. She is now raising her three grandchildren on top of her six boys and girls who live with her and are not yet working. One of her daughters, twenty-four, has a son and daughter she looks after alone. When that new workload was imposed on Rosa, she had to give up her job as a farmworker at a distant property (where she was paid 16 rands a day, corresponding to 400 rands a month) because of the frail condition of the baby boy. From then on she devoted herself exclusively to her eleven children and grandchildren. Nevertheless, she was able to cope with the situation provoked by the death of her daughter thanks to her own mother's old-age pension of 700 rands per month. But the week before our visit, her mother too had died, and that financial loss was not yet compensated for by the foster care grant she had just applied for. She would not be getting the first installment for several months at best. An impossible situation: with no resources, she must raise eleven children, which is what precisely is preventing her from going out to earn a living. "Now I'm going to depend on my brothers and sisters," she said.

"Whatever they will give me I will be very grateful." Unfortunately, the other family members' situation is hardly any better.

Rosa had four brothers and a sister. An older brother died, of diabetes they say, leaving a wife and two school-age children. A younger brother, John, is forty-nine and worked as a house painter in the region or in Johannesburg. When times were good he earned up to 400 rands a week, which allowed him to take care of his children, seven from two different wives; four are still at home, and his second wife, with whom he now lives, does not work. During the interview, it appears, however, that the description of his activity must be written in the past tense, because four years ago he fell sick and was taken to the hospital. They found tuberculosis and treated him. Though he only alludes to it in passing, it seems clear from his present physical appearance that his infection is related to AIDS. This impression is apparently confirmed by the fact that he just obtained a disability grant. The 700 rands he now receives is half of what he earned when he was working. A second younger brother, Paul, forty-six, is a glazier. He works in town and does not live with the rest of the family. He is married, his wife is unemployed, and they have three children still in school. A younger sister, Mathala, thirty-one, is a student in Johannesburg. She is married to a schoolteacher and has a son and daughter who live with her husband in a little town in the region. As to Rosa's older children, they are hardly in any position to help. The eldest girl, thirty-three, lives alone with her three children from two different fathers; she does not work and only has her son's grant to live on. The second is the one who just died of AIDS. The third lives in town and does odd jobs. The fourth is put up by his older sister and is out of work. The fifth is also jobless and has two very young children for whom the father sends about 100 rands a month. The next two are no longer in school but still live at home. The last three are still in school.

The family tree I sketched as we talked with the various members is composed of the deceased and the survivors (actually, this is the word John used when he mentioned one of his nieces: "She survives with the grant of her youngest child"). Of the five adults living on the concession—Rosa, John and his wife, Paul's wife, and Rosa's fifth daughter—none works. Rosa no longer has any resources, John gets his disability grant, Paul sends a little money to his wife, as does the husband of Rosa's daughter. In other words, twenty people (five adults, two teenagers, thirteen children—among whom are three orphans) live on approximately 1,500 rands, depending on Paul's irregular earnings. Less than 80 rands, or U.S. $10, per person monthly. An unstable situation too. When I return a year later, Rosa has started working on the farm again; she stays overnight because it is too far and only comes home on weekends with her weekly salary of 100 rands. The children are more or less left alone all day, with their sick uncle and three women busy with housework. The grant to raise the children has not arrived yet, and she expects to have it soon if her grandson does not die of AIDS in the meanwhile. For the illness is there, no doubt about that, given the uncle's poor physical state and the frailty of the little orphan, but it is inscribed within the larger landscape of misery and misfortune. Seen from this concession, how vain the controversy about virus or poverty seems, how out of place the polemic on antiretroviral drugs and food! Should one be treated or get enough to eat? For this family, as for so many others, neither is possible anyway.[10] AIDS is just one more calamity in their existence menaced by social disorder and economic instability. It transforms fatherless children into orphans and precarious workers into welfare cases. "Those who remain, may God help them to have good families!" said an AIDS patient, also in Tickyline. For those, especially the widows and widowers, on the one hand, and the orphans, on the other, life is often made even more difficult.

Losing one's spouse is not only a tragic personal experience; it is also a problematic social fact. About women whose husbands were killed under apartheid, Ramphele (1997: 99) wrote that "political widowhood raises questions of importance about the extent to which social space is created or denied for the public expression of pain, loss and suffering of individual social actors." Becoming a widow or widower due to AIDS is an ambiguous and painful status. Ambiguous, because the victim often becomes the accused: thinking of the disappearance of the deceased in terms of sexual transmission or witchcraft casts suspicion on the mourning spouse. Painful, because relatives do not hesitate to take advantage of the situation: the dead person's belongings and even his or her children become objects of greed and heartbreak.

For Betty, the young woman from Tickyline, life after her husband Abraham's death was certainly worse even than during his illness. When I first saw them they were a peaceful couple in spite of their mutual misfortune. They married in 1995. Two years later, a child was born. The little boy was often sick, and when he was in the hospital they discovered he was HIV-positive. When they got tested, the parents discovered they too were infected. It was clear to both of them that Abraham had infected Betty and, indirectly, their son. But with the help of religion, they managed to face the tragedy that could have torn them apart. They joined NAPWA, he as an employee, she as a volunteer. At the end of 2003, Abraham's health went rapidly downhill. As he lay dying, the brothers and sisters he had never gotten along with came to the house and in front of his wife and child took all the furniture, claiming it was theirs. The day after he died, they went to the bank and emptied the account, taking the 10,000 rands that were his lifelong savings and that he intended to go to his wife and especially to his child: when we had spoken a few months prior to this, he had confided to me that since he saw many orphans through his work in the association, he worried a lot about what was to become of his own son. Part of the money taken by the family went to pay for the funeral, but they bought a cheap coffin to limit the expense. The brothers and sisters were able to act this way because the couple were not married, either according to South African law (they only had a simple verbal agreement but no contract stipulating joint ownership of goods) or according to Sotho tradition (the *lobola,* or dowry, that clinches the union between the families had never been paid). Robbed of their savings, no longer receiving her husband's salary, and with only a disability grant of 170 rands for her son, Betty found employment in town with a fruit and vegetable wholesaler. She now leaves the house at 7:00 A.M. and comes home at about 6:30 P.M. six days a week. She earns 200 rands weekly. She takes care of three of her sister's children at the same time as her own son. He worries her because since his father died he looks depressed, sleeps during the day, has problems in school. In spite of everything, Betty says she feels strong, and in her soft voice she tells me, "I think I will be for the next ten or twenty years." A few months earlier, Abraham had shown the same self-confidence.

For the one who remains after the partner's death, the distress caused by the loss is only one of the ordeals. The disappearance of the deceased's earnings that are not compensated for by welfare, the symptoms of the illness that often then invade the surviving spouse, the worrying about the children one knows will be left alone, sometimes the greed or accusations of relatives (especially in-laws)—these are just so many extra reasons for despair that the widow or widower has to deal with. Given this painful reality, it is remarkable that, contrary to the situation of orphans that has been studied by several surveys and for whom initiatives have been launched all over the African continent, research and actions by the international institutions, NGOs, and local authorities aimed at widows and widowers should be so rare.[11] Clearly, social judgments produce moral hierarchies in the evaluation of suffering.

From this perspective, orphans are indeed a target for special solicitude.

Specifically, one should speak of "AIDS orphans" as they are internationally referred to in the abundant reports and papers, biographical pieces and statistical projections that reveal both compassion and anxiety. This legitimate interest in children who are victims of the epidemic is all the more remarkable as for a long time what prevailed was almost total indifference to their lot. As Pamela Reynolds (2000: 141) noted, during apartheid "the South African state committed systematic violence against the institution of the family among the Africans," and "a consequence for many people was a dramatic disjuncture between the ideals and the experiences of family life," with forced displacements and separations and a great amount of family and conjugal disruption. In her survey, for example, half the young people questioned had not been raised in their nuclear families, a third had never lived with their fathers, a third had spent less than half their childhood with their mothers, nearly all had known family breakups. But these negative effects were practically ignored in statistical studies, academic research, and public policies.

In fact, it is AIDS that brought interest in childhood from the perspective of loss of family ties and, more precisely, parental ties, as if it were a totally new reality. The seriousness of the problem remains difficult to evaluate, however, given the few studies (only two concern the country as a whole), the diversity of criteria (absence of one or both parents or of only the mother), the variability in age limits (under fifteen or under eighteen), and a certain tendency to dramatize a situation obviously already tragic.[12] According to the Human Science Research Council's survey named after Nelson Mandela, 13 percent of children under 15 had lost one or the other or both of their parents, among whom 3 percent no longer had their mothers and 8.4 percent their fathers (the cause of death was not specified). According to the projections of the Centre for Actuarial Research of the University of the Cape, the number of children under 18 who were motherless in 2003 reached one million, of whom 200,000 no longer had either parent (2 million had lost only their fathers). In comparison, the same year the Department of Social Development counted 173,000 beneficiaries of the foster care grant (the allowance was given to the orphans' tutors).[13] Finally, in the area in the north where we did our own investigation, a local survey carried out in the Lenyenye school by the director and her staff yielded the following results: of 1,008 pupils, 150 were counted as orphans (of father and/or mother), among whom only 13 received the corresponding grant and 300 were considered vulnerable (neither parent working). The figures are impressive, but again the issue of "AIDS orphans" needs to be evaluated thoroughly. First, the present reality should be considered in relation to the social history of South African families: in our interviews, many adults said they had been raised by a grandmother at a time when AIDS did not yet exist and when little interest was shown in these situations. Second, the statistics obviously do not only reflect the impact of the epidemic, as it is supposed: thus, the far greater number of fatherless children is more likely linked to the frequency of homicides and accidents, a fact very rarely mentioned.

The question of custody is no less complex than the question of how to interpret statistics, for it mixes family practices and social policies in sometimes contradictory fashion. On one side, a tradition exists that consists in entrusting children to relatives when one is unable to raise them, for economic reasons or because of a remarriage; that is also true if the mother dies, in which case, the grandmother usually takes in the orphan. But on the other side, a welfare system has grown up that provides financial assistance to people who decide to raise a child that is not their own within the administrative framework of the foster care grant: the sum allocated to the relative represents a large amount, especially given the low incomes in rural areas, and has become the object of rivalry within families. In other words, what was supposed to come from generosity and solidarity henceforth stirs up envy and jealousy. Thus a woman who had taken in her deceased sister's children suddenly becomes aware that other family members have developed—once the grant is obtained—a sudden affection for the little orphans. A grandmother raising the three children of her own daughter who recently died of AIDS similarly tries to put her hands on their grants but finally has to accept using the money for the children's benefit as the social worker threatens to withdraw her tutorship.

Thus, in a context of often extreme poverty, government subsidies are both significant contributions to the household budgets and new reasons for infighting among relatives.[14] Beyond the tension created by the effects of a doubtlessly generous system, one can question the more fundamental ambivalence concerning the reasons for treating children so specifically in the time of AIDS. This favor rests on a double moral peculiarity: the fact that childhood is linked to innocence (as opposed to the supposed fault of adults); and the fact that AIDS induces specific responses (nobody had really bothered about the orphans of violence). The exceptional regime of compassion for AIDS orphans is thus part of the discomfort that for many South Africans surrounds the management of the epidemic that mixes good intentions and social inequality, concern for childhood neglected until then and forgetting injustices inherited from the past. An unspeakable discomfort—for in the name of what could one blame the attention accorded the most vulnerable victims of the epidemic? An extrahistorical category, pure sufferers, these orphans embody the ambiguous misfortune of those who remain.

BORN AGAIN

This then's survival
not passive drift, nor fear,
but jaunty, sword-edge joy,
extempore:
this
balancing on air.

LYNNE BRYER

"Balancing on Air"

"I get the / result / I'm HIV / positive / I'm proud / of that / Because as / from now / I'm going to / change and / I know where / I'm / I admit that / I'm alive / Nothing can't / happen to me / Unless if / there is something / could happen to me / Maybe I can / started to solve / But not me / I accept that / I'm HIV / positive." At the page labeled March 5, 2003, from the diary of the young woman from Lenyenye, these words that resemble the lines of a poem are the trace of the illness announced. The only trace, for Olga tells us she does not keep a diary and will not write anything else. A tenuous trace, therefore, but in which one can catch a glimpse of her emotion and her resolve, her acceptance of the news and her affirmation of life in a sort of fever of revelation. She comments: "I'm going to change. I was fast, I had many boyfriends. I would change every month. Now it's over." Many narratives attest the same transformation in the way of life at the moment when the illness is discovered or in the time that follows. A painful change, sometimes preceded by a phase of denial but which at the same time heralds a new life, a sort of resurrection. Not only will nothing ever be the same again, but the inner revolution commands a strength that manages to stave off the announced death: "As long as I am living nothing will happen to me," she adds in a sort of magical tautology. Of course, we know since Michael Bury's (1982) pioneering work that serious illness constitutes a "biographical break," brings on a "critical situation," and implies an after where nothing is as it was before. In the new life that begins, the pathology is both a burden and a resource for the reconstruction of the self and one's relation to the world. Its omnipresence as a permanent reminder of the finitude of existence supposes forms of adjustment. The patient puts his or her life in order. This is how we can read the note concluding the diary of another AIDS patient in Alexandra who had also begun to write eight months earlier when first told she was HIV-positive: "Most important about my HIV: it has taught me to plan my life." But in Olga's quasi-verses, as in the experience of many of the other patients we met, there is more. A form of mystic exaltation that is also the religious experience of African churches where trances are omnipresent in all the ceremonies and pave the way to public invocations, as reported by Jean Comaroff (1985) in her study of the Zion Christian Church.[15] Reading the young woman's inspired and fragmented text reminded me of another illumination, Blaise Pascal's in "the year of grace 1654," on the day of the revelation from which he drew his *Thoughts:* "Certitude. Certitude. Feeling. Joy. Peace. / God of Jesus Christ . . . . Jesus Christ. / Jesus Christ. / I left him, I ran away from him, renounced, crucified. / May I never be separated from him. / He can only be preserved by the means taught in the Bible. / Total and sweet renunciation. / Total submission to Jesus Christ and my director. / Eternally in joy for one day of exercise on earth. / *Non obliviscar sermones tuos.* Amen." What Csordas (2004) calls the "intimate alterity," typical of the mystical emotion, is here expressed at its highest point in the hermetic quality of the inner experience and transcribed into a language that is choppy, allusive, violent. Olga's words thus speak of the reconstruction of the self, of the new identity (though illness) holding the old one (before the discovery) at arm's length. What one usually associates with AIDS are its deathly features, which are indeed its most manifest and tragic characteristic. But one must also, in the light of individual and collective experiences, try to grasp its properly vital dimension as it is expressed in the discourse of the African Renaissance and in practices of moral regeneration, but also finally in that modest ambition: wanting to live.

An African Renaissance

At the International Conference on the African Renaissance organized by Malegapuru William Makgoba and inaugurated by Thabo Mbeki,[16] held in Johannesburg on September 28–29, 1998, Bernard Makhosezwe Magubane (1999: 13–19), member of the Human Science Research Council of South Africa, put the idea the conference intended to celebrate into historical perspective: "The concept of renaissance has received its name from those who thought of the Middle Ages as a dark, trance-like period, from which the human spirit had been awakened. Before the Renaissance, Europe—like Africa—experienced a great instability. From 1300 onwards European society lived through a period of social turmoil that makes Africa's recent troubles seem mild in comparison." After recalling the various forms of this upheaval, he came to the central event, the plague known as the Black Death in the mid-fourteenth century: "Any account of the waning of the Middle Ages must therefore start with the horrors of the Great Plague or Black Death, which reached Europe in 1347. It kept recurring, striking blindly and inexorably for almost fifty years. In the process, the old moorings of society were weakened, as the old certainties lost meaning. It was an episode of exceptional catastrophe that reminds us of AIDS." And he explained further: "You may be asking yourself: What has this to do with the African Renaissance? It seems to me that to understand the idea of the African Renaissance we must take stock of the crises to which the European Renaissance was an answer. Like Europe in the fourteenth century, Africa today is faced with disintegration resulting from the exhaustion of the capitalist mode of production. Our people are bewildered, tormented and suffering. It sometimes seems as though Satan is triumphant. At the end of the millennium, characterized by collapsing assumptions, it is reassuring to know that the human species has lived through worse before." It is probable that Paul Veyne (1971) would find in this peculiar exercise of comparative history an unexpected actualization of his own definition of it: a "heuristic comparison." For the African historian, the European Renaissance makes it possible to formulate the African Renaissance. A particularly performative type of utterance, given the realities of the continent: to speak like J. L. Austin (1970), one can do the latter with the words of the former. The demonstration is entirely centered on the contrast between the dark ages and the luminous tomorrows, on the one hand, and the parallel between the tragedies of medieval Europe and the dramas of contemporary Africa, on the other. In this reasoning the horrors of the present attest the renewal in the future. With a central place given to the illness in its pandemic and murderous form: yesterday the Black Death; today AIDS.

The African Renaissance no more corresponds to a precise political program than to a coherent ideological vision. If this rhetoric is omnipresent in the contemporary South African public arena, it does not, however, deliver a homogeneous discourse about Africa. In fact, it is composed of two quite distinct arguments. The first one is traditionalist and insists on eternal African values, summed up in a word that has become a leitmotiv in contemporary South Africa and well beyond the intellectual circles: the notion of *ubuntu,* reputed to be specifically African, synthesizes a certain sense of humanity and community, a preeminence of the group over the individual. It is to those ancestral resources that national reconstruction appeals, and the mobilization of volunteers in home-based care for AIDS patients, in particular, explicitly refers to these shared traditional values.[17] The second one is modernistic and proposes an economic and political African plan for the world with socialist variations (proposed by a minority) or liberal ones (supported most notably by the president). Its most striking concrete manifestation, though it is still only embryonic, is the New Partnership for Africa's Development (NEPAD), an economic policy embracing several African states. At any rate, it expresses the idea that Africa generally and South Africa in particular have a major role to play in reshaping the global order and, with regard to AIDS, finding African solutions that include setting up an ambitious national research project for a vaccine.[18] Though theoretically opposed, the two orientations are not mutually exclusive in practice: traditional African values sometimes harbor discourses of modernization. But beyond these differences in approach, what unites the various ways of interpreting the African Renaissance is grounded on two elements: resistance to an all-pervasive Afro-pessimism; desire to acknowledge African specificities. The first does not always steer clear of a romantic view of the continent. The second rarely avoids the pitfall of essentializing Africanity. Both, however, participate in a project with which many of the actors I met during my field studies identify and in the name of which they act. Caricatures of this discourse hardly mention this social reality that in fact exceeds the mocked rhetoric (sometimes heavy, one must admit). The African Renaissance certainly is an "Afrocentrism."[19] But compared to the figures that Stephen Howe (1998) has subsumed under the expression "strong Afrocentrisms," especially following the ideas of Cheikh Anta Diop or Martin Bernal, the African Renaissance presents two important differences: the first concerns the relation to time, the second the relation to praxis.

On the one hand, whereas "strong Afrocentrisms" are centrally preoccupied with genealogy, seeking the origins of humanity or civilization in Africa, the African Renaissance is above all, as Lydia Samarbakhsh-Liberge (2000: 390) has put it, a "discourse about history." True, it is speaking of a time immemorial when people lived in blissful communities, but much more than that golden age, what motivates most of those who adhere to it is the reminder of a far less placid past, when African peoples were subjected to oppression and exploitation. No text embodies it better than the famous "I am an African" speech given by Thabo Mbeki in Cape Town on May 8, 1996, before the Constitutional Assembly.

> I owe my being to the Khoi and the San whose desolate souls haunt the great expanses of the beautiful Cape. They who fell victim to the most merciless genocide our native land has ever seen. . . . I am formed of the migrants who left Europe to find a new home on our native land. Whatever their own actions, they remain still part of me. . . . In my veins courses the blood of the Malay slaves who came from the East. Their proud dignity informs my bearing, their culture is a part of my essence. . . . I am the grandchild who lays fresh flowers on the Boer graves, who sees in the mind's eye and suffers the suffering of a simple folk, death, concentration camps, destroyed homesteads, a dream in ruins. . . . I am the child of Nongqause. I am he who made it possible to trade in the world markets in diamonds, in gold, in the same food for which my stomach yearns. . . . I come of those who were transported from India and China, whose being resided in the fact, solely, that they were able to provide physical labour. . . . Being part of all these people, and in the knowledge that none dare contest that assertion, I shall claim that—I am an African.[20]

For Thabo Mbeki, the history of Africa is a tragic one—which is why it must be born again. But Afro-pessimism links the past and the future in the same catastrophic vision. The discourse of African Renaissance on the contrary starts from the historical dramas to imagine a better future based on its own resources.

On the other hand, whereas "strong Afrocentrisms" have a theoretical and ideological foundation, the two being irreducibly connected, the African Renaissance is above all—contrary to what Lodge (1997) would have us think in his systematic critique of its "ideas"—a political praxis. Though it possesses a conceptual apparatus and is embedded in academic discussions, with references to significant twentieth-century African and African American literature, the crux of the matter is its concrete project. Its pragmatism can best be seen in the mixture of talk about tradition and modernity, cultural identity and economic reasoning, national reconciliation and positive discrimination that justify the rise of African capitalism. In concluding the speech on the African Renaissance Thabo Mbeki delivered at the United Nations University in Tokyo on April 8, 1998, he stated the objective: "The first thing we must do, clearly, is to succeed. We must succeed to strengthen and further entrench democracy in our country and inculcate a culture of human rights among all our people, which is indeed happening. We must succeed to rebuild our economies, achieve high and sustained rates of growth, reduce unemployment, and provide a better life to the people, a path on which we have embarked."[21] Thus, for many South Africans who promote it locally and globally, the success of the African Renaissance is to be measured in terms of how much the gross national product has increased or in terms of the social progress accomplished through social justice, much more than in terms of any abstract theory or ideology that a few intellectuals try to develop.

Two weeks before the African Renaissance conference, held in the Johannesburg Hotel Karos Indaba under the auspices of some of the largest South African companies and banks, the Symposium on Social Science and Globalization in Africa took place in the same city at the University of Witwatersrand. If there was a coincidence in the fact that the two events were scheduled almost at the same time, it is certainly revealing of competing paradigms at work in South Africa and more broadly on the continent.[22] In the hotel conference, Africa—analyzed mainly by African scholars—was presented in its historical and cultural singularity; its contribution to the global world could only be imagined on that basis. In the university symposium, Africa—in the view of researchers from throughout the world— was seized in a far more sweeping movement; globalization informed and shaped it while taking from it some of its economic and cultural resources. Between the two intellectual communities, dialogue was impossible. It did not take place then, and it has not since. African Renaissance was construed against a certain world division of power and knowledge.

This opposition takes on two distinct meanings, generally confused in the discourse of its promoters as well as in the refutations of its detractors. On the one hand, it is about the distribution of power in the world, in particular the huge inequalities that can be translated in terms of quantity and quality of life. This is what Thabo Mbeki is saying when he denounces the global imbalance, the plundering of the African continent, the undue profits of the pharmaceutical industry. On the other hand, the conflict is about the universal order of knowledge, in particular, the validity of unanimously accepted explanations and solutions. This is what the president is saying when he rejects the viral theory and sexual transmission in favor of poverty as the explanation for the epidemic. In his first combat, he is backed by the progressive forces that include the activists of the Treatment Action Campaign; in the second, his followers are mainly Afrocentrists and dissidents.[23]

The fact that in this controversy the two figures who best embody the African Renaissance opposed each other so vehemently shows the difference that exists between the two ways of resisting the world order: for Malegapuru William Makgoba, who attacks the power relations existing in the scientific world but not its knowledge, to resist is to produce an African vaccine; for Thabo Mbeki, who interprets knowledge as an expression of power struggles, resistance is inventing an African science.

Thus the exclusive insistence on the question of dissidence has caused many analysts to lose sight of the fact that the African Renaissance is a political mystique far more than a scientific heresy. Even if there are currents of scientific heterodoxy in its midst—on the question of AIDS naturally but also in the field of history and in the social sciences generally—the common denominator for all those who participate in that movement is their faith in the capacity of Africans to surmount their present difficulties. If one considers the lack of interest in Africa by the international community, foreign investors, and pharmaceutical companies, it would be unfair to see in the renascent ideology only an identity closure (though undeniably it is the case for some) while forgetting what it represents above anything else: a refutation of the morbid ideology that is crushing Africa. In the political mystique of the president and of the elite as in the mundane experience of ordinary citizens, to be reborn means resisting death. To use Benedict Anderson's phrase (1983), the "imagined community" of the African Renaissance is less the ethnic or racial community that observers insist on most of the time (and that its promoters also willingly defend) than a community of destiny and of perspective. A community of destiny that means seeing the past as a story of affliction and desiring the future as a promise of resurrection. A community of perspective that emerges in reaction to the pessimistic vision of the other and opens up a horizon of possibles.

A Moral Regeneration

Thabeng and Phumzile met in the support group of the association in the Soweto neighborhood where they live. About twenty AIDS patients come together there every day to exchange local news, share a meal, sometimes schedule activities: right now, the project to create a vegetable garden is on their minds. They are among friends and talk about what cannot be mentioned outside these walls.

Thabeng is twenty-five. He discovered he was HIV-positive a year ago. "Before, I used to drink, to smoke ganja, to take Mandrax. I discovered I was positive last September. From then, I stopped everything." As he recalls, changing his way of life has been a complex process. Shortly before learning about his illness he lost his six-month-old child. The little boy had problems as soon as he was born, and Thabeng and his girlfriend had consulted several healers. The day he died, Thabeng was drunk. He was sleeping, and nobody could wake him up. He did not realize what was happening. At dawn he found his girlfriend and family weeping around the small coffin. Of this scene that had taken place without him he keeps painful memories. When his girlfriend died a few months later, he was at her bedside. He utters this ambiguous phrase: "I was with her all the time to forgive her for all the trouble she had put me into. Meanwhile I was asking myself, 'What is it she wants to say to me?' It was during the funeral that I finally understood: she wanted me to change my life." A few days later, he does the test, discovers he is infected, and decides to lead a new life. He reveals his illness to a close friend and joins the support group. He says he no longer drinks, smokes, or takes drugs.

Phumzile is a little older; she is thirty. She met her first boyfriend when she was seventeen, and they had a child. Then she met another man with whom she had a second child. Her second companion fell ill and died. She then returned to her first boyfriend so as not to stay alone, she explains. They separated once again, and she went back to her mother's place. This is when her first symptoms appeared. She was twenty-five at that time. For several months she remained prostrate, no longer leaving the house or seeing her friends. She hid her condition from everybody. She had a boyfriend but did not dare tell him the truth: "I did not disclose to him. I just asked him to use condoms. But he did not want to." One day, while watching a television program on AIDS, Phumzile saw a young woman who was explaining that she is infected: "I saw this beautiful woman. She stands up and says she's positive. I told myself, 'There's life there.' After the show, I called to get information and they told me about support groups. From then my life changed. My family did not know about my condition. I went to my mother and told her everything about it. And I started a better life. I became pretty myself. You must respect yourself so that people respect you. In funerals, for example, you shouldn't be drinking. When I go out, people I haven't seen for some time tell me, 'You are beautiful!'"

For Thabeng and Phumzile, being together means sharing their illness. They do not have to explain; they know. They understand each other. They remind each other to take their pills. "I am very happy with him," she explains, "because when I feel bad I can talk with him. Each and every pain I can share with him." And Thabeng adds, "It's easier when both are positive because you have the same problems. We even make jokes out of it. When one is having trouble, the other laughs, 'It's that AIDS of yours which is starting again.'" Their plans are first of all to find work in a home-based care organization and make themselves useful to others, because for the time being they are surviving on their disability grant; then they want to marry and have children but through adoption, so as not to take any risks. "I know they will find a cure and we want to be here for it," they say. At the time of this interview, the government was on the point of making antiretroviral drugs available in the public health care system. I ask them if they are going to go to the hospital to ask for them. They answer, "We won't go there, because these treatments have side effects." They establish a clear distinction between the "cure" that gets rid of the disease and the "treatments" that only prolong life. They eagerly await the first but are suspicious of the second. Both died a few months later without having received either of them.

In the many narratives collected in Soweto and Alexandra or in Limpopo, it is remarkable that when AIDS sets in—or rather, when people discover they are HIV-positive—their normal life is totally disrupted. This change may seem obvious with respect to the gravity of the prognosis and given the absence of treatment. The disruption means more, however, than simply looking forward to suffering and death. For precisely in view of that outcome, a different life is in fact about to begin, conceived of as a new life in the strongest sense. The existence of persons living with AIDS is based on a set of new values: truth, faithfulness, dignity, respect, solidarity. Each of these values deserves comment. One no longer hides one's diagnosis but confides in close friends, and sometimes even discloses it publicly. One no longer has multiple love affairs but builds a future with a partner, who frequently is also HIV-positive. One no longer lets oneself go to drinking or taking drugs but becomes virtuous, even a model for others. One is no longer ashamed of the sickness but accepts it, going to support groups where everyone shares the same experience. One is no longer immured in one's misfortune but becomes compassionate to others' affliction and sometimes volunteers to work in home-based care. Of course, these are norms, and they are not necessarily respected.

Mesias, who hid his illness for several months from his companion and future spouse, Phindile, explains it: "After disclosing my status to my dearest wife, I started a new life. I realized it was a new life, because I was living in a free world where I knew there will be no more heavy questions for her." Shortly after, he manages to convince her to be tested also: "I assured her if you become positive in your mind you won't die and you will live long. So after that assurance she took it seriously and she went to the test and she was positive and the real life started from there." For him as for many others I met, the disruption brings liberation from the old life and conversion to a new life. The revelation of the illness is their road to Damascus. The dual phenomenon of liberation and conversion is deeply moral. The person's scale of ethical values is turned upside down. One becomes another man or another woman. And where the illness is concerned, one expects a concrete benefit from that metamorphosis. "Healing is performative," writes Gay Becker (1997: 153). This individual transformation I have described is, however, embedded in a collective movement. There are two sides to the social discourse expressing the moral revolution: the first one is religious, the second one political.

The "born again" experience is deeply anchored in the South African Christian churches, from the Zion Christian Church (ZCC) to the Apostolic Faith Mission through the Pentecostals and several others.[24] Many patients describe a conversion that is both religious and moral, like Mesias, whom Phindile convinced to accompany her to the ZCC so he would find inner peace, return to the straight and narrow, and perhaps receive an effective treatment for AIDS. This is how Astrid, a young woman living with AIDS in Alexandra, expresses rebirth: "The time will come when people will know. The Bible tells us that incurable diseases will come in the last days. The way you believe is a booster of your immune system. God said: be strong. I am strong. I am not going to die. I am a real fighter. I am not of the dying type [she laughs]. Those drugs will prolong my life and I will live, live, live. It's in my mind. You must have a new identity. I tell my church: I'm the child of God. I'm a new person. I'm the child of God." The relationship between religion and morality is more complex than is often supposed. It cannot amount to the simple idea that religious conversion is the source of moral regeneration. It would probably be closer to the truth to see religious practices and moral values as the common inheritance of a missionary culture that Comaroff and Comaroff (1991) have analyzed.

It is in that sense that a volunteer for an Alexandra home-based care organization declared that to face the hardship of their work with the sick, they had sessions of "religious debriefing" three times a week: it consisted in "praying, singing, and reading the Bible," she explained. I found the expression a remarkable hybrid that reworks a psychological notion in the language of religion to express the local management of the "trauma."[25] Psychology as a lay religion or maybe, conversely, religion as practical psychology: it is easy to see that beyond the historical differences, this has to do with global configurations that allow an interpretation of the local worlds. This pragmatism is attested by the ease with which many of my interviewees changed churches, sometimes for geographic reasons, often because they came across zealous priests promising a cure, but almost never seeing anything more to it than the effect of circumstances. Making an effort to live one's life morally becomes meaningful when held up against the whole set of religious dispositions that are relatively independent of the activities of African churches. Conversion somehow updates religious culture and illness justifies its moral dimension. But they are also confirmed by another, secular type of discourse.

The political division of ideological labor in South Africa has it that former Deputy President Jacob Zuma was charged with voicing moral regeneration and the president with promoting the African Renaissance.[26] The official history of what in 2002 became a national action under the banner of the Moral Regeneration Movement began in 1998 with the Moral Summit called for by then-President Nelson Mandela that brought together spiritual and political leaders. Following that initiative, workshops, publications, and a national referendum preceded the creation of the movement led by Jacob Zuma. As the former president defined it, the message of moral regeneration depends on collective ethics more than on individual behavior. Already on December 16, 1997, in the famous Mafikeng policy speech marking the fiftieth anniversary of the ANC, Mandela had called for "moral renewal," justifying it in the following terms: "It is out of the great human tragedy which marked the period of the colonial and apartheid domination in our country, superimposed on and integrated within the universal impact of the modern market mechanism that we have inherited what we see on the surface of human activity in our country, including the corruption of civil servants by the private sector, the low level of tax morality, white-collar crime and the subversion of business ethics, venality, theft and fraud within the public sector, the uninhibited commitment to unbridled self-gratification which underlies such crimes as rape and child abuse." Two characteristics clearly distinguish this discourse from the corresponding religious ideology: its historical inscription and its political implications. The facts being challenged are the result of a past of oppression and concern the common good of the nation. Even the acts that can be given a more psychological and especially individual dimension, such as murder or rape, possess a social dimension. It is a militant discourse marked by the struggle for freedom and democracy.

The direction subsequently taken by that mobilization (which also included traditional authorities) was to absorb some of the cultural overtones of the African Renaissance: the idealized community and *ubuntu*. But it also changes with the problems of society, as was clear in the speech Jacob Zuma gave at the Moral Regeneration Movement's rally on May 12, 2000: "As we appeal to our people to lend a hand for the betterment of the lives of those affected by the HIV and AIDS epidemic, we also want to make a call to all South Africans to behave in a manner that would not endanger their lives." Aside from the specific phraseology, it is tempting to see in this speech a type of discourse not too removed from that employed in other places and other times (by international backers, development agency directors, or heads of state in their ritual invocations destined to assuage the collective conscience). There is something more here, however, and the interviews carried out with men and women who have lived through the two or three past decades show that the rhetoric and the promises it contains truly echo the spirit of the "new beginnings" Philip Bonner and Lauren Segal (1998) wrote about in their social history of Soweto. For many of those who were or dreamed of becoming the militants in the project for a new world, political morality is not an empty notion.

This all signifies that what might simply appear as patients' good intentions when they discover their illness—reminiscent of the way the European heart or lung patient decides to stop smoking less for the physical than for the moral benefit he or she hopes to derive from that decision—takes on a much more important social meaning due to the double ideology, religious as well as political. There is, if one can put it that way, an atmosphere of moral regeneration to which the actors are subscribing when inventing their new lives, and ostensibly individual decisions thus join the mainstream. Where AIDS is concerned, however, it would be a mistake to exaggerate the practical effects of such moral transformations, and it is not certain that health education specialists should hasten to include moralistic discourse in their programs. A young woman from Lenyenye who declared she had decided to live differently, especially to stop having multiple lovers, explained her evolution much more pragmatically than ideologically: "I don't have somebody to support me, so I have to find men to support me. When I jump to the next one, I know this one does not have money anymore. Recently I met a man who was rich enough. I'm with him since last October. He's a contract person on the tar roads. He's got the latest BMW. I go once a month to his place. He lives in town. He's married. I didn't tell him I'm positive, but I ask him to use condoms." Her new fidelity is less the result of the moral choice it is claimed to be than the product of circumstances that allowed her to find a rich protector (who probably had similar affairs in several cities). If circumstances change—if her boyfriend stops seeing and helping her—she will naturally have to adapt. She says furthermore: "There is no difference between my present boyfriend and my previous ones. Except that as I saw he was coming regularly and had money, I decided to stop seeing the others." Morality and pragmatism are not mutually exclusive.

An even clearer illustration of the precariousness of such conversions can be seen in Pearl and Mbembathisi's story. When I first met them in their Alexandra apartment they were not only the most romantic and tender couple one could imagine but also the most resolute about the radical changes they planned. Pearl said she had lived an easy life in the township where her grandparents owned a bar and were well-off. In the 1990s, she explained, one could have fun with boys. It is in that context that she discovered she was HIV-positive. From that moment on, she was tired of a life of pleasures and only found comfort with her boyfriend. "I want to marry him before I die," she would say. Mbembathisi recounted he had known the indistinct borders separating the struggle with his comrades and committing crimes with the *tsotsis* of the 1980s. He had thus participated in the murder of persons suspected of collaborating with the white regime and in the arson of a house where a young woman accused of being a policeman's mistress had perished along with her children, her dogs, and her cats, as he put it. Thrown in jail for having shot a policeman who was paralyzed as a result, he was infected by a cellmate who raped him. "Since I discovered I am positive," he tells me, "I have started to live positively." When he said he wanted to become a minister, get married, and have a child, Pearl laughed and said she was afraid of dying from complications if she got pregnant (to dissuade HIV-positive women from becoming pregnant, nurses tell them that their bodies will not be able to take it). Pearl and Mbembathisi spent a great deal of time together speaking of their illness, and she confided that if their state worsened they wanted to die together. A year later, when asking about them, I learned they had separated. She had become a prostitute in a bar in the township; he had joined his delinquent friends. Both had gone back to their old ways.

Life as Survival

In an interview given when he was seriously ill, Jacques Derrida made this profound comment that had both ontological and personal meanings:

Long before the experience of survival which is now mine, I indicated that surviving is an original concept, the very backbone of what we call existence. We are structurally survivors, marked by the structure of the trace, of the testament. But having said this, I would not like to leave myself open to the interpretation of survival as being on the side of death and the past more than on the side of life and the future. Everything I say about survival as being a complication of the opposition between life and death stems from my unconditional love of life. Survival is life beyond life, life more than life, and my discourse is not aimed at death. On the contrary, it is the affirmation of a live person who prefers to live and thus to survive rather than to die, for survival is not only what remains, it is living the most intensely.[27]

He died a few weeks later.

Sociological and anthropological literature has made much use of the word *survival* to account for the living conditions and resistance strategies in the ordinary context of poverty or in the exceptional circumstances to which displaced or oppressed populations are exposed. The word *survivor* itself, which originally indicated that one had come through an extreme situation such as a concentration camp, has become banal to the point of signifying the time after any traumatic event. In the first case, one speaks of strategies of survival; in the second, of the survivor's resilience. But however the word is used, it functions as an objectification. To speak of survival means to speak of the basic needs that must be met—this is what I myself have done in describing the sexual transaction of women who sell their bodies for a meal or for shelter. To speak of survivors means speaking of living after a critical event—and one uses the term *survivors* to describe rape victims. Words create a distance here between the observer and the subject. But objectification is done without really knowing what it means to survive. That is what Derrida is talking about: of a subjectivity that is both shared by all human beings and unique to each, which is both the ontological experience of being "survivors structurally" and the personal experience of the "affirmation of a live person who prefers to live and thus to survive rather than to die." Works in the social sciences rarely mention subjectivity. But there is more. The experience that I am discussing here is different from what is usually said about it. In common sense as in scientific discourse, to survive means—one supposes—to undergo suffering. Both terms are important: "to undergo" implies passivity; "suffering" has a negative connotation. In this sense, surviving is a passion. Breaking with this approach consists on the contrary in saying that "survival is not only what remains, it is living the most intensely." It transforms surviving into action. This active subjectivity is what I encountered in the townships of Alexandra and Soweto, sometimes too in the villages of Limpopo.

Echoing the philosopher's words, Mesias had told us, "The only thing is that the challenge of life will be when you wake up in the morning, that will be a great thing, that will be a challenge of life—as long as you wake up in the morning. Because, you know, our process is to be born and to die—but in between that is life." When I asked him to explain what life meant to him now, he answered simply, "It's just normal life. Normal life is what people live out of it. That is normal life: Having food in your stomach, having somebody next to you, being respected in your community." What he was describing was precisely what he possessed: the pension that allowed him not to depend on his family; the presence of his wife with whom he had finally settled in a little house; the respect won in the eyes of others, if not for success at least for courage in face of the illness. Nothing very much, all told, and probably his life was more than that (he sometimes conducted health education work in the neighborhood, participated from time to time in the activities of a patients' association, kept busy looking for work that he ended up finding), but the existence without qualities that he described had become the center around which he had built his life (or better, rebuilt his life, as it was the exact opposite of what it had been before: alcohol, girl-friends, violence). He concluded, "I am always free, you know, always free. If I think of coming home, I feel like I am going to heaven."

Coming from this still young man who did not consider taking anti-retroviral drugs (though he knew his immune defenses were very low) and who spoke about what he must do before he died (finish paying for the land he had bought and build a house for his wife), coming therefore from this man who had no illusions about the time he had left, those words contained the essence of the meaning of survival. When trying to define happiness, which in his *Ethics* he identifies with the supreme good, Aristotle distinguishes three dimensions of existence: the physical, the sensitive, and the moral.[28] It seems to me that those are the three dimensions we find in Mesias's words, and, moreover, in the testimony of many AIDS sufferers I met during my years of research. Living once death has been announced means ensuring the continuity of the living body (by being careful, by watching what one eats, by taking certain medicines and not others); it also means enjoying life (by limiting pain, looking out for the simple pleasures, surrounding oneself with loved ones); it means, finally, being virtuous in the remaining time (being faithful to one's spouse, caring for one's children, saving up for one's own funeral expenses, showing consideration for those who will be left behind, sometimes still participating in the collective life such as a patients' association or a support group). Needs, pleasure, and virtue: the three define a practical ethics of life I often encountered in South Africa.

For Aristotle, however, the moral existence is the only one that truly corresponds to happiness and therefore to the supreme good, because, as he says, it is "specific to man." A long philosophical tradition inspired by the Greek philosopher, from Walter Benjamin to Giorgio Agamben through Hannah Arendt, opposes biological or physical life (*zoē*) and moral or political life (*bios*), praising the latter to the detriment of the former. From this perspective, life in the *polis* represents a higher ideal than existing *per se*. The South African experience of AIDS—and this probably transcends one single context—nevertheless invites us to reevaluate the "simple fact of living," in Walter Benjamin's words. Survival, for the stricken individuals and also perhaps for the whole nation shaken by the epidemic, means finding meaning in the finitude of existence, a meaning of which healthy individuals and richer nations have lost the trace. That life deserves to be seen as something else other than what does not distinguish us from other animals, as a little more than what typifies a slave's destiny, which is how Aristotle refers to *zoē* as opposed to *bios* characterizing the free man. For those who live it, it does indeed possess the meaning of a moral and political subjectivity. To echo Michel Foucault (2001), who formulated this idea precisely at the end of his life, the "care of the self" is also a care for others: in short, an ethics. It seems to me that if we read Aristotle's *Politics* carefully, we discover that he himself was not insensible to that sort of subjectivity: "It is also with the simple aim of living that men join together and maintain a political community: for doubtless there is already something morally admirable in the sole fact of living, at least as long as the difficulties of life are not too excessive. Besides, one sees the majority of men endure much suffering in their passionate love of life, as if it contained a certain calm and sweetness in its very nature." If we disregard the somewhat condescending "already," we see the contours of what can be considered an ethics of survival.

Survival, therefore. Requalifying what has often been disqualified and being attentive to what it means to live on the edge of death implies inscribing the simple fact of living on the political agenda. But it also implies giving back to the agents who are at that point in their life the subjectivity of which they are frequently deprived when their experience is translated into the supposedly objective terms of analysis. Of course, it is always perilous—epistemologically first, then ethically—to pretend one can talk about the subjectivity of others. What do we know, in the end, of the other's actual experience? Since Wittgenstein ([1953] 2004: 136), we understand there is something insurmountable there: "How do words refer to sensations?" he asks. And further on: "How can I go as far as to want to intervene by means of language between pain and its expression? I am the only one to know if I really suffer; another person will merely suspect it." Thus is it at this outer limit that anthropologists can operate—that is, not only by imposing their own thoughts as they analyze the words of their subjects which have become their object of study but also by making their subjects' voices audible and clarifying the significance they attribute to their actions and words. It would be extremely dangerous in this regard to consider that an AIDS patient's survival is a life no longer worth living because it is only pain, misery, degradation. My interviewees say otherwise. They do otherwise. They survive otherwise. When one patient speaks about living "a normal life," and when another says she "wants to die once married," they assert they belong to the world of the living. When one chooses to use the meager disability grant to pay her mother's debts and help her younger brother, and when another takes a rich lover to be able to continue dressing elegantly and raising her children decently, they are confirming their attachment to this life, not only because it is good, but also because it is dignified to live it. In exchange for the stories they have received from them, anthropologists should consider they owe them to say so.

In his reflection on suffering, Stanley Cavell (1997: 98) makes an interesting distinction: "The difference between natural and social science is not that one is interpretive and the other is not, but that in one case conviction in its objectivity is continuous (except in intellectual crises) and that in the other conviction may have to be won afresh in each project (as if there were nothing but crises)." The anthropologist must take the risk of objectification, even going so far as to explore the other as subject. Pursuing his idea, the philosopher adds: "My knowledge of myself is something I find, as on a successful quest; my knowledge of others is something that finds me." Hence, the little—and least—one should expect from the anthropologist is to account for that something: "It seems reasonable to me, and illuminating, to speak of that reception of impression as lending my body to the other's experience. The plainest manifestation of this responsiveness may be taken to be its effect on a body of writing." It is in this body of writing that the words of the philosopher of deconstruction and the words of the AIDS sufferer, Derrida and Mesias, can legitimately come together—in what they are saying about their mutual survival. It is in this body of writing that the anthropologist seeks the meaning of his work.

PROPOSITION 6: POLITICS OF LIFE

In South Africa, AIDS biopolitics have often seemed like "necropolitics," to use Achille Mbembe's (2003) expression. While modern forms of "governmentality" consider life the main target for government action, while the "technologies" of living organisms are the primary characteristic of normalization systems, while "the disciplines of the body and the regulation of populations," following Foucault (1976), sum up the state's mode of intervention par excellence, South Africa—and along with her, the whole of the African continent with its civil wars, ethnic conflicts, and exterminating deliriums—has been portrayed as an exception in the supposedly universal process of civilization—to sound this time like Norbert Elias (1982), who tried to test his theory in Africa at the end of his life.

In the polemics triggered by AIDS, the government's policy, particularly insofar as the delays in implementing the prevention of antenatal transmission is concerned, has been termed a "genocide" by some—such as the satirist Pieter-Dierk Huys or the research scholar Malegapuru William Makgoba—a "holocaust" by others—such as Judge Edwin Cameron or the activist Zachie Achmat.[29] These politics of death are equally reflected in the intellectuals' more analytic but no less dramatic reasoning, as in the following text by Ulrike Kirstner: "In Mbeki's logic of governance, the right to life and the right to life-saving and life-prolonging drugs, comes under the sovereign power of state officials. It brings to mind the original definition of absolute sovereign power: namely the power to let live and make die."[30] In the interviews I carried out with residents of Soweto as well as with academics in Johannesburg, it was a recurrent theme, like a dreadful and prophetic refrain of which an inhabitant of the townships gave the following version: "When we are sitting down in the support group, we discuss. This is what we say. The ANC wants us to die. Most people with HIV are unskilled, uneducated, unemployed. *We* are unskilled, uneducated, unemployed. How will the government benefit from us? The more numerous we are, the more problems we cause. If they can get rid of us, there will be less unemployment, less crime. Let them die." The tragic interpretation of politics espouses Zygmunt Bauman's (2004) depiction of contemporary societies in which he denounced the production of "wasted lives." Another aspect appears, however, in this man's words: their extermination, not actively through physical violence, but passively by therapeutic abstention.

The parallel with apartheid is the backdrop for this vision, a parallel that was first used, as we saw, to express the principle of the new struggle. Chris Hani used it in his famous speech in 1990 in Maputo, saying in substance: we have rid ourselves of the scourge that we supported for decades, let us not allow ourselves to be caught short by the one that is coming. It is also in that spirit that the Treatment Action Campaign launched its prevention program in 2001 during the twenty-fifth anniversary of the Soweto uprising: the posters showing yesterday's and today's victims side by side underlined the message. But then the comparison progressively shifted from the struggle as such toward the object being combated: "AIDS is our new apartheid" is a phrase coined by Archbishop Desmond Tutu and often heard afterward. And finally, from the combated object we pass to the combated subject: the government of today has thus been likened to the government of yesterday in a rhetoric that covers far more than AIDS and has become a leitmotiv expressing the public's dissatisfaction with the authorities: "It's even worse than during apartheid," one often hears or reads. National officials and representatives are not exempt from this escalation, with the difference that criticism there turns into accusations of racism, systematically used to discredit opponents, including references again to the argument that the adversaries want to exterminate the African population, an argument that the president implicitly and the health minister explicitly have publicly employed.

"Power over life" and "race war": the two Foucauldian themes of his 1976 lectures at the Collège de France (1997) have merged in the South African public arena. We know that for Foucault, the two characteristics of Western politics of modernity are, on the one hand, the transition from "sovereignty" (the right to "make die and let live") to "biopower" (the right to "make live and let die") and, on the other, the transformation of "race war" from a conflict naturalized within a state to "state racism" that implements nonbelligerent forms of eugenics.[31] The point where these two transformations meet, between the power of life and state racism, depends on where the break is made: "the break between what must live and what must die." This policy takes the form of the elimination of the weakest, the "abnormal," the "degenerate," in order to make "life generally more healthy and pure." Whence "the importance of racism," which is "the condition permitting one to exert the old sovereign right to kill." In other words, state racism is what has been left over from sovereignty in contemporary biopolitics. The thesis is forceful but problematic, especially because it claims to apply to all contemporary configurations regardless of their historical context or political project: "There is hardly any modern state functioning that at a given moment and within certain limits, in certain conditions, does not experience racism." That lack of differentiation in the South African discourse is what causes the polemic to swell and finally politics to dissolve. It is, on the contrary, differentiation that I wish to place in the foreground.

Because the apartheid regime postulated the social and political inequality of a priori racially defined, in other words, biologically qualified, groups,[32] it succeeded fully and completely—like the Nazi regime in another context—in superimposing power over life and state racism: if eliminating the enemies and even eradicating the black race were a possibility on the horizon that certain groups in the state margins tried to realize (for instance in the chemical and biological warfare but also in a whole series of other projects), fundamentally the dominant principle was one of separation and exclusion. Politics in Arendt's (1995) sense, that is, living together in "human plurality," was twice rejected: ideologically and practically. One might therefore say that the racist biopolitics of apartheid were the negation of politics. Better yet: they represented the end of politics, to use the idea put forth by Agnes Heller (1996: 3), for whom "politics begins where biological ties and determinations cease to be overarching, where the membership in a common political body takes precedence over the solidarity with biological body." Apartheid ended the possibility of politics.

On the contrary, the postapartheid regime rests not on the equality of racial groups but on their nonpertinence: races do not exist; therefore, there is no reason to proclaim them equal. National reconstruction is at that price—at least according to official ideology. But it hits up against the reality principle, on the one hand, which claims that each individual, group, and institution has been raised and socialized into thinking in terms of race, and, on the other hand, the history backlash, for, independently of all reality, the past never ceases to surge and stir people up. Once it is stated that races do not exist, contradictions appear whether in statistics, if only to measure inequalities, or in the policies of affirmative action, consisting precisely in correcting them. Invoking race in the public debate, when it is not simply a question of cynical calculations, means that what exists no more in the law does exist in society, in people's minds and bodies. So "postapartheid" condemns racist biopolitics yet conserves its trace. This is what justifies the prefix *post-*, for it is an afterward that intimately preserves the imprint of the before. In that way too, postapartheid is a return to politics, in its Arendtian sense: a difficult return, in suffering, contradiction, and conflict, but a return nevertheless. Its horizon is a common humanity. But a humanity that does not forget.

AIDS, however, causes the biological question to crop up once again in politics. Yet, except if one blatantly misinterprets the facts, it must be admitted that the politics of life being played out around the epidemic have nothing to do with the racial biopolitics of the ancient regime, except that they are its heritage, as postapartheid is apartheid's heir. The unequal socioracial distribution of the infection attests to it as much as the violent controversy that has been its hallmark. But what is today's politics that point in two radically different directions—that of the government and that of the activists—and in the name of which the most violent battles the South African nation has known since its liberation are being fought? Are they but one in two opposite forms or, as the government's opponents claim, a politics of death versus a politics of life? To answer that question, we must go back, once again thinking with Arendt [1959: 85], to the more or less clear distinction established between two words that in ancient Greek texts (Aristotle in particular) mean life: *zoē,* the physical life "driven by the motor of biological life which man shares with other living things"; and *bios,* the social life specific to human beings "full of events which ultimately can be told as a story, establish a biography." This opposition was radicalized by Agamben (1997), who speaks of "bare life"—the one inscribed in the body—and "political existence"—the one created by language; for him, modernity is characterized by the fact that "the space of bare life, situated at first in the wings of political organization, progressively ends up coinciding with political space." But in the South African history of AIDS, far from merging as his theory would have us expect, the two politics—of *zoē* and *bios*—collide.

On the one side, the activists and with them those fighting to gain access to treatment in all its forms (prophylactic for the newborn and for rape victims, therapeutic for patients) inscribe their crusade in the register of biological existence. Their slogan in this respect is clear: the right to life. For them, every life saved is valuable in and of itself and the unceasing proclamation of figures recalling the thousands of children it would theoretically be possible to spare thanks to antiretroviral drugs is above all the expression of a sum of physical existences. Hence their incomprehension when the risk of increasing inequalities in the face of illness and death is invoked by the government, since given the economic and health realities of the country, some will receive medicine and others will not: to a certain extent, for them, that criticism cannot object to saving lives, however few. I have proposed we speak in this case of biolegitimacy.[33] On the other side, not considering the strictly heterodox positions that quite obviously appeal to different logics, the government (through its fight against poverty and discrimination) brandishes another form of common good, in the hope of reducing inequalities in access to food as much as to treatment. Its slogan would more likely be: the right to justice. The life it is defending is political. To do this, it depends on the legitimacy it received, and is still receiving, from its constituency, but also, and this is too often forgotten, the polls in which unemployment and violence are far ahead of AIDS among the preoccupations of South African citizens. I suggest that we interpret this perspective as the traditional expression of sovereignty.[34] Of course, the conceptual opposition I have drawn here is too cut-and-dried. First, the activists, who when interviewed admit their fight is based on the principle of biolegitimacy as presented here, also—rightly—affirm that they progressively took their opponents' arguments into consideration, to integrate the question of equity in the problem of access to medicine. Second, the government, which never stops referring to the people as the incarnation of sovereignty, is also in its own way—and legitimately—defending a form of bare life, the one of basic needs, and of enough food to begin with. Nevertheless, in this confrontation between two politics of life—and certainly not a politics of life versus a politics of death—I see the theoretical heart of the controversies that have torn the country apart for a decade now.

Yet that opposition is not insurmountable. Several elements show that it is already concretely being challenged in people's daily acts and commitments. That is the meaning of the prevention and care programs that have never stopped functioning even at the highest point of the polemic and more recently of the roll-out of antiretroviral drugs decided by the government at the same time as the increase in social grants, especially for patients and orphans. But perhaps the confusion between the two forms of life has never been as evident as when the agents expose it and in fact play on it, in the strong sense of the term. By refusing to take antiretroviral drugs as long as they were not available to everyone in the public sector, at least in principle, TAC chairperson Zachie Achmat courageously and publicly threw his own physical existence into the balance and introduced bare life into political action, just as Supreme Court judge Edwin Cameron did by being the first important person of the South African state to announce that he was HIV-positive and gay.[35] Such gestures illustrate in the most convincing way possible what the new politics of life is becoming, what Nikolas Rose (2001) calls, after Adriana Petryna, a "biological citizenship," that is, "a universal human right to protection, at least of the bare life of the person and of the dignity of their living body." In such a regime, "all human lives have the same value" at least in theory, because in practice we very well know that on the contrary "biological lives of individual human beings are permanently submitted to judgements of value." Nikolas Rose is referring here especially to the domains of medicine, genetics, and ethics. But the remark touches on more than the realm of biomedicine.

The affirmation that all lives have the same value—on which, taking off from very different premises, both the activists seeking to save those who can be saved and the government trying to defend an ideal of social justice may agree—is belied by the biological evidence of premature deaths (young adults and their children as AIDS victims, but also as victims of other illnesses, homicides, and accidents); it is also contradicted by the political evidence of lives that have never really counted (for a long time, even their deaths went unrecorded under the apartheid regime). The inequality of lives, biological and political, local and global, is perhaps the greatest violence with which anthropologists are confronted in the field, as they daily prove the truly existential and vital distance that separates them from the men and women whose histories and lives they encounter.

CONCLUSION

This World We Live In

This world needs a wash and a week's rest.

W. H. AUDEN
The Age of Anxiety

ON APRIL 17, 2004, South Africa celebrated the ten-year anniversary of the end of apartheid. General elections were held that very day, and the ANC won a landslide victory that was also a personal triumph for its leader, Thabo Mbeki. His party took more of the vote than it had with Nelson Mandela directly after the fall of the hated regime. Few observers noted, though, that in the vast opinion poll conducted a few weeks before, 86 percent of Africans said they would vote for the ANC, 0 percent for the Democratic Alliance, the main opposition party, and the figures were almost exactly reversed for whites: 1 percent and 69 percent respectively. There were huge celebrations in the various spheres and levels; in Pretoria, forty heads of state and approximately ten prime ministers attended a ceremony in the presidential gardens (France was represented only by its foreign minister), and on the city's public lawns tens of thousands of South Africans, most just ordinary citizens, gathered to express their emotion (little notice was taken again of the fact that there were hardly any whites among them). A few weeks earlier, the roll-out of antiretroviral drugs had begun in all the country's major hospitals, putting an official end to the long controversy over AIDS treatment. These events did not draw much international media attention, however. America was discovering with horror that its soldiers regularly practiced torture in Iraqi prisons and that it was known and had been covered up at the highest military levels. The European Union was electing representatives for the first time as a twenty-five-member entity, a process for which there was little enthusiasm among either old or new members: voter turnout proved unprecedentedly low. France was reassured to see itself unified in its protest against the anti-Semitic acts being committed on its soil while continuing to ignore the daily ordeal of racial discrimination in its poor segregated neighborhoods. During the weekend preceding the South African election, all the major French television stations, both public and private, had joined together to organize a televisual demonstration focused on the AIDS cause; the point was to remind viewers that infection was still a threat. The programs spoke little of Africa, where it is hardly necessary, however, to recall this obvious fact. Only the controversial presentation of a documentary on the origin of AIDS in which it is maintained that Africans were accidentally contaminated by polio vaccines in the 1950s provoked some discontent, which the filmmakers then responded to with various arguments and self-justifications.

In the prologue to *The Age of Anxiety,* W. H. Auden (1991: 449) writes of moments "when the historical process breaks down," "when necessity is associated with horror and freedom with boredom." It seems fair to say that today's world is undergoing such a moment, between "times of peace," when "there are always a number of persons who wake up each morning excited by the prospect of another day of interesting and difficult work, or happily certain that the one with whom they shared their bed last night will be sharing it with them again the next," and "war-time," when "everybody is reduced to the anxious status of a shady character or a displaced person," when "even the most prudent become worshippers of chance." This observation is not mere doomsday prophesying. The "age of anxiety" we are living in can indeed be conceived of as a kind of intermediary period in which, at both the national and planetary levels, the security of a minority is bolstered and fueled by the insecurity of the majority and order reigns at the center to the detriment and disordering of the periphery. Ours is an age of anxiety precisely because of the tension that exists between what is being protected and what is being abandoned, what is being fought for and what is given up for lost. In a world of inequality and violence, we can only be reassured on condition that we conceal from ourselves the price that must be paid for such reassurance.

In this respect, the history of AIDS in South Africa can be read as paradigmatic of the world we live in today. It was reassuring yesterday to be able to describe the controversy surrounding the etiology of the disease and the suspected dangers posed by treatments as nothing more than a marginal phenomenon, the misguided notions of a discredited group of dissidents and the whim of a paranoid president. So we did not seriously consider the meaning of an interpretation that put social concerns at the core of the AIDS epidemic, and we did not value the social relevance of this interpretation. It is reassuring today to learn that antiretroviral drugs are at last available and arrangements for home-based care are in place. But we are not asking about the objective conditions in which men and women continue to become infected, the conditions in which they are given access to therapeutic drugs and are followed for their side effects, the conditions in which, very simply, patients work, eat, live. It was perhaps reassuring to think that there are sexual behaviors and cultural representations that favor the spread of the disease. So we did not evaluate how heavily the historical realities of racial disparities, gender inequalities, and production relations weigh in the spread of the disease, or look into what has happened to people in the mines and on the farms, in the townships and former homelands. It is reassuring to see civil society organizing to fight AIDS as it did to fight apartheid. But we are not attending to the deep wounds, rancor, resentment, and suspicion left by the many years of struggle. Moving beyond the framework of AIDS, we are relieved to see this decidedly strong, dynamic democracy take action, just as we were relieved recently to see peace return and reconciliation under way. But we are no more ready today than yesterday to see the presence of the past in the present, a past that will obliterate the future as long as it is not recognized as such; that is, as long as it is recognized not only as memory to be honored but also as present in which the past is reactualized.

A few years ago, Orin Starn (1992: 152) raised the question of why and how anthropology had "missed the revolution" in Peru, letting itself drift along using old traditionalist or populist approaches to the Indians, failing to see the economic and social distress of the Andes peasants, which was facilitating the rise of armed movements, first among them Shining Path. Perhaps we should ask if today we are not missing other revolutions, less audible and visible but undoubtedly violent to judge by the estimated number of victims and above all the sweeping changes these revolutions foreshadow. Social science researchers, who have tended to dismiss social theories about the AIDS epidemic and those who promote them, denouncing more quickly than they analyze, should not feel they are exempt from this doubt, particularly when they set out to construct the AIDS epidemic. I do not wish to err on the side of pessimism with such probing, particularly since I am convinced by South Africa's demonstration of the ability of its political and intellectual elites and population to cope with this great challenge while maintaining its democratic values. But it is not my purpose here to assess this historical success, which seems to me undeniable; rather, it is to grasp what the South African experience of AIDS can tell us about some of the most crucial issues in today's world. What I have described here of inequality in the face of death, which is first and foremost inequality in life, and of sexual violence, which is also social violence, exemplifies the inequality and violence that affects bodies and afflicts the weak everywhere in the world. Controversies and rumors, distrust of medical treatments and reluctance to believe in medical experts' impartiality, the idea of a national or an international plot—these phenomena attest to the logic of suspicion and resentment that can prevail in situations of domination, and they offer a stunning demonstration of how knowledge and power are intimately related. Interpretations of the world in terms of race and accusations of racism, the feeling of a common cause uniting all black people regardless of national borders or continents, reference to genocidal projects or intentions—these phenomena suggest a full-blown imaginary of race war rooted in the harsh reality of racial discrimination and conflict.

The "pathologies of power" that Paul Farmer (2003) writes of extend beyond the material dimension of social determinations of the disease to the discursive dimension of political interpretations of it. They exceed the limits of the physical body and affect the social body as a whole. Moreover, local space is porous, open to global realities, just as it can itself shed light on global realities. These facts suggest that it is useful and worthwhile to relate the ethnography of South Africa to world history. Media-reported facts about the rest of the planet take on different meaning in light of information collected in the field. We can no longer take lightly the graffiti on Alexandra township walls that glorifies "Bin Laden" scrawled next to calls to "Kill the Boers," any more than we can underestimate the meaning of the contrast so often noted in South Africa between the compassion shown to the United States by Western countries after the attack against the twin towers and those same countries' indifference to the destruction of a building in Nairobi, when both events were due to terrorism and only the victims—Americans, Africans—were different. We cannot understand the South African president's unbending support for Jean-Bertrand Aristide, which moved him to offer the Haitian leader asylum after he was thrown out of power, if we do not understand his sense of South Africans' and Haitians' shared destiny: enslaved, the Haitian people were able to liberate themselves, just as black South Africa, persecuted by apartheid, was able to defeat its oppressors; Haiti was the first country to be decimated by AIDS, while South Africa is the most recent and dramatic nation case; and both heads of state have been demonized by the international community. People in South Africa and elsewhere in the Third World were critically attentive to the fact that anthrax, the deadly bacteria that gripped the headlines of the terrorism chronicle in North America in 2001, was precisely the germ used a few years earlier by the apartheid regime in its biological warfare programs against black opponents, and that in order to obtain sufficient quantities of an antianthrax antibiotic, the United States activated an exception-for-health-purposes clause it had refused to ratify a few months earlier, during the World Trade Organization round, in connection with making AIDS drugs available in developing countries. The Nigerian religious authorities' 2004 decision to prohibit a polio vaccination campaign that would have used a product made in North America suspected of being used to sterilize women may be seen, together with the discovery published in the most serious international scientific journals that the disturbing spread of hepatitis C on the African continent might be due to shots given in a program for combating schistosomiasis during the colonial period, are ambiguous echoes of the largely contested thesis that a polio vaccine was responsible for the genesis of AIDS half a century ago. Here phantasmatic production and historical reconstitution seem to make sense in terms of each other. The history of AIDS in South Africa constitutes a web of meaning that extends well beyond country borders and the disease itself. It recounts a political world order composed of both social configurations and symbolic arrangements, relations of knowledge and power, representations of the self and discourses on the other.

In a long and impassioned article published in the *New York Review of Books,* Helen Epstein (2000) suggested there is a "mystery of AIDS in South Africa" that she considered it her duty to elucidate. It was of course her prerogative to see the situation that way. But why not consider the possibility that the problem lies not only in the existence of a mystery but also in our inability to penetrate it? What we do not understand about South Africa and the AIDS epidemic there may have to do with our not caring enough to understand. The journalist spent three weeks in South Africa—not, she says, enough time for her to grasp the complexity of what she compares to "some mystical Hebrew text" or indeed to meet and speak with all the persons she had hoped to. The fact that some of them were unavailable to see her seemed to her a further indication that she had "come to land in a fairy tale, where everybody is evasive and ignores appointments." It both made her indignant and set her to wondering if she herself had not been touched with "South African paranoia." She does, however, draw a few strong conclusions about this "vaguely postwar atmosphere, in the self-imposed curfew, the corruption and crime," noting that the South African head of state, whom she had glimpsed on television during an interview shown in the United States, "seemed to be hiding something." In her conversation with a young white South African manager on the flight out of South Africa, she says she is finally given this decisive clue: "It's all political. Everything is political in South Africa." The fact that such a short visit was not enough to elucidate the "mystery"—to understand a social world in light of its history—is hardly surprising to anthropologists accustomed to thinking and working in the long term—a practice for which they are often criticized because it goes against the imperious necessity to act in the world. For them, however, the AIDS epidemic and controversy in South Africa may not just be an object of knowledge that can only be understood gradually, slowly, but also a question of ethics, to be conceived in terms of respect for the other. And they may even think it quite all right for a society not to be immediately transparent to a foreign observer, especially since it is hardly transparent to itself. Suspending judgment for a moment, reining in the sense of urgency that compels us to speak out, taking the time to observe and listen, preferring critical reflection to hasty denunciation—these are the intentions, the premises, on which this book is constructed. And they are perhaps the loftiest demands made on us by this world we live in.

Demands that it is no simple matter to respond to. "The structure of modern sensory experience is inherently ironic. The sensory sphere is experienced in such a manner that profound transformations occurring in it or imposed on it are rendered imperceptible to the individual eye. This is precisely why everyday life in modernity has become the site for far-reaching historical transformations. For it is there that the historical unconscious is most powerful," observes Nadia Seremetakis (1996: 19). In the "polarity between the sensational and the mundane," which is also the "dichotomy between the sensational and the sensory," the latter is "left unmarked, unvoiced and unattended to." We readily talk about the AIDS controversy in South Africa and its most striking moments of clash and conflict, just as we readily talk about September 11 and other history-making events. But we are often silent about the ordinary experience of AIDS, the most personal, intimate suffering, just as we are often silent about the most entrenched injustices in the world and how they are perceived by the people who suffer them. In light of the history of AIDS in South Africa but from a wider perspective, let me then attempt a last analysis of the "profound transformations" that generally remain "imperceptible." Poverty and violence, discrimination and exclusion—the matters of this study—have surely always been present everywhere. However, in contemporary societies these realities are characterized in a heretofore unknown manner by two inseparable facts: differences among people have never been so great, nor have they ever been so clearly and fully perceived. In other words, inequalities have become both objectively and subjectively patent.

Inequalities have increased. Disparities in life expectancy mean that the worst-off people on the planet may live only half as long as the best-off. The same iniquitous relation exists within certain nations. More subtle but no less cruelly effective is the difference in value attached to the lives of some compared to the lives of others. Highly similar moral assumptions account, on the one hand, for accepting the idea that the majority of third world AIDS victims not be treated when the most sophisticated, costly treatment is made available to sick persons in rich countries, and, on the other, for the practice in contemporary warfare of having bombers fly at altitudes that will protect the lives of Western pilots when this necessarily causes "collateral damage" in the form of hundreds of deaths among precisely those indigenous civilians the bombers are supposedly defending. This polarization can increasingly be discerned in the global space. Certain territories are protected from poverty and violence; economic and civil security is the rule there. Others are left to the ravages of poverty, brutality, misery; in those places, acute material insecurity is people's daily lot. The South African space inherited from apartheid and then recomposed according to the same logic of protection-abandonment is a particularly expressive form of this reality, which is less manifest elsewhere but just as operative. At the scale of the planet, protected regions such as those encompassed by the European Union can only maintain themselves by applying the principle of restricted access, as is attested by recent developments in immigration and asylum policies. In contrast, abandoned zones are developing and growing. In some cases they represent entire countries, where the best that people can hope for is intervention by international peace-keeping forces and humanitarian organization teams.

Meanwhile, inequalities are being felt more strongly perhaps than ever before. This is of course explained in large part by media attention to misfortunes and suffering throughout the world, above all by the power of the media images of those misfortunes and that suffering. Poverty is more likely to be seen as an injustice the more unequally distributed it is discovered to be. Violence is more likely to be thought of as intolerable the more conscious viewers are that elsewhere there is peace. But the changes I am speaking of are more fundamentally anthropological, and they entertain a twofold relation with identity and time. First, construction of the self involves recognizing that one is a member of a community with a shared destiny—the community of the dominated and oppressed. It should be noted that this identity lexicon differs sharply from the earlier one, where the key term was exploitation. Political and moral self-identification of this sort transcends national borders and often takes on a racial dimension, precisely the dimension along which the African continent and its American diaspora are coming closer today, in particular. But such self-identification does not neglect broader loyalties encompassing other victims, as is shown by the reception of the Palestinian cause in such culturally and historically dissimilar contexts as South African townships and poor French suburbs. Second, self-construction now implies a reappropriation of the past, which in turn reveals the historical continuity of oppression and domination. The present only makes sense because it is linked to what preceded it, to that which *was* and has been forgotten, to buried humiliations, and to silenced resistance. Today's numerous reparation demands—reparation for apartheid in South Africa, elsewhere for slavery or for genocide—cannot be dismissed as mere cynical calculation or political manipulation. They are an entirely new expression of the embodiment of time, at once intensely personal and more broadly reflexive. In this sense, the particular ways the dominated and oppressed understand facts and their experience—interpreting their misfortunes and suffering in terms of victimization, grasping certain facts as if they pointed to conspiracy—are indicators of contemporary types of subjectification.

The age of anxiety we live in is characterized by tensions generated by the harshest inequalities ever known, inequalities that are also the most profoundly felt by the men and women who suffer them. It is also an age in which the sufferers are invisible to the men and women who profit from these inequalities. The well-off may deny the existence of the badly off, seeing the disparities in contemporary South African society as amounting merely to the rise of a black bourgeoisie, for example. Or they may misread them, seeing the afflicted as responsible for their affliction, as in behavioral or culturalist approaches to AIDS. Or they may simply not take any interest in them. Considered from this perspective, the age of anxiety Auden wrote of is one of rumor and disavowal, blindness and silence, injustices deepened by denial.

But there are other horizons, other possibilities. For "anxiety" we might substitute "uneasiness," which John Locke understood as a feeling of intellectual discomfort that comes over us when we consider the state of the world and which he saw as a necessary cause of voluntary action. Uneasiness, or better, *inquiétude,* as it is translated in French, which gives it a sense more active than affective. An age of anxiety is blind to inequalities, their causes and consequences: hurrying from commemoration to commemoration, it is without memory. An age of uneasiness is sensitive to inequalities and tries to grasp them as both condition and experience: attentive to the embodiment of memory, it works to apprehend the present as a moment within a history. While an age of anxiety divides the world and produces two contradictory, opposed orders of intelligibility, an age of uneasiness calls for a shared world that nonetheless remains open to different readings, divergent understandings. Anxiety, because it is linked with disinterest in others, paralyzes. *Inquiétude,* when it is associated with concern for others, moves people to act. It is a challenge for anthropologists. And a duty for the citizens of the world.

NOTES

INTRODUCTION

1. See "Why South Africa Matters," special issue of *Daedalus: Journal of the American Academy of Arts and Sciences* 130, no. 1 (2001).

1. AS IF NOTHING EVER HAPPENED

1. For a presentation and discussion of the Maputo conference, see Zwi and Bachmayer 1990. For a view of that conference as it fits into the history of the epidemic in South Africa, see Marais 2000; van der Vliet 2001.

2. Data are from the following reports: UNAIDS, *AIDS Epidemic Update,* Dec. 2000; RSA Department of Health, *National HIV and Syphilis Sero-Prevalence Survey in South Africa,* 2001; Medical Research Council, *The Impact of HIV/AIDS on Adult Mortality in South Africa,* September 2001.

3. Among them the political scientist Tom Lodge (2002: 255): "When historians assess the democratic credentials of Thabo Mbeki's government in future, it is likely that their most critical attentions will focus on its response to the HIV/AIDS pandemic, surely its most formidable developmental challenge."

4. In his preface to John Kani's play, *Nothing but the Truth* (Johannesburg: Witwatersrand University Press, 2002), the great novelist Zakes Mda warns, "There is a demand from some of my compatriots that, since we have now attained democracy, we should all have collective amnesia, because memory does not contribute to reconciliation. We should, therefore, not only forgive the past,

we should also forget it. However, it is impossible to meet this demand, for we are products of our past. We have been shaped by our history. Our present worldview and our mind-set is a result of our yesterdays."

5. My colleague Jean-Pierre Dozon, with whom I have long been discussing AIDS in Africa within this program and many others, was with me on this occasion.

6. In the French-language version of Mbeki's speech that the South African embassy made available a few days later, at an AIDS information day event that tried to explain national policy, the word *fool* was translated into the French as *idiot*. The term seems well chosen if one thinks of Dostoevsky's Prince Mychkin: an ostensibly "simple-minded" man speaks the truth, alone against all. Nevertheless, it does not sufficiently consider the irony of the leader designating himself as such, the king being his own "fool" in front of the "wise men" of his panel.

7. The AIDS in Context conference, held 4–7 April 2001, was jointly organized by the University of Witwatersrand History Workshop and Center for Health Policy, the AIDS Consortium, Soul City, GALA, and the CSIR. A selection of the talks given was published in two special issues: *African Issues* 61, no. 1 (2002); and *African Journal of Aids Research* 1, no. 1 (2002). Apart from the opening speech by Judge Edwin Cameron, who was personally involved in the polemic against the president, the only people who discussed it in their presentations were Costa Gazi, an opposition politician, and the public health specialist Helen Schneider. Doctors, activists, journalists, and health officials also participated in the concluding roundtable discussion that was heated on this issue. But no historian, sociologist, anthropologist, or political scientist made it the main focus of his or her presentation.

8. There is an interesting parallel with the Dreyfus case in the late 1890s in France, which was called "l'affaire par excellence" by Pascal Ory and Jean-François Sirinelli (1986). As I have suggested (2004), the controversy on AIDS has played a comparable role in the constitution of civil society in South Africa as the Dreyfus affair did for the invention of the intellectual in the French public sphere.

9. The letter can be read on www.washingtonpost.com; the text of the opening speech, on www.anc.org.za. For a detailed analysis of these two documents, see my article in a special issue of *Les Temps modernes* (2002).

10. Like other members of political parties banned by Pretoria from 1960 to 1990, Thabo Mbeki has experienced apartheid, whether directly during his adolescence, in particular when he was expelled from college for his organization of a class boycott, or indirectly but not less real during his exile in Europe and Africa, through reported facts about the situation back in South Africa, through collective humiliations and raised hopes, through the story of comrades shot, including his own brother in 1987, or imprisoned, like his father, Govan Mbeki, a

leader of Umkhonto weSizwe, who spent twenty-seven years in jail. See Hadland and Rantao 1999; Jacobs and Calland 2002; Lodge 2002.

11. I was engaged in a research program aimed at apprehending the historical conditions and structural processes underlying the heretofore unknown epidemic spread of the disease in southern Africa. With Michel Kazatchkine, director of the Agence Nationale de Recherche sur le Sida, I called for just this kind of approach in *Le Monde,* 16 May 2000, republished in English on 23 June in the South African *Weekly Mail and Guardian.*

12. For a sociohistorical analysis of anthropological studies of AIDS in Africa in the 1980s and 1990s, see Fassin 1999a; also Treichler 1999 on the history of the epidemic.

13. During my first meeting with Puleng, in addition to the volunteer, Regina Makwela, who had organized it, I was accompanied by Frédéric Le Marcis and Tod Mashape Lethata, from the anthropology department of the University of Witwatersrand.

14. Using Pierce's analytic distinction, Valentine Daniel (2000) proposes that for the purposes of anthropological discourse, violence should be conceived as the intersection of three terms. "Mood" corresponds to "a state of feeling—usually vague, diffuse, enduring, a disposition toward the world at any time yet with a timeless quality to it." "Moment" entails "the sense of a unique fact or event, a here-and-nowness, a selective narrowing of possibilities to just one actuality." "Mind" refers to "the tendency to generalize, to reason, to take habit." The three together account for how the mood gives meaning to the moment and is analyzed by the mind.

15. An important literature was developed in the 1990s around "social suffering": in France, it was mainly a sociological production, precisely in Pierre Bourdieu's group at the Collège de France; in the United States, it was rather an anthropological enterprise, especially with Arthur Kleinman's program in the Social Science Research Council. For an analysis of this field, see my article in *Critique* (2004a).

16. Talking about oneself, telling one's story, is not a trait inscribed from the beginning of time in human activity but a historically constructed activity. Jean-Pierre Vernant (1989: 215) outlines its archaeology in the Western world, distinguishing between the three figures the Greeks used to present the self: "the individual, in the strict sense, his/her place, role, group, the value he/she is recognized to have"; "the subject: an individual speaking in the first person in his/her own name and presenting certain features that make him/her appear a singular being"; and last, "the self, the person, the complete set of practices and psychological attitudes that give the subject inwardness and unicity and thereby constitute him/her as a real, original, unique being, a singular individual whose authentic nature lies entirely in the hidden recesses of his or her internal life." To

the individual corresponds biography; to the subject, the autobiography or memoirs; to the self, the confession and diary. While for the anthropologist these category definitions are debatable and the borders between them difficult to establish, this analysis at least enables us to more accurately date preoccupations we tend to think of as inventions of modern man.

17. A small book of the exhibition was published: *Living Openly: HIV-Positive South Africans Tell Their Stories* (Pretoria: Department of Health, 2000). In the midst of a gallery of unknown faces are the emblematic figures Nkosi Johnson and Zachie Achmat, charismatic president of the Treatment Action Campaign.

18. As Philippe Denis and Nokhaya Makiwane recalled in their talk at the international Aids in Context conference, the practice of "memory boxes" was developed in South Africa by the AIDS Counseling, Care, and Training Association, active in Soweto. They took their inspiration from a program developed in 1997 in Kampala and used in 2000 by the Oral History Project of the University of Natal School of Theology. Initially founded to reconstitute the histories of Christian communities under apartheid, the project had to adapt to the grim new fact that one-third of adults in KwaZulu-Natal province were HIV-positive. One of the most important changes introduced at this juncture was having historiographers collect biographies.

19. Significantly, most of the life stories collected and reported on in these studies on contemporary forms of social violence are women's. As Brooke Grundfest Schoepf (1992) has shown on the basis of Zairean life stories, gender-related inequalities are manifest both in women's objectifiable risk (namely, material survival through sex commerce) and the ideological discourse on it (responsibility or even sin).

20. The first such works, some written by physician-anthropologists such as Daniel Hrdy (1987), author of the main synthesis on the matter in the early years of the epidemic, mix psychologism, often rife with prejudices about Africans' presumed "sexual promiscuity," and culturalism, detailing exotic "ritual practices."

2. AN EPIDEMIC OF DISPUTES

1. This opinion may appear unfair or peremptory, and I have developed a more circumstantial argument elsewhere (2001a). It certainly deserves to be put in perspective by mentioning exceptions, which is what I will do as I go along, referring to the studies of health policies that have been particularly helpful in the research presented here.

2. Concerning the Western world, one can refer among others to the work of Carlo Cipolla on the plague (1976) and of Allan Brandt on syphilis (1985); concerning the colonial empires, see Megan Vaughan's work on Africa (1991) and

David Arnold's on India (1993). A more detailed bibliography is available in Paul Slack's introduction to a collection of essays on epidemics (1992).

3. This statement by Frederick Tilney is placed at the front of the volume that Elisabeth Fee and Daniel Fox (1988) dedicated to the "burdens of history" that weigh on AIDS.

4. Written after my investigations in Senegal in the mid-eighties, the book (1992) includes a number of such stories, in which I hope my positivist approach is not too blatant.

5. Seeming to echo twelve years later a phrase by virus coinventor Robert Gallo who, when asked in 1988 what he thought of Peter Duesberg's thesis, answered that there was nothing to discuss. "Call five thousand scientists and ask them," said he. Taken from an interview published by *Spin,* the phrase is quoted by Steven Epstein (1996). Consensus is a good way to define the way the community sees itself.

6. The history of the disputes presented here is based on a survey of the articles that appeared in the press between 1995 and 2004 in the country's main newspapers and on the few available works signed by researchers, mainly Hein Marais (2000), Virginia van der Vliet (2001), and Helen Schneider and Joan Stein (2001). It also includes formal interviews and informal discussions with several of the actors who were directly involved, including Olive Shisana, former director general of the Health Department; Nono Simelela, former director of the National Program on AIDS; William Pick, former director of the School of Public Health at the University of Witswatersrand; Helen Schneider, former director of the Center for Health Policy; Max Price, dean of the Faculty of Medicine at the University of Witswatersrand; Justice Edwin Cameron, member of the Constitutional Court; Mark Heywood, spokesman for Treatment Action Campaign; activist and journalist Timothy Trengrove-Jones; Peter Duesberg, leading dissident at the University of California, Berkeley; members of the French embassy in Pretoria and of the South African embassy in Paris; officers from international agencies in South Africa; medical doctors, hospital nurses, field activists, patients.

7. Newspaper references for the history of the *Sarafina II* scandal are mainly *Weekly Mail and Guardian,* "Health Minister Defends AIDS Musical," 9 February 1996, "Two Arms of Government in a Tangle," 1 March 1996, "Zuma's Revenge," 26 July 1996, "Vested Interests Backed Zuma Criticism," 13 September 1996; *The Star,* "Zuma Draws Final Curtain," 6 June 1996; *Saturday Star,* "Seeds of Sleaze Bearing Bitter Fruit," 25 May 1996.

8. The sharp-tongued reporter and politicians' portraitist Mark Gevisser reported enthusiastically on this speech: "Finally the state gets serious about AIDS," exclaimed the title of his article in the *Weekly Mail and Guardian* of 22 July 1994, which went on to compare its action with the previous policy: "After years of official foot-dragging and negligence, the government has finally en-

dorsed an AIDS programme." At that time, not only was mentioning the absence of the possibility of treating the sick not criticized, but it appeared justified: "Despite a high HIV-infection rate (550,000), there is not yet an undue strain on health care services: currently, there are only 10,000 people with AIDS needing medical treatment as opposed, for example, to 11,000 killed on the roads each year." A few years later the epidemiological situation had dramatically changed, and so had the health dogma: prevention, which had been the end-all for the international organizations, became secondary; therapies, which had been refused because of their cost, became the new priorities worldwide.

9. According to Christopher Saunders and Nicholas Southey (2001), the National Party founded in 1914 to represent the Afrikaners split in two in 1934 and the most extremist fraction created the Purified National Party. Led by D. F. Malan, it carried the elections of 1948 and established the apartheid regime. Once again called the National Party, it ruled for nearly half a century. With Peter Botha, then Frederik de Klerk, it became somewhat reformist and negotiated the democratic transition. During the presidential elections of 1994, it came in second with 20 percent of the voters and participated in Nelson Mandela's Government for National Unity. Two years later it left the government to join the opposition to the ANC. The Democratic Party, founded in 1989, brought together three small parties made up mainly of former National Party moderates. It played an important part in the transition but obtained mediocre results in the 1994 elections. With few representatives, it actively opposed the government and approached de Klerk when the latter quit the government. Together they founded the Democratic Alliance in 2000 and formed the main opposition in Parliament until its dissolution in 2003. Both parties are today multiracial in theory but nonetheless made up mainly of whites, with a relatively important proportion of coloureds in the National Party.

10. Quoted by Marais (2000) in his review of the first years of the struggle against AIDS. The point of view confirmed by Helen Schneider, who directs the Center for Health Policy at the University of Witwatersrand and is quoted in the same volume: "Maybe if Zuma wasn't so visibly under pressure from the Sarafina scandal, then perhaps it could have just slipped away and we could have gone on with other things."

11. See Jim Day's article, "Zuma's Remarkable Road to Recovery," in the *Weekly Mail and Guardian*, 23 May 1997. Gary Adler and Nkosazana Zuma quotations come from the study by Hein Marais (2000), who added that after the *Sarafina II* scandal, several NGOs decided to stop attacking the minister of health since that made them objective allies of the opposition. But that decision went largely unnoticed to say the least.

12. Newspaper references for the Virodene story are in particular *Cape Argus*, "SA Scientists Claim AIDS Drug Breakthrough," 22 January 1997, "Is It April

Fool's Day?" 23 January 1997, "Zuma Slated over AIDS Drug Fiasco," 6 February 1997, "Why the Violent Attacks on Virodene?" 5 March 1997, "Deliver and I'll Be Loyal to ANC, Says Winnie," 26 April 1997, "New Volleys Fired in Virodene War," 4 March 1998, "Lessons from the Virodene Saga," 22 December 1998; *Cape Times*, "Despair as Hopes of Miracle Cure Fade," 24 January 1997, "Mum's the Word for Health Dept Officials," 28 January 1997, "AIDS Community Torn Apart by Virodene Scam," 28 February 1997, "Medicines Control Council Has for the 4th Time Denied Researchers Permission to Conduct Human Trials with Virodene P058," 3 February 1998, "ANC Stood to Gain Millions from Virodene," 3 March 1998; *The Star*, "No Approval Granted for New AIDS Drugs," 24 January 1997, "Let the Sufferers Use Virodene, Pleads Zuma," 2 December 1997; *Weekly Mail and Guardian*, "Unhealthy Example," 24 January 1997, "AIDS 'Breakthrough' Broke All the Rules," 24 January 1997.

13. This situation is perhaps less radically unheard of than it may at first appear, however, as we will see later. In France, in October 1985, Minister of Health and Social Affairs Georgina Dufoix had anounced, in the presence of Professor Even (one of the chief physicians of the Laënnec Hospital in Paris who had led the experiment) that a medication called cyclosporine, usually administered to transplant patients to reduce the risk of rejection, was also effective against AIDS. She was basing her opinion on the partial results of a clinical test conducted among a few patients and as yet unpublished in the scientific journals. The affair had made the front page of the newspapers, raising great hopes among patients before it was corrected: the product was not effective. Claudine Herzlich and Janine Pierret (1988: 1126), in their study on how the media built up the illness in the 1980s, write: "In the entire history of AIDS in France, the event most built up by the press was that official announcement."

14. In this context, the Tyberberg Hospital of Stellenbosch University also released the news of the miracle drug. In an article titled "Cheap Local Drugs Offer Fresh Hopes for Patients with AIDS or Other Immune Problems," the *Saturday Star* of 8 March 1997 gave a detailed report on Professor Patrick Bouic's results: "An affordable, non-toxic drug that bolsters the immune system and helps to fight HIV more effectively will be available to consumers from 1 April. The drug, based on extracts from the indigenous African potato has been tested on HIV and AIDS patients in approved clinical trials since 1992 and has been found to boost the immune system to such an extent that the quality of patients' lives improves markedly." This time, the local ethical committees had been asked for their opinion and the Medicines Control Council had given its go-ahead. While Virodene, called an "industrial," obscure, and dangerous product that had never been evaluated according to the rules, appeared more and more as an evil intruder in AIDS treatments, the African potato, said to be a "native," absolutely harmless, and duly approved substance, became the positive and legitimate point

of reference, glorifying the encounter between nature and tradition under the reassuring auspices of official medicine. A moral and political landscape of the nonconformist pharmacopoeia was in the making.

15. The minister of health was supported by the president of the Women's League of the ANC, Winnie Mandela, who congratulated her during the association's general assembly for her fight against AIDS and asked "the White-controlled press to stop discrediting black female politicians."

16. The article was published in March 1998 on the ANC web site: www.anc.org.za/ancdocs/history/mbeki. In defense of the research team, he writes, including the health minister and himself in the comment: "In our strange world those who seek the good for all humanity have become the villains of our times."

17. In September 2001 Zigi Visser was thrown out of Tanzania where he had been secretly experimenting with Virodene on AIDS patients. It then transpired that the new health minister Manto Tshabalala-Msimang had shortly before visited the clinic where the researcher worked. In June 2002 financial revelations about the company producing the drug threw light on connections with the COSATU and a newspaper inquiry showed that Visser had continued advising Thabo Mbeki on various health questions at least until 2000. See *Weekly Mail and Guardian,* "Tanzanians Used as Guinea-Pigs," 7 September 2001; and "Who's Bankrolling Virodene?" 28 June 2002.

18. See my article on the AIDS policies implemented in the Congo (1994). On the front page of the country's major newspaper, *La Semaine africaine,* of 26 November 1987, ran the following headline: "Fight against AIDS. Two Africans Discover a treatment: MM1. May It Cure!"

19. The history of the drug is recalled by Chris Hall in "AIDS Scam: Kenya Had One Too," published by the *Weekly Mail and Guardian* on 6 March 1998. The North American tests were reported in short pieces in two of the major scientific journals: "Kemron's Secret: It Does Not Work," *Nature* 356, 23 April 1992, 648; and "USA: NIH Reopens the Kemron Case," *Lancet* 340, 31 October 1992, 1087–1088.

20. See the document published by the magazine *Transcriptase Sud,* 2001, 7, especially the articles by Pialoux, " 'Affaire Therastim': l'espoir et les doutes"; Philippe Msellati, "Un risque pour la prévention"; and Jean-Pierre Dozon, "Que penser de la publicité faite à l'invention d'un remède anti-sida en Côte d'Ivoire?"

21. Citations and facts are taken from the following newspaper articles: *Cape Argus,* "Government Withdrawal of Drug Angers Those with AIDS," 11 February 1998, "Can We Afford Not to Use AZT?" 16 October 1998; *Cape Times,* "Babies' Lives in Balance as Zuma Zaps AIDS Drug Trial," 22 February 1999; *Saturday Star,* "Suffer the Little Children," 30 January 1999; *Weekly Mail and Guardian,* "Babies Too Poor to Live," 16 October 1998, "We Can't Not Afford

AZT," 4 December 1998, "The High Cost of Living Babies," 14 May 1999. And also Pat Sidley, "Mbeki Claims That AZT Is Dangerous," *British Medical Journal* 319 (1999): 1522; "South Africa to Tighten Control on Drug Trials after Five Deaths," *British Medical Journal* 320 (2000): 1028.

22. Data are taken from two reviews of medical literature compiled by Diana M. Gibb and Beatriz H. Tess, "Interventions to Reduce Mother-to-Child Transmission of HIV Infection: New Developments and Current Controversies," *AIDS* 13, Suppl. A (1999): S93–S102; and Lynne Mofenson and Mary Glenn Fowler, "Interruption of Materno-Infantile Transmission," *AIDS* 13, Suppl. A (1999): S205–S214, as well as from the most significant articles published on the subject through 1999. The idea is to mirror as closely as possible the state of the art at the time of the South African controversy, thus avoiding the anachronisms that have often biased analyses and sometimes legal decisions in the history of AIDS.

23. The investigation weekly *noseweek* was to become the media's Trojan horse for the dissident ideas in South Africa. Two journalists play a major role in this respect: Anthony Brink, whose article "AZT: A Medicine from Hell," published on 17 March in *The Citizen,* sums up the dissidents' complaints about the drug; and especially former scientific reporter of the important Johannesburg daily *The Star,* Anita Bell, who was said to have easy access to the chief of state and the health minister.

24. The terms of course implicitly refer to Thomas Kuhn's (1962) theory of scientific revolution. In the present instance, however, the crisis may be read in two distinct ways: from the orthodox point of view, it simply indicates we are leaving the scientific field; from the unorthodox point of view, it blazes the trail for a new paradigm. In the first perspective, Duesberg is a charlatan; in the second, an innovator of genius. Nostradamus according to some, Galileo to others. But whereas Kuhn envisages exclusively the case where science wins out, we must also try to account for the case where she loses.

25. The new terms chosen in the controversy, the demonization of the adversaries and of the products, the use of divine or satanic metaphors, and finally the reference to heresy, suggest that it is less through the sociology of science than through the sociology of religions that one can make any sense of it. See especially the seminal article by Pierre Bourdieu (1971) on the "religious field."

26. Titled "Challenged by Our Times," *Weekly Mail and Guardian,* 14 December 2001. Sipho Seepe writes: "If anything, South Africa has become, at government level, a purveyor and compost heap of discredited ideas."

27. See especially the open letter that the head of state sent to the president of the Medical Research Council, Malegapuru William Makgoba, in February 2000, advising him to read an article published in the June 1999 edition of *Current Medical Research and Opinion* by one of the most active dissidents, Eleni Papadopulos-Eleopulos, and the invitation he publicly extended to the head of

the opposition coalition Democratic Alliance, Tony Leon, in July 2000, quoting large excerpts from *Mortality and Morbidity Weekly Report* of the Centers for Disease Control in Atlanta.

28. This story has been told and analyzed in great detail by Steven Epstein (1996), especially in the first part of the book, "The Politics of Causation."

29. The group's theories are on www.virusmyth.com: "It is widely believed by the general public that a retrovirus called HIV causes the group diseases called AIDS. Many biochemical scientists now question this hypothesis. We propose that a thorough reappraisal of the existing evidence for and against this hypothesis be conducted by a suitable independent group." Most of the persons signing this declaration are biologists or physicians in the United States. Not least among their ranks is Kary Mullis, who won the Nobel Prize in chemistry and invented the PCR (polymerase chain reaction) permitting the amplification of ADN, thanks to which the presence of the AIDS virus can be easily detected. Among the first to answer the call was Paul Rabinow, the only social science research scholar who had carried out an anthropological investigation on the discovery of PCR (1996). In fact, he was linked to Peter Duesberg through the seminar he had at Berkeley in collaboration with Nancy Scheper-Hughes.

30. For a recent update of the dissident stand, see the article by Peter Duesberg and David Rasnick, "The AIDS Dilemma: Drug Diseases Blamed on a Passenger Virus," *Genetica* 104, no. 2 (1988): 133–142. The two scholars, though allied against scientific orthodoxy, do not seem to share exactly the same view: for Duesberg, AIDS exists but is not due to HIV; for Rasnick, AIDS does not even possess empirical reality.

31. The undated nine-page document bears the title, *HIV Blamed for Poverty: South Africa's Racism and Apartheid Absolved. Critical Remarks on the 'Orthodox' Biomedical Science of HIV/AIDS.*

32. Excerpts from the diary were published in the *Weekly Mail and Guardian* of 8 September 2000 under the title "All the President's Scientists: Diary of a Round-earther." It should be noted that the press ombudsman considered that the publication of this text did not respect the principles of honesty and impartiality and obliged the weekly to print a right of reply from the panelists in its next issue.

33. The press and even those who stand by official science willingly repeat this presentation, and though they do so in interrogative form, it still obtains performative effects. In an opinion column of the *Weekly Mail and Guardian*, Sean Davidson, head of the microbiology department at the University of the Western Cape, a confirmed orthodox, wondered, "When Galileo declared, in the fourteenth century, that the Earth revolved around the sun, they laughed at him. We therefore must ask ourselves today, with an open mind, if what the dissident scientists say, that HIV is not responsible for AIDS, does not come from mis-

understood geniuses." The article goes on to show the contrary, but the question was nevertheless put.

34. The details of this controversy come mainly from the following articles: *Sunday Star*, "Young, Gifted and Dead," 9 July 2000; *The Citizen*, "Accidents, Violence 'Main Killers,'" 11 July 2000, and "AIDS, HIV Statistics Must Be Carefully Scrutinized," 28 September 2000; *Weekly Mail and Guardian*, "Lies, Damned Lies and *noseweek*," 6 October 2000, and "We Make Mistakes but We Do Not Lie," 20 October 2000; *noseweek*, Editorial, no. 30, 2000.

35. A glance at the entire front page of the paper gives a general though sketchy idea of what was going on on that memorable day and how it was being rendered. It shows how national questions are made to fit the global scene. In counterpoint to the dreadful information, "Young, Gifted and Dead," one finds in smaller letters another trilogy about youth, exactly symmetrical to the main headline: "Sexy, Savvy and Sensitive." Below the headline is the picture of a young woman, announcing the first issue of a supplement coaxing young people to lead a "healthy lifestyle." Death from AIDS is counterbalanced by a healthy life that protects. Two other articles share the front page. On one side, the "Judas of the South Sea Islands" being handed over to public condemnation, alluding to the New Zealander whose vote had decided which country would be selected to host the 2006 World Cup; mandated by the South Sea Islanders to support South Africa, he had committed treason by abstaining, which allowed Germany to win. To see, so close to victory, the world event slip out of their hands had elicited bitter and violent reactions all over the African continent; once again, it was said, the West had united against Africa and, by buying the vote of a little country, stolen what was rightfully theirs, since they had never hosted the World Cup. On the other side, came the announcement that a summit meeting of chiefs of state was to be held to transform the old Organization for African Unity into the African Union, a dynamics comparable to the European Union; but South Africa was already the locomotive of another ambitious program, NEPAD, the New Economic Pact for African Development.

36. The duel was as much about the epidemiological arguments (pessimistic or optimistic) as about choice of vocabulary ("HIV seroprevalence" suggests that data are representative of the general population, whereas "antenatal survey" reminds one that it concerns a specific population): R. E. Dorrington et al., "HIV Seroprevalence Results: Little Grounds for Optimism Yet," *South African Medical Journal* 90 (2000): 452–453; and L. Makubalo et al., "HIV Antenatal Survey Results: Little Grounds for Pessimism," *South African Medical Journal* 90 (2000): 1062. Three years later the same protagonists were once again face-to-face about data for 2002, which this time showed an increase of 26.5 percent as against 24.8 percent in 2001. See *The Star*, "Concerns over Secrecy about HIV Figures," 3 July 2003.

37. Of course, this is not only true of South Africa. We know that in France, toward the end of the 1990s, the National Health Observatory (Institut National de Veille Sanitaire) had undergone some severe attacks on the part of certain associations, especially Migrants against AIDS (Migrants contre le sida), which had invaded its offices to force them to divulge statistics on the epidemic by nationality and origin that had not been issued for nearly twenty years. See my article on this theme (1999b). It is more generally integration policies that can be read between the lines in French health information.

38. Malegapuru William Makgoba wrote in his preface, "This report is a frightening reminder of how social prejudice has contributed to create the most explosive epidemic in the history of our country." See R. Dorrington et al., *The Impact of HIV/AIDS on Adult Mortality in South Africa*, Medical Research Council, September 2001.

39. Besides, the data are not only indicators of an epidemiological situation or even of a social reality. They are also, as the government is well aware, weapons. Thus, in July 2003, the mathematical model used by the Medical Research Council to set up its projections was used by the Democratic Alliance to base its announcement of an impressive million deaths due to AIDS since 1985 and to consequently organize demonstrations in memory of the victims, just so many more opportunities to attack the government. See *The Mercury,* "Will Secret AIDS Report Get a State Response?" 14 July 2003.

40. The quote is taken from an article by Belinda Beresford in the *Weekly Mail and Guardian* of 14 September 2001: "AIDS Suit: State's Reply." The articles mainly consulted and quoted for this period are *City Press,* "Now, Mrs. Minister, Does HIV Cause AIDS?" 15 September 2000; *Sowetan,* "Under Fire: Constitutional Court Judges Put Government's AIDS Policies to Severe Test," 4 April 2002, "AIDS Drug Gets OK," 17 April 2002; *The Star,* "New Efforts to Ensure Cheaper Drugs," 14 July 2000, "AIDS Panel's Report Reveal Divergent Views," 5 April 2001, "AIDS-Drug Ruling Hailed," 15 December 2001, "Yes, You Will, Dr No," 5 April 2002; *Weekly Mail and Guardian,* "AIDS Activists to Challenge the State," 8 September 2000, "Just Say Yes, Mr President," "Cabinet on AIDS: Ja, Well, No Maybe," 15 September 2000, "Drug Giants Prepare for War," 2 March 2001, "Not Even the Horror of AIDS Can Temper the Greed for Profit," 16 March 2001, "Drug Giants Back Down," 20 April 2001, "State Faces New HIV Battle," 24 August 2001, "Death of an Activist," 19 April 2002.

41. A drawing in the *City Press* of 17 September 2000 by the humorist Findlay derides the government's judgments thus: the president and the health minister are in the company of a third character, wearing a Ku Klux Klan hood (Manto Tshabalala-Msimang had circulated the book denouncing an AIDS world conspiracy by an American author who had been connected to that organization) in the television game "Who Wants to Be a Billionaire?" All three answer the first three questions (do apples fall from trees? is the pope Catholic? do

snakes have armpits?) without hesitation. Then comes "the billion-dollar question": is HIV the cause of AIDS? The three characters are seized by profound doubt and must forgo winning the jackpot.

42. See Didier Fassin and Helen Schneider, "The Politics of AIDS in South Africa: Beyond the Controversies," *British Medical Journal* 326 (2003): 495–497. To give more impact to the positions the article endorsed, the journal put the title on the cover, presented it as "editor's choice," and defended its perspective under the title "AIDS in South Africa Is More than Polemics." But neither the controversies nor the polemics stopped. See, for the answers to our paper, http://bmj .bmjjournals.com/cgi/eletters/326/7387/495.

43. Read in particular *Jump and Other Stories* (London: Bloomsbury and Penguin Books, 1992). From "The Ultimate Safari" to "Comrades" and "Amnesty," she draws, little by little, the twilight of apartheid.

3. ANATOMY OF THE CONTROVERSIES

1. One week before Trengrove Jones's article, in the same newspaper, an article by Paul Kirk, "Govt AIDS Nut Linked to Ku Klux Klan," had revealed that Cooper, called a "fraud, liar and charlatan" in the article, was closely connected to the racist organization that originated in the southern United States, whose rallies he often attended. William Cooper's texts are on the web sites www.hid denmysteries.com and www.thewatcherfiles.com. On the latter, one discovers that "A.I.D.S. is Man-made," with an epigraph by Peter Duesberg claiming that "AZT is AIDS by prescription." The illustration on the web site's homepage shows the White House being benevolently gazed upon by a macrocephalic creature from outer space.

2. From the many examples of this mixture of indignation and sarcasm especially prevalent among certain editorialists, one might pick out in the South African press the long article "The Triumph of Unreason," *Weekly Mail and Guardian,* 19 April 2002, and from the international press, Helen Epstein's study, "The Mystery of AIDS in South Africa," *New York Review of Books,* 20 July 2000.

3. Publishing the two lectures that Max Weber gave in 1919 (1959) side by side in the volume that goes by that title has established a duality that has become paradigmatic today but is nonetheless misleading. In reality, each text was asymmetrically constructed. In *Wissenschaft als Beruf,* the author defines his norm as the relationship entertained by the scientist with the politician; in *Politik als Beruf,* he submits politics to his own scrutiny as scientist. The first text is mainly prescriptive, the second essentially descriptive, which is the most usual: the scientist wonders about the politician much more often than the other way around. The South African government's position disrupts this norm, and that is one of the reasons the controversy is so disarming.

4. See George Annas, "The Right to Health and the Nevirapine Case in

South Africa," *New England Journal of Medicine* 348, no. 8 (2003): 750–754. Excerpts are taken from this article.

5. "Considering the progress of science in this field, the National AIDS Council feels it has become unacceptable to make pregnant women and contaminated children run this risk now that the possibility of proposing efficient ARV treatments is opening up" (Conseil national du sida, *Promouvoir l'accès aux antirétroviraux des femmes enceintes vivant avec le VIH/sida dans les pays du Sud*, République française, 24 June 2004). See also World Health Organization, *Antiretroviral Drugs and the Prevention of Mother-to-Child Transmission of HIV Infection in Resource-constrained Settings. Recommendations for Use*, 2004 revision, WHO2004.PMTCT ARV, www.who.org.

6. "AIDS Scientists Were Laughing at SA," *Cape Times*, 28 July 2004. During a speech in Bangkok, TAC president Zachie Achmat denounced the attack, calling it a "sideshow" and a "tragedy." In South Africa the newspapers gave it only passing mention, and no lesson was taken from it.

7. See, for example, the reviews of the literature proposed by L. Mofenson and J. A. McIntyre, "Advances and Research Directions in the Prevention of Mother-to-Child HIV-1 Transmission," *Lancet* 355, no. 9222 (2000): 2237–2244; and by K. De Cock, M. G. Fowler, and E. Mercier et al., "Prevention of Mother-to-Child HIV Transmission in Resource-Poor Countries: Translating Research into Policy and Practice," *JAMA* 283, no. 9 (2000): 1175–1182.

8. The new doctrine was recognized mainly after a test carried out in Uganda. See the pioneering article by L. A. Guay, P. Musoke, and T. Fleming et al., "Intrapartum and Neonatal Single-Dose Nevirapine Compared with Zidovudine for Prevention of Mother-to-Child Transmission of HIV-1 in Kampala, Uganda: HIVNET 012 Randomised Trial," *Lancet* 354, no. 9181 (1999): 795–802; and its equally positive reevaluation four years later: J. B. Jackson, P. Musoke, and T. Fleming et al., "Intrapartum and Neonatal Single-Dose Nevirapine Compared with Zidovudine for Prevention of Mother-to-Child Transmission of HIV-1 in Kampala, Uganda: 18-Month Follow-Up of the HIVNET 012 Randomised Trial," *Lancet* 362, no. 9387 (2003): 859–868. At this time, however, the wheel was beginning to turn for nevirapine and its scientific "champions."

9. "AIDS Activists to Challenge the State," *Weekly Mail and Guardian*, 8 September 2000. The picture accompanying the article shows a newborn African baby in a crib with a nurse standing by. As sole commentary, the caption reads: "No treatment."

10. "Death of an Activist," *Weekly Mail and Guardian*, 19 April 2002. The first words of the article are: "The last days in the life of a young mother have shown up the power and the dangers of antiretroviral drugs." Government spokesman Parks Mankahlana's death, thought to have been brought on by the same side effects, was also especially delicate to broach publicly, since it involved a man who not only had never admitted he had AIDS but who also accused the

international pharmaceutical industry of getting rich on the backs of African patients. See "Parks' Funerals Fail to Stop AIDS Rumors," *Sapa*, 4 November 2000; and "AIDS Drugs Killed Parks, Says ANC," *Weekly Mail and Guardian*, 22 March 2002.

11. "The Regime vs. the Regimen," *Weekly Mail and Guardian*, 28 March 2002. Belinda Beresford, author of the editorial, rightly notes that "the tragedy is that real debate is being killed and issues lost in a fog of confusion."

12. "It's the Trials, Not the Drugs," "Furor over Testing on Humans," "AIDS, a Threat to Democracy," *Weekly Mail and Guardian*, 7 April 2000, 5.

13. In the "pirated" account of a meeting of the ANC's parliamentary group, Howard Barrell claimed that Thabo Mbeki had said that that CIA was behind the promotion of the viral etiology of AIDS, since it served the interests of the pharmaceutical companies, *Weekly Mail and Guardian*, 6 October 2000. Journalists laugh at the reference to the American secret service, seeing it as just one more of his ridiculous ideas. It was nevertheless echoed much later when it was revealed that there was a real connection between the U.S. Central Intelligence Agency and South African Military Intelligence under apartheid and during the international embargo; this time, the same paper congratulated itself for owning the electronic files that prove it: "The CIA Connection," *Weekly Mail and Guardian*, 13 June 2003.

14. See Marcia Angell, "The Ethics of Clinical Research in the Third World," *New England Journal of Medicine* 337, no. 12 (1997): 847–849. The fact that this journal represents scientific authority and possesses the greatest impact of all the medical press worldwide lends legitimacy indeed to the debate and the terms in which it is expressed. It nevertheless has received many reactions, especially from the people responsible for the criticized studies.

15. South Africa's position in these tests is not neutral. At the end of the poll of sixteen studies carried out in the third world by Peter Lurie and Sydney Wolfe, "Unethical Trials of Interventions to Reduce Perinatal Transmission of the Human Immunodeficiency Virus in Developing Countries," *New England Journal of Medicine* 337, no. 12 (1997): 853–856, the authors wonder: "What are the potential implications of accepting such a double standard? Researchers might inject live malaria parasites into HIV-positive subjects in China to study the effect of the progression of HIV, even though the study protocol had been rejected in the United States and Mexico. Or researchers might randomly assign malnourished San to receive vitamin-fortified or standard bread." And they add: "These are not simply hypothetical worst-case scenarios; they have already been performed." The second was published in the *South African Medical Journal* in 1996. The parallel between China and South Africa is suggestive. And the conclusion allows for no answer: "Residents of impoverished, postcolonial countries, the majority of whom are people of color, must be protected from potential exploitation in research."

16. As she explains, the formula was borrowed from a quote by the famous South African satirist Pieter-Dirk Uys: "In old South Africa, they killed people, today they just let them die."

17. See Solomon Benatar, "Health Care Reform and the Crisis of HIV and AIDS in South Africa," *New England Journal of Medicine* 351, no. 1 (2004): 81–92. The author ends his article thus: "In reflecting on the first decade of South Africa's transition to democracy, it is necessary to strike a fair balance between justified criticism and deserved praise for a government faced with the overwhelming burden of a major political transformation and the simultaneous challenges posed by a devastating disease."

18. At the end of 2003, six and a half million people in South Africa were receiving allowances instituted in 1998, including 2 million retired persons who received 700 rands a month from the Old Age Grant and 3.4 million children who received 700 rands from the Care Dependency Grant. See *South Africa Yearbook 2003–2004,* www.gsci.gov.za.

19. Reprinted in the *Acts of the AIDS in Context Conference* (2002), then in a series of publications developing the same "witchcraft paradigm," it followed a monograph on a case of withcraft in a Soweto neighborhood (2000).

20. Listening to their anger, I thought of what Chinua Achebe (1988) wrote as he read a British critic who reproached him with not knowing his place. He said he remembered the colonial phrase: "I know my natives."

21. Another example of academic "scandals" concerns an exhibit of photographs of naked African homosexuals during a lecture titled "Sex and Secrecy" at the University of Witwatersrand in June 2003. The young woman anthropologist, Nokuthula Skhosana, complained indignantly about the "fascination" with black bodies and alluded to the way Sarah Baartman's had been treated over a century ago. In its 27 June 2003 edition, the *Weekly Mail and Guardian* somewhat complacently dedicated its front page to this scandal, ambiguously illustrating it by a selection of photos under the title "Are Black Bodies So Fascinating?"

22. Significantly, aside from the classical references to Evans-Pritchard (but none to the many publications of the School of Manchester that as is well known were the first to be interested in sorcery among the urban working class of southern Africa precisely in a perspective of social change (see Marwick 1987), the only authors quoted by Adam Ashforth (2002) for their contribution to the analysis of the relationship between AIDS and witchcraft are John and Pat Calwell who, as will be seen below, are the paragons of culturalist essentialism in the history of AIDS.

23. An author such as David Hammond-Tooke (1970) proposed analyses of witchcraft in the urban Eastern Cape that went in this direction already over a quarter of a century ago.

24. Even if that does represent a very real issue, as Isak Niehaus (2001) re-

minds us in his study of the procedures and practices of witchcraft control in the Limpopo before and after 1994.

25. On the "applied culturalism of Public Health," see my article (2001) in which I discuss the reasons for the attractiveness of cultural approaches in medicine.

26. See "Sex with Virgins to Cure AIDS," www.truthorfiction.com/rumors. The petition too is on the web site. The document presenting the rumor mentions the existence of this myth in other African countries as well as Cambodia, India, and Jamaica.

27. See L. M. Richard, "Baby Rape in South Africa," *Child Abuse Review* 12, no. 6 (2003): 392–400. The fact is also reported by the Integrated Regional Information Network of the United Nations: "Focus on the Virgin Myth and HIV/AIDS," 25 April 2002, www.aegis.com/news/irin.

28. See R. Jewkes, L. Martin, and L. Penn-Kekana, "Virgin-Cleansing Myth: Cases of Child Rape Are Not Exotic," *Lancet* 359, no. 9307 (2002): 711. The authors mainly use data from an unpublished report by L. Penn-Kekana and R. Jewkes, "Child Sexual Abuse in Mpumalanga," mimeo., 55 pp.

29. The absence of signature has obviously raised conjectures and brought on policelike investigations. It was especially noted that the electronic file contained an inscription "suggesting it had been written on Thabo Mbeki's computer," but according to the experts, "that was not conclusive evidence." See "Would the Real AIDS Dissident Please Declare Himself," *Weekly Mail and Guardian*, 19 April 2002; and "ANC Divided over Dissident AIDS Report," *Sunday Independant*, 23 March 2002.

30. In the case of Parks Mankahlana and Peter Mokaba, it is remarkable that their premature deaths (in 2000 and 2002 respectively) were unofficially attributed to AIDS: "Pressure on ANC to Know if AIDS Killed Parks," *Independent*, 26 October 2000; "Mokaba Had Acute Pneumonia—ANC," *Sapa*, 10 June 2002; "Standing Ovation for Kente," *The Star*, 21 February 2003.

31. Comparing the various prevention strategies in Africa, a WHO cost-efficiency study shows that the cost per year of life gained ranges from $1 for the combined programs to promote condoms and treat venereal diseases to $1,800 for the antiretroviral therapies for adults; to prevent perinatal transmission, the single doses of nevirapine come to approximately $10, but adding artificial milk to avoid contamination by breast-feeding adds $200. Without being able to draw a final conclusion, the authors proposed that these elements be taken into account when making the choices which clearly put the drugs at a disadvantage: A. Creese, K. Floyd, A. Alban, and L. Guinness, "Cost-Effectiveness of HIV/AIDS Interventions in Africa: A Systematic Review of the Evidence," *Lancet* 359 (11 May 2002): 1635–1642.

32. See D. McCoy, "Back to Basics for Health Care," *Weekly Mail and Guardian*, 4 May 2001. Conscious that the prevention of mother-to-child trans-

mission is on the verge of becoming reality, he suggests a program be implemented, "but it must be done in a way that will ensure rapid and continued health infrastructure development, keep equity high on the agenda and not inadvertently cause more harm than good."

33. "How Pityana Buckled," *Weekly Mail and Guardian,* 30 November 2001. The article speaks of a "capitulation" that "raises questions as to the Commission's independence."

34. "Minister Blasts Shilowa," *The Star,* 13 February 2002; and "How Mbeki Snubbed Madiba," *Sunday Independent,* 7 April 2002. We discover that the ANC asked Nelson Mandela not to intervene again on the question of AIDS and nevirapine on his own initiative without first referring to the Party.

35. To add to the confusion of his itinerary and the complexity of the scene, this activist was convinced that all patients should be able to access antiretroviral therapy yet refused it for himself when his diminishing state of health required it on the basis of its possible side effects. Orthodox for others, he became heterodox for himself.

36. "The Heart of the AIDS Protest," *Weekly Mail and Guardian,* 12 April 2002. "For the entire world TAC is the duo Markandzackie [Mark Heywood and Zachie Achmat]."

37. In his inaugural speech at the AIDS in Context conference in April 2001. He considers arguments opposed to the implementation of treatments "morally undefendable."

38. According to the Health Systems Trust, 62 percent of the family doctors and 77 percent of the specialists are in the private sector; these figures were respectively 53 percent and 66 percent ten years earlier. Of the 7,600 physicians in the public sector, 21 percent come from abroad, mainly from central Africa, eastern Europe and Cuba; this proportion is up to 43 percent in the Limpopo, 44 percent in the Mpumalanga, and 54 percent in the Northwest. See *South Africa Survey 2000/2001,* South African Institute of Race Relations, Johannesburg 2001.

39. "Hospital Staff Victimized by Department," *Weekly Mail and Guardian,* 16 November 2001; and "AIDS Angel Faces 'Dr. Death' Witch-hunt," *The Star,* 4 March 2002.

40. In an admittedly difficult context constituting the suffering of some and the helplessness of others—as one of them testified in an anonymous diary of which excerpts appeared in "Scent of the Plague," *Weekly Mail and Guardian,* 29 June 2001. This clinical ethos is not always the case. Our surveys show that differences in status, social class, and racial category not only continue to influence the daily practice of the profession; the development of the epidemic has been a boon for some doctors in the public and private sectors who claimed they had treatments to propose or resold drugs. For a case study of the hospital world, see Loveday Penn-Kekana 2004.

41. See Jon Cohen, "South Africa's New Enemy," "A Research Renaissance,

South African Style," and "Confronting Conference Complexities," *Science* 288 (2000): 2168–2170.

42. "Mbeki-Leon: The Gloves Come Off," *Sunday Independent,* 12 August 2000; "What Leon and Mbeki Had to Say," *Weekly Mail and Guardian,* 6 October 2000; "Mbeki, Leon Row Is Harming Race Relations," *The Star,* 11 October 2000.

43. "AZT Doctor Turns Minister into Disrepute," *The Star,* 10 January 2000; "AZT Doctor Aims to Sue Health Minister," *The Star,* 5 March 2000; "Gazi Ready to Pay up for AIDS Drugs," *Sapa,* 24 March 2000.

44. "AIDS Test for De Lille," *Sowetan,* 5 April 2004; "Fiery De Lille Softens on Visit to Her HIV Baby," *Cape Argus,* 14 October 1998; "De Lille's AIDS Soiree Turns Sour," *The Star,* 16 May 2000.

45. "Departmental Muddle Causes AIDS Drugs Delay" and "AIDS Babies' Fate Now Lies in Cabinet's Hands," *The Star,* 3 and 10 April 2001. The especially acute tension just then was due to the fact that after a long period of hemming and hawing and recantations in this affair, the health minister seemed on the verge of giving the green light for treatments to commence. Bureaucratic complications and last-minute political blocks seemed to be compromising the finalization of the evaluation process.

46. A TAC officer with whom I talked this over expressed no regret whatsoever. For him, Nono Simelela was indubitably an honest and dedicated person, but "she should have quit." Many others I spoke to thought on the contrary that precisely because of the polemics surrounding the issue, her efficiency and discretion had allowed several others, including the most sensitive, to advance.

47. "The Madness of Queen Manto" recalls Nicholas Hytner's film *The Madness of King George,* which came out in 1994 and told the tale of the last years of King George III of England at the end of the seventeenth century.

48. Somewhat later, he declared to the press that the minister had even offered him a hug of reconciliation, which he refused. See "TAC Disrupts Manto's Speech," *Sapa,* 25 March 2003; and "Time for Hug Is Over, TAC Tells Manto," *Mercury,* 26 March 2003. In a commentary published in the *Weekly Mail and Guardian* on the following 4 April under the title "The Long Walk to Civil Disobedience," Zachie Achmat excused himself for his personal attacks against the minister but repeated that he condemned her politics.

49. A full-page advertisement titled "Questions and Answers on TAC's Civil Disobedience Campaign" presents the argument given by the major South African dailies toward the end of March 2003. Reactions to this campaign were published mainly in readers' columns (*Sowetan,* 4 April 2003). The ANC was granted the right of reply to Achmat's commentary: "Confidence Moloko: 'This Is Everyone's Fight,'" *Weekly Mail and Guardian,* 11 April 2003.

50. Tom Lodge (1983) reminds us that this form of protest, first theorized by Thoreau and then applied by Gandhi was used by Africans to combat the first

apartheid laws in 1952 under the leadership of Walter Sisulu. It meant defying legislation by committing small crimes in order to swamp the police precincts, the courts, and the prisons, a tactic that gave the ANC its broad-based popularity.

51. In contrast, NAPWA (National Association of People Living with AIDS), closer to the government and TAC's great rival in the fight against AIDS, chose exactly the same time to apply a very different strategy. The Black Easter campaign's official objective was to force the pharmaceutical companies to give in on the prices of antiretroviral drugs by having demonstrators block their main offices. The enemy here was not the South African government but the drug multinationals. The campaign got under way on 17 April but was interrupted on 29 April when negotiations began between the association and the large firms (Merck-Sharp-Dohme, Glaxo-Smithkline, Bristol-Myers-Squibb, Boeringer-Ingelheim, and Roche agreed to negotiate). See "Napwa Suspends 'Black Easter' AIDS Campaign," *Sapa,* 29 May 2003.

52. Charged by the Centre for the Study of AIDS with editing *AIDS Review,* the researcher and journalist close to TAC's Tim Trengrove-Jones (2001) regrets that "the idiom of war persists with its unfortunate connotations of conflict, control, enemy, body as battlefield." Knowing the warlike style of TAC, the comment is remarkable.

53. As journalist Belinda Beresford (herself connected to the activists) puts it in the *Weekly Mail and Guardian* of 12 April 2002: "In three years, TAC has succeeded in humiliating repeatedly the government." The price for the efficiency of the movement was to stiffen social relations around the AIDS issue.

54. This is what the director general of the Health Department, Ayanda Ntsaluba, explicitly told the *New York Times* on 31 March 2002, following leaks about dissident documents going the rounds of the ANC: "In a practical way the debate within the ANC really does not affect what we are doing."

55. That is what a professor of medicine in a high academic position at the University of Witwatersrand meant, having publicly called for the rapid implementation of antiretroviral drugs, when he told me, just after the public announcement of the national rollout of drugs, "Now real difficulties will start. We had pretended they did not exist, but we must confront them now." On this point, see also Schneider 2004.

56. The story of an HIV-positive child born to seronegative parents reported in the papers gives one an incidental but nevertheless significant idea of this system. If the "mystery" did not confirm the dissident theses (what some people did not fail to point out), it at least seemed to show that AIDS remained a strange and little-understood affliction. See "Mystery over HIV Baby," *Sowetan,* 8 January 2003; and Penn-Kekana 2004.

4. THE IMPRINT OF THE PAST

1. See especially "What Leon and Mbeki Had to Say," *Weekly Mail and Guardian,* 6 October 2000; and "Two Views on AIDS and AZT," *City Press,* 8 October 2000.

2. Zachariah Keodirelang Matthews (1901–1968) was the first African to obtain his B.A. degree and become principal of Adams College (in the Natal). He taught social anthropology at South African Native College in Fort Hare, the first public university for Africans, and then in 1945 became head of the Department of African Studies before joining the ANC. His political career ended in exile after his acquittal at the treason trial of 1959 (see Saunders and Southey 2001). The full text of Thabo Mbeki's speech can be found on www.anc.org.za.

3. Pierre Nora's ambitious undertaking of the "lieux de mémoire" (1984–1992) demonstrates the contemporary reconfiguration of the relationship between these two ways of experiencing the past. In it, memory becomes an object to be worked on by the historian. Simultaneously, the growing appeal to history to understand, judge, and confirm the facts of the present reveals what François Hartog and Jacques Revel (2001) call the "political uses of the past." There, the historian becomes the subject of the workings of memory.

4. The seminal work of linguistic research carried out by Reinhardt Koselleck (1997) on the German distinction between *Historie* and *Geschichte* in particular allows us to construct a history of the concept of history, while the detailed survey by Michael Herzfeld (1991) on the differentiations in the relation to historical temporality in a village on Crete demonstrates the existence of a timeless production of memory.

5. James Clifford (1988) and George Marcus (1999) and in their wake a whole critical movement in anthropology took a stand precisely against this first version of hermeneutics.

6. One can note here the critique formulated by Michel Callon (1999) of the sociology of unveiling developed by Pierre Bourdieu, to which he opposed his own sociology of translation.

7. Borrowing Martyn Hammersley's (1993) term as he contests the fact that "the acknowledgment of the rhetorical dimension of ethnographic descriptions puts a term to the project of representing reality." According to him, on the contrary, "the objective of truth must prevail." This is what he has termed "fallible realism."

8. This is particularly the case—whatever their merits—of the work of Hein Marais (2000), Philippe Denis (2001), and Helen Schneider (2002) that bears on the history of AIDS but also of Tom Lodge's (2002) writings or the texts collected by Sean Jacobs and Richard Calland (2002), which broach this policy within the more general frame of the changes taking place in South African society. One no-

table exception: Virginia van der Vliet's (2001) article, which talks about the beginnings of the epidemic during the apartheid era.

9. This is what transpires from the voluminous unpublished documentation also of publications such as Walker and Gilbert 2002 and Eaton, Flisher, and Aaro 2003. Among the exceptions one can especially mention the psychosociological study by Catherine Campbell and Brian Williams (1999) on the risky practices in the mines as well as the historical surveys by Robert Morrell (2001) on the changes in masculine identities and by Peter Delius and Clive Glaser (2002) on the sexual socialization of young men.

10. Going back to the end of the nineteenth century, a time when urbanization and industrialization were developing and with them the politics of segregation and exploitation of the black populations, might seem as if one were looking too far for the keys to the South African society of today and the elements permitting us to understand its difficulties in facing the AIDS epidemic. Nevertheless, it is indispensable, if one wants to avoid the biases pointed out by Packard (1989: 20) in a set of works on African epidemics, which, as he writes, "in limiting their time frame have been unable to describe how these linkages have evolved over longer periods of time and how realignments in specific sets of political and economic interests have shaped the longer history of both health and health care." He himself starts his history of tuberculosis in South Africa at the end of the nineteenth century.

11. The authoritarian grouping of the black populations in the homelands was accompanied by a redefinition that was not only racial ("Whites," "Coloured," "Indians," and "Africans") but also ethnic (for "Africans" only). According to Leonard Thompson (2000: 190), "The white racial group formed a single nation, with Afrikaans- and English-speaking components, while African belonged to several (eventually ten) distinct nations or potential nations—a formula that made the white nation the largest in the country." The imposition of these categories was artificial, but it contributed to making ethnic identities exist, a powerful mode of preventing uprisings against the regime.

12. See especially "Greater Tzaneen Sub-District," mimeographed document of September 2002, 45 pp. This superimposition of systems ill fitted among themselves had already been severely criticized by the Gluckman Commission in 1942, as De Beer (1984) reminds us.

13. It would be interesting, and doubly edifying, to complete the comparison in absolute terms with a comparison in relative terms, that is, of the rates. First, the frequency rate: the number of cases during that period compared to the density of population is 25 per 1000 and 7 per 1000 respectively among Africans and whites. Second, the death rate: the number of deaths compared to the number of cases reported is respectively 33 and 44 percent. In other words, there are fewer cases among the Africans, who are, however, three and a half times more exposed to infection and one-third more likely to die once they have fallen ill.

This is a sign both of the objective relativity of the danger and of the considerable inequality that exists between Africans and whites in the face of the epidemic.

14. Posel (1987) shows this for the period preceding the institution of apartheid, that is, toward the end of the 1940s. Though the Afrikaner nationalists held a theory of white supremacy and racial separation, it was competing with the practical constraints of capitalism, including British capitalism, especially concerning workforce availability. It is interesting to note that this tension can be observed even in intellectual circles, where, as in a game of mirrors, they try to account for apartheid largely through Marxist analysis that is attentive to class interests but also an analysis, then called liberal, that foregrounded the effects of ideology.

15. As Thompson (2000: 203) puts it, "The government did not keep detailed medical statistics for the Africans." In particular: "Official life expectancy figures for Africans were not available."

16. In reporting this episode, De Beer (1984: 70) adds: "But people do not choose to live under unhygienic conditions. They are condemned by political and economic factors to live in areas where healthy living is impossible."

17. On sanitarization as a double process of the medicalization and politicization of social objects, see Fassin 1997 on the politics and practices of public health.

18. This was especially true of the first national campaign in 1988, as shown by Louis Grundlingh in "A Critical Historical Analysis of Government Reponses to HIV/AIDS in South Africa as Reported in the Media, 1983–1994," AIDS in Context Conference, Johannesburg, 4–7 April 2001.

19. In fact, as Jochelson (2001: 87–88) has demonstrated, after an authoritarian phase of population control through quarantine, which at first drew mainly a social line (between the poor, partly made up of "poor Whites," and the rich), prevention programs (on the model of what elsewhere in the world was known as "new public health"), a more pedagogical orientation judged to be less restrictive and more respectful of the individual was put into practice. In this new frame of intervention, the messages that were supposed to be better adapted to the populations being addressed revealed the ordinary prejudice of society but also its political orientations: whites were expected to be as desirous of building a healthy nation as they were of conforming with religious ideals, syphilis being not only a sign of individual immorality but also a cause of collective degeneration; blacks, on the other hand, were ineluctably "becoming rotten with disease and a menace to civilisation," in General Jan Smuts's words in 1937 (quoted in Jochelson 2001: 93).

20. Other representations are in competition with anthropophagy, namely, sorcery, but the complex connections between the two are well known. Elaine Katz (1994: 191) reports these remarks by a South African merchant: "The native shivers to-day at the idea of the cold morning in the compound and talks with

his fellows about the 'mlugu 'tgate'—the witchcraft of the white man—which has led to the death of many of his brothers in the mines."

21. For René Dubos (quoted by Marks and Andersson 1992: 104), this disease, which he calls the "white plague," is "perhaps the first penalty that capitalist society had to pay for the ruthless exploitation of labor."

22. Pursuing the urban segregation implemented by "native locations" and anticipating what the "homelands" would be under apartheid, "reserves" had been created by the Native Land Act of 1913. This act limited the land that the native populations could claim and that the white farmers were not allowed to buy. However, as Harold Wolpe (1995) has shown, the fact that Africans were prohibited from acquiring land outside these "reserves," given the demographic growth and the unforeseeable climatic circumstances, transformed them into a "cheap workforce" for industry.

23. The report of the Commission for Research on Tuberculosis of 1932 (quoted in Packard 1989: 206) is especially explicit in this regard: "The biological lack of resistance exists quite apart from any risk incurred in the mining industry or in any other industries." Of course, this does not prevent one from considering that improving living and working conditions plays an important part.

24. In a survey on tuberculosis among 28,522 men working in four gold mines in the province of the Gauteng (around Johannesburg), 425 were considered to have tuberculosis because of the presence of the Koch bacillus in their spumen; of these, 49 percent were HIV-positive. However, a sample of the total population shows 21 percent HIV-positive. In other words, HIV is a risk factor for tuberculosis among this population, since it occurs twice as often among those who have tuberculosis as among other miners; but it must be pointed out that half the individuals who have tuberculosis are not HIV-positive and that the vast majority of HIV-positive people do not have tuberculosis. See P. Sonnenberg et al., "Risk Factors for Pulmonary Disease due to Culture-Positive M. Tuberculosis and Non-Tuberculous Mycobacteria in South African Gold Miners," *European Respiratory Journal* 15 (2000): 291–296.

25. Long before the South African controversies began and with no connection to dissident ideas, Packard and Epstein (1992) stressed the fact that, several decades later, the same interpretive keys were being used, such as explaining sexual practices through naturalization of people and culturalization of their behaviors. Criticizing the fact that the same significant omissions were being repeated concerning the search for social and economic causes, they mentioned the role of infections or malnutrition but also of iatrogenetic transmission.

26. In this respect, the very fine analysis proposed by Butchart (1998) hardly justifies his criticism of Packard and Marks, as if political and moral economics were mutually exclusive, as if a central locus of power embodied by the apartheid state, and a reticular system of powers insinuating themselves into the cracks of the social space could not exist in South Africa.

27. Taking their cue from the Black Power movement in the United States, African intellectuals led by Steve Biko developed a new form of resistance toward the end of the 1960s based on the denunciation of the "inferiority complex" inculcated by whites and on promoting "self-esteem" as a means of fighting against the oppression of blacks, meaning all racially dominated people whether African or not (Saunders and Southey 2001).

28. Land in South Africa represents the Afrikaner Motherland and is thus a central stake in the project of apartheid. Arriving in Pretoria on 1 June 1948 after the National Party won the general elections, the new prime minister, D. F. Malan (quoted in Thompson 2000: 186), declared: "In the past we felt like strangers in our own country, but today South Africa belongs to us once more. For the first time since Union, South Africa is our own. May God grant that it remains our own."

29. Interview published in *Le Monde,* 28 November 1987, with the title, " 'The Epidemic Will Be the First of Major Changes in African Society,' Professor Clumeck Declares."

30. See UNFPA, *AIDS Update 1999,* prepared by Joseph Sioncke and available at www.unfpa.org. The quotations are taken especially from the section "Promiscuity and the Primacy of Cultural Factors: A Lethal Mixture in Africa," p. 6.

31. The Australian couple redirected their research during the 1990s so as to make the observation of low heterosexual transmissibility compatible with the observation of high African seroprevalence. Their model distanced itself from the cultural paradigm of the preceding decade, and they started promoting the notion that circumcision protects against AIDS and that, on the contrary, uncircumcised men are a very high risk group whose presence defined the "AIDS belt," that is, the central arena of the infection in Africa (Caldwell and Caldwell 1996). In conformity with this new lead, anatomical this time, circumcision programs were launched in various parts of the continent.

32. This focus took place very early and was rarely refuted. In "The AIDS Problem in Africa," *Lancet* (11 January 1986): 79–82, the first important review published on the subject, the epidemiologist Robert Biggar of the National Cancer Institute of Bethesda wrote on the basis of the survey's first results: "Hypotheses that implicate non-sexual forms of parenteral transmission, such as reuse of inadequately sterilised needles or insect vectors such as mosquitoes are untenable."

33. Among many other examples covering the whole African continent one might quote, in the Congo, D. Ngoie-Ngalla's short pamphlet in the *Semaine Africaine* of 18 February 1988: "The black man was not only in their eyes the incarnation of evil and sin for Christians, but also a creature whose physical aspect inspired repulsion, who probably smelled, and whose physical appearance announced a depraved morality. AIDS and its origins said to be Negro by a science

that does not dare say its name came just in time to deliver the civilized nations from the nightmare of a Negro invasion."

34. A former slave in the Cape colony, she was taken to London in 1810 where she was exhibited in fairs for her callipygian anatomy. The "Hottentot Venus" was transferred to France and died there in 1819. An autopsy was performed by Georges Cuvier and her genital organs presented to the Academy of Medicine and kept in the Museum of Mankind until 1985. When Nelson Mandela was elected president, he asked France to authorize the repatriation of her remains. The ceremony in honor of their homecoming took place on 9 August 2002, National Women's Day. As Sander Gilman (1986) has shown, she is the symbol of the sexual violence perpetrated against Africa.

35. Reported by van der Vliet (2001). Citations taken from the official minutes recorded in the *Debates of Parliament*.

36. The observations were published the following year: G. J. Ras et al., "Acquired Immunodeficiency Syndrome: A Report of Two South African Cases," *South African Medical Journal* 64, no. 4 (23 July 1983): 140–142. Two years later, the first seroepidemiological study led the authors to declare that the virus "HTLV-III is not endemic in southern Africa" except among homosexuals: S. F. Lyons et al., "Sero-epidemiology of HTLV-III Antibody in Southern Africa," *South African Medical Journal* 67, no. 24 (15 June 1985): 961–962.

37. These citations are taken from the lecture given by Louis Grundlingh, "A Critical Historical Analysis of Government Reponses to HIV/AIDS in South Africa as Reported in the Media, 1983–1994," AIDS in Context Conference, Johannesburg, 4–7 April 2001.

38. See especially, R. Sher et al., "Lack of Evidence of HIV Infection in Drug Abusers at Present," *South African Medical Journal* 70 (1986): 776–777; and B. D. Schoub et al., "Absence of HIV Infection in Prostitutes and Women Attending Sexually Transmitted Disease Clinics in South Africa," *Transactions of the Royal Society of Tropical Medicine and Hygiene* 81, no. 5 (1987): 874–875.

39. As Anthony Zwi and Deborah Bachmayer (1990) wrote when reporting on these statistics. They show that fragmentation of health services has resulted in extremely poor coordination.

40. See the blood bank survey published by D. B. Schoub et al., "Epidemiological Considerations of the Present Status and Future Growth of the Acquired Immunodeficiency Syndrome in South Africa," *South African Medical Journal* 74 (1988): 153–157. The study on antenatal visits is reported in M. Shapiro, R. L. Crookes, and E. O'Sullivan, "Screening Antenatal Blood Samples for Anti-Human Immunodeficiency Virus Antibodies by a Large-Pool Enzyme-linked Immunoabsorbent Assay System," *South African Medical Journal* 76 (1989): 245–247.

41. See Louis Grundlingh, "A Critical Historical Analysis of Government Re-

sponses to HIV/AIDS in South Africa as Reported in the Media, 1983–1994," AIDS in Context Conference, Johannesburg, 4–7 April 2001.

42. See especially, D. Seftel, "AIDS and Apartheid: Double Trouble," *African Reports,* November–December 1988, 17–22; A. T. Viljoen, "Apartheid and AIDS," *Lancet* 8674, no. 2 (25 November 1989): 1280.

43. Some speak of "deportation," as demonstrated by the title of this article published in one of the major international scientific journals: Michael Cherry, "South Africa Uses Deportation in the Battle against AIDS," *Nature* 31, no. 332 (March 1988): 386.

44. And sometimes tragic expulsions, such as the one that cost the life of 150 Zaireans who in March 1993 were forcibly loaded onto a barge supposed to carry them to the other side of the Congo River to Kinshasa, which sank a few hundred meters from the pier at Brazzaville (Fassin 1994).

45. These pieces of propaganda are cited respectively by Zwi and Bachmayer 1990; van der Vliet 2001; Jochelson 2001.

46. These facts are reported by van der Vliet 2001. Mzala's article, "AIDS and the Imperialist Connection," published in *Sechaba,* can be found at www.disa.nu.ac.za.

47. His article, "Potential Decimation of the Eve of Liberation," published in 1990 in the journal *Progress,* is one of the first to announce the imminence of a health catastrophe (cited in van der Vliet 2001).

48. In the collection of short stories evocatively titled *Post-traumatic: New South African Short Stories,* ed. Chris van Wyk (Joubert Park: Botsotso Publishing), pp. 198–207.

49. About the Swapo soldiers, former South African army officer Johan Theron admitted in May 2000 that he had obeyed Basson's order and with Basson's help administered deadly injections of myorelaxants to hundreds of prisoners who were then thrown into the ocean from military planes. See especially *Sowetan,* 4 May 2000, and *Weekly Mail and Guardian,* 26 May 2000. The judge subsequently dropped the charges alleging a secret agreement, letting off former army members who had fought in the South African province that after independence in 1990 became Namibia.

50. Taken from the microbiologist Mike Odendal's hearing: "So you personally put drops of anthrax onto these cigarettes?—Yes.—And what would have happened to the person who smoked these cigarettes?—Well, it's difficult to speculate, but I can imagine that might have fatal results.—Were you aware of that at the time you did it?—Yes" (Truth and Reconciliation Commission, CBW Hearings, p. 83). Anthrax had also been put in chocolates and on envelopes. For the laboratory researchers, it was nevertheless considered much less efficient than substances such as paraoxon.

51. See in particular the well-documented book by the journalist Charlene

Burger and the researcher Chandré Gould (2002). The transcripts of the commission can be consulted at Truth and Reconciliation Commission Hearings, www.doj.gov.za/trc. Many newspaper articles tell the story of Project Coast and its director, among them, *Weekly Mail and Guardian,* 18 Feburary 2000, 26 May 2000, 10 August 2001; *Sowetan,* 8 November 1999, 3 May 2000, 4 May 2000, 25 May 2000, 12 April 2002; *Sunday Independent,* 8 October 2000; *Sunday Times,* 14 April 2002; *Sunday World,* 17 October 1999, 14 November 1999; *Citizen,* 25 May 2000, 12 April 2002; *Star,* 10 April 2002, 12 April 2002. There are at least two documentaries on Wouter Basson and Project Coast: one produced by the BBC and directed by Peter Molloy; the other coproduced by French television France 3, written by Tristan Mendès-France and directed by Jean-Pierre Prévost.

52. Taken from Daan Goosen's hearing: "In 1983–1984, I am not too sure when Dr Basson presented me with a scenario and a document. This document contained a proposition from someone in Europe and this guy says he's got a bacteria which has the possibility of only affecting, making sick and killing pigmented people" (Truth and Reconciliation Commission, CBW Hearings, p. 201). The same person mentioned later that in a discussion with the director of Project Coast, the question was raised as to the substances that might produce cancer in Nelson Mandela so that if he came out of prison "he shouldn't make problems."

53. This article was preceded by another one on 2 September 1999, also in the *Weekly Mail and Guardian.* It already mentioned this story, basing itself on research carried out by Dr. Robert Shell, director of the research unit on population at the University of Rhodes, and widely circulated in southern Africa in a document called "Trojan Horses: HIV/AIDS and Military Bases in Southern Africa," 18 pp. Using a mathematical model, the demographer showed that if askaris had contaminated four prostitutes in a population of one million inhabitants until then free of AIDS, deaths from now until the year 2021 would number 365,788.

54. See especially, "South African Doctors Demand Action on 'Unethical' Colleagues," *British Medical Journal* 319 (1999): 514; and "Why Is Dr. Death Still Busy in the Wards?" *Sunday Independent,* 7 May 2000.

55. The Mexican historian Miguel León Portilla ([1959] 1989) was the first to reverse the historiographic gaze by showing how the Spanish conquest had been experienced by the Indian populations of Mexico: "the vision of the vanquished" has become a generic expression of this other way of writing history. The title of his work and the principle of his analysis were taken up a few years later by Nathan Wachtel concerning the Indians of Peru.

56. It can hardly be otherwise when one has lived through the Alexandra of the 1960s and 1970s that Mark Mathabane, the child of the township become tennis champion, described in *Kaffir Boy: Growing out of Apartheid* (London: Bodley Head, 1986). Segregation and misery, arbitrary arrests and public humil-

iations were part of everyday life. The opening scene of this book of memories describes a police raid in the township at nightfall. His father, who does not have a work contract and therefore a pass is in hiding. When he is discovered, he is interrogated and humiliated naked in front of his children—"a pitiful sight" that makes him "gasp with horror" (p. 21). When he comes out of prison, "a vindicative hatred for white people, which was soon to become the passion of his life, had crept into his speech and as he spoke haltingly, his words ringing with anger, he punctuated each reference to white people with a four-letter word" (p. 50).

57. See Susan Booysen, "History Weighs More than Reality," *Star,* 8 April 2004: "Political past and present have combined to forge a collective, cross-class political identity among the majority of South Africans. In the study of elections, the voting choice is portrayed as an overlay of sociocultural identity, issue preference and party identification. Yet none of these explanations cater for the effect of past and present experiences of oppression, liberation and liberation movement government on voting."

5. THE EMBODIMENT OF THE WORLD

1. The open letter addressed to NAPWA in March 2003 inquiring into the opacity of its finances and denouncing its aggressive campaigns was signed, however, by a collection of actors from different associations—including members of NAPWA who were in disagreement with their national leaders. See "Aids Activists Take on One of Their Own," *Weekly Mail and Guardian,* 7 March 2003.

2. For instance, she could have acknowledged an affinity with the other woman inasmuch as both are physicians employed in the public health sector. During the major political crisis provoked by the 15,000 senior citizens who died during the heat wave in France in August 2003, the health minister and the doctor representing the emergency medical specialists who had just accused (in the media) the Health Department of incompetence, were reconciled when they found themselves at the negotiations table for, as a senior civil servant explained, "they are both first and foremost doctors." In the South African case, they are less united by their professional history than divided by the color bar.

3. In the present case, the director was adopting a reflective stance allowing her to distinguish analytically her own perception from the other's, respectively the "objective" from the "emotional" way of seeing things. Though she excuses the latter, she nevertheless places it lower down on the scale of understanding the world.

4. Incidentally, the example he gives is that of the black doctor: at the time Hughes was writing, being a black doctor presented two not very compatible main characteristics, his occupation (associated with a privileged white milieu) and his color (associated with low-ranking and little-valued occupations). The

surprise that a doctor can be black attests to the fact that the second characteristic clearly has precedence over the first. Socially, he is treated like a black before being considered a doctor or a member of the middle classes. Thus it is effectively his racial ascription that defines his status.

5. Racially construed identities obviously do not necessarily determine the terms of the opposition in this way, though the case in point seems to be the most frequent. A "Black" may deny there are any racial connotations in his speech by objectifying social relations as being due to class, for instance, whereas a "White" may on the contrary openly express his racism, including by using socially condemned language.

6. From this point of view, see the criticism Laurent Vidal (1995) leveled against the KABP (Knowledge-Attitudes-Beliefs-Practices) surveys that are the paradigm for the risk studies concerning AIDS carried out by international institutions.

7. "Nearly Half of Mine Workers Have HIV," *Business Report,* 24 November 1999. One can imagine the anguish caused by such a news item relayed by the press. The percentages announced at the time were probably overestimated, however. A survey done in 2003 in the mines of all southern Africa came up with an average rate of 14 percent seropositivity and 18 percent for South Africa alone. This rate breaks down to only 4.5 percent for management, mainly white, but soars to 23 percent for the contracted workers, nearly all African. See "AIDS Taking a Massive Toll on Mining Industry," *Pretoria News,* 23 February 2004.

8. "Mines Accused of Conducting Covert AIDS Tests," *Reuters,* 17 August 2000. The tragic repatriation of one thousand foreign miners is reported in "South Africa Uses Deportation in the Battle against AIDS," *Nature* 332 (1988): 386.

9. "SA Mining Firms Test Workers for AIDS," *Reuters,* 13 February 2001; "De Beers Starts to Test Miners for HIV/AIDS," *Reuters,* 1 March 2001; "Companies Unite to Fight HIV/AIDS," *Sunday Business Times,* 29 March 2002.

10. "Anglo American Announces HIV Plan," *Mercury,* 6 August 2002; "Anglo Deal Paves Way for AIDS Drugs," *Weekly Mail and Guardian,* 26 August 2002.

11. As Shula Marks noted about Anglo American's indignation against South African AIDS policies: "There was some irony in the Corporation's grandstanding in relation to the government's tardiness in providing antiretrovirals for HIV/AIDS sufferers." And she adds, "In 1932, the Committee on Tuberculosis formed jointly by the state and the Chamber of Mines, pointed to the contrast between 'the generous provision of hospitals and efficient whole-time medical staffs by the mining industry for its native workers on the Rand with the almost complete absence of a public medical service of any kind for the natives throughout South Africa' and pointed to 'the fact that industrial concerns often set an example to governments in the care of their dependents.'" See Shula Marks,

"The Silent Scourge? Silicosis, Respiratory Disease and Gold-Mining in South Africa," unpublished document, 22 pp., www.wiser.wits.ac.za.

12. "Multinational Revolt," *Weekly Mail and Guardian,* 11 April 2003; "Mbeki Rejects Reparations Tax Proposal," *Business Report,* 16 April 2003; "Tutu Rejects Guilt Money" and "Lawyer Ignores Mbeki," *Sowetan,* 17 April 2003.

13. Of course, company logic does not exclude its employees' feelings. We do not doubt the sincerity of the lecturer and more generally the fact their doctors and nurses were devoted. We could even say, following the analysis by Luc Boltanski and Eve Chiapello (1999), that contemporary capitalism derives a profit from all this goodwill to boost its moral prestige. The best illustration of this convergence of interests *bien compris* is former president of Anglo American's Gold and Uranium Division, Clem Sunter, today president of the foundation and coauthor with economist Alan Whiteside of one of the first books on AIDS and one of the creators of the South African Business Coalition on HIV/AIDS. See "Companies Unite to Fight HIV/AIDS," *Sunday Business Times,* 29 March 2002.

14. On the management of risk and stress linked to working conditions in the mines, one can also read the testimonies gathered by Matsheliso Palesa Molapo (1995) in Western Deep Levels, the deepest mine pit in the world, 3,600 meters underground.

15. Elaine Katz (1994) used a cartoon from the newspaper *Die Vorlooper* of 12 June 1913 as a frontispiece for her history of silicosis. It shows the front of a mine pit piled up with skulls, with the caption: "Silent cause of the strike. During the last ten years 52,205 natives have died in the mines; 16,556 accidents took place and about 60,000 were sent home as invalids."

16. "Health, Human Dignity and Partners for Poverty Reduction," *ANC Today* 2, no. 14 (5 April 2002), at www.anc.org.za.

17. J. M. Coetzee, *Elisabeth Costello* (London : Secker & Warburg, 1999). "The Problem of Evil" is the sixth of eight lectures given by the heroine of the novel.

18. Of the big countries, only Brazil, with a Gini index of 60, slightly outstrips South Africa. The other most unegalitarian nations are the Central African Republic, Sierra Leone, and Guatemala. In comparison, the United States has an index of 40.8, France's is 32.7, and Denmark's is 24.7. See World Bank, *World Development Report 2000/2001: Attacking Poverty* (Oxford: Oxford University Press, 2001).

19. The data are taken from the *Poverty and Inequality Report* of the Central Statistical Service and from *October Household Survey* of Statistics South Africa. See *South Africa Survey 2000/2001,* South African Institute of Race Relations.

20. A current form of this denial consists in asserting that henceforth disparities in positions and remuneration are no longer the result of "open discrimination" but of "differences in levels of education and competence, of urban

or rural localization and of economic sector" (Nattrass and Seekings 2001), apparently forgetting that such "differences" precisely concern the fields in which a century of racial segregation has construed inequalities in the most efficient way possible, by developing an educational system with several tiers, forcing people to live in separate locations, and limiting access to most occupations.

21. The data presented here are taken from the calculations of life expectancy done by the Institute for Future Research and from the figures for infant mortality of the Health Systems Trust. See Mokate 2000; and *South Africa Survey 2000/2001*, South African Institute of Race Relations. The historical indications are taken from the article by Beryl Unterhalter, "Inequalities in Health and Disease: The Case of Mortality Rates for the City of Johannesburg, South Africa, 1910–1979," *International Journal of Health Services* 12, no. 4 (1982): 617–636.

22. Olive Shisana and Leickness Simbayi, *Nelson Mandela/HSRC Study of HIV/Aids* (Pretoria: HSRC, 2002). This survey unfortunately does not give any factorial analysis that would allow comparing the different factors studied in relation to one another.

23. Leigh Johnson and Debbie Budlender, *HIV Risk Factors: A Review of the Demographic, Socioeconomic, Biomedical and Behavioural Determinants of HIV Prevalence in South Africa* (Cape Town: Centre for Actuarial Research, 2002). The survey covering the industrial sector is presented in this report.

24. "A Society of Rapists" and "How Lucky I Am to Be Heard," *Weekly Mail and Guardian*, 7 April 2000. Charlene Smith writes: "The elimination of AIDS will not happen through condoms and vaccines. It has everything to do with the attitudes of the men and boys who rape; who believe they can have sex with anyone they want, whether it is a woman walking in the street, their non-consenting wife or their daughter."

25. This correspondence was published with the consent of the two protagonists in "Mbeki versus Leon: SA President Debates AIDS," *Sunday Times*, 9 July 2000; "What Leon and Mbeki Had to Say," *Weekly Mail and Guardian*, 6 October 2000; "Two Views on AIDS and AZT," *City Press*, 8 October 2000.

26. See the programmatic preface to Lewis Nkosi's *Making Birds* (Cape Town: Kwela Books, 2004).

27. Which Bourdieu (1980) condemns as the symmetrical dangers of the "realism of structure" derived from excessive "objectivism" and of the ideal vision of the agent in the name of "subjectivism."

28. For Soweto, it is Sipho Sepamla with *A Ride in the Whirlwind* (1981); for Sophiatown, Don Mattera with *Gone with the Twilight* (1987). For District Six in the Cape, Richard Rive with *Buckingham Palace* (1988).

29. The heroine in Coetzee's novel *In the Heart of the Country*, published in 1977, has the same first name. A century later and on either sides of the color line dividing South Africa, the young Sotho woman of Alexandra and the young Afrikaner woman from Karoo both experience physical and sexual violence,

threats and imagined murders, unequal relations between the sexes and the generations.

30. It is significant that one of the most important studies on women during apartheid, by Belinda Bozzoli (1991), only treats sexuality according to two very specific angles: one is moral, referring to the commonplaces about women and the city's capacity to corrupt; the other is political, mentioning the memory of women showing their breasts to provoke the white police. Neither the corporeal nature of sexuality nor its violence was considered at that time in South African social sciences and the public arena.

31. See Zazah Khuzwayo, *Never Been at Home* (Claremont, South Africa: David Philip, 2004). The dedication reads: "[This book is] dedicated to two women who were both victims of abuse mentally, physically, and sexually: my mother, Nokuthula Anastasia Khuzwayo, and my sister, Thembi Patricia Khuzwayo."

32. Chis Menges's film *A World Apart* received the Jury's Grand Prize at the Cannes Film Festival in 1988. It revealed both apartheid and the resistance it elicited.

33. An old woman told us how the village was displaced: "In those years, Ramalema was under Chief Makee. We had a piece of land where we could be self-reliant. Our family had some sheep, goat and cows, but our father had to work on a farm. We were forced from our lands to here. The chief was instructed by the Boers to do so. It was very hard to be removed like that. But nobody could refuse, since there was the chief's word. We walked from there with our animals, but there was no room for them here. Before, we had a large piece of land. Here we were given just a plot to build the house. The animals we had to keep outside the village." It is estimated that between 1960 and 1982 in South Africa, about 3.5 million people were affected by the apartheid regime's expropriation policy. It should also be remembered that in 1994, on the eve of the first democratic elections, whites, who represented only 11 percent of the population, owned 84 percent of the private lands (Aliber and Mokoena 2003).

34. This impression certainly should be put into perspective. As Delius (1996: 3) wrote in his chronicle of the Sekhukhuneland (the former Pedi kingdom in the first half of the twentieth century), one should beware of the "dominant narrative of conflict and change" that looked condescendingly on the villages because they are supposed to have participated less than the townships in the emancipation of the African populations and reduced them to the status of "helpless victims caught up in uncontrollable currents." All recent historiography has shown, on the contrary, that the reserves, then the homelands, "have been fundamentally fashioned by the intersecting forces of racism and capitalism" and that "their struggles have in turn helped to shape the particular nature of both rural and urban society."

35. As Leslie London (1999) has shown, alcohol is part of the traditional eco-

nomic organization on farms and is even a common way of remunerating farm-workers, known as the "dop system."

36. South African literature does not really give an inside view of these stories. Though an African literature of the townships exists, from the *Drum* generation to Njabulo Ndebele's short stories, there is no literature of the homelands or more generally on the rural world. Novels on country life are essentially the province of white authors, from Alan Paton to Nadine Gordimer and J. M. Coetzee who report that experience by re-creating it from the point of view of the black populations.

37. Elsa Joubert's most famous novel, *Die Swierfjare von Poppie Nongena,* was first published in Afrikaans in 1978 and translated into English as *The Long Journey of Poppie Nongena* in 1980.

38. The law of 1994, named the Restitution of Land Rights Act, has as its objective the return of property to the legal owners who have been displaced since 19 June 1913, the date of the Natives Land Act, which was the first of a long series of laws that founded a racially discriminatory legislation. It has brought forth 63,000 demands of restitution concerning nearly 80,000 properties (*Survey 2000–2001,* South African Institute of Race Relations). In September 2002, 34,365 of these demands had been granted to 73,662 families, or 394,442 persons. Compensation for the 505,000 hectares concerned cost the South African state 1.8 billion rands (South Africa Yearbook 2003, www.gcis.gov.za). The restitution policy is one of the two main parts of South African agrarian reform, the other being the policy of redistribution through which the government subsidizes those who want to buy land from owners willing to sell it. In both cases, we are far from the situation in Zimbabwe that the opposition constantly waves as a bogeyman.

39. I take the liberty of referring here to my own text (2004b: 27) concerning the articulation between *condition*—an "operation of objectification" by which "social structures and norms translate into daily life, ordinary acts, the way of being in respect to oneself, to others and to the world"—and *experience*—an "operation of subjectivization" by which "people give shape and meaning to what they are living, to the relation they make between their present and their past, between their present and their future."

40. See Achmat Dangor, *Bitter Fruit* (Cape Town: Kwela Books, 2001). Significantly, "memory," "confession," and "retribution" are the three parts of the novel.

6. LIVING WITH DEATH

1. The intuition of this sort of double talk came to Freud during the following event. A seer had told a man that the psychoanalyst treating his brother-in-law would die during the summer, poisoned by shellfish. "At the end of summer,

the patient declares approximately this: I know that my brother-in-law is not dead, but still this prediction was remarkable." And Octave Mannoni, who cites this episode (1969: 12), adds, "There must be something of the belief, supported by the seer, which remains and is recognized, transformed, in this absurd feeling of satisfaction."

2. Rob Dorrington, Debbie Bradshaw, David Bourne, and Salim Abdool Karim, "HIV Surveillance Results: Little Grounds for Optimism Yet," *South African Medical Journal* 90, no. 5 (2000): 452–453; Lindiwe Makubalo, Nothemba Simelela, Rose Mulumba, and Jonathan Levin, "1999 HIV Surveillance Results: Little Grounds for Pessimism," *South African Medical Journal* 90, no. 11 (2000): 1062.

3. "Concerns over Secrecy about HIV Figures," *The Star,* 3 July 2003; *National HIV and Syphilis Seroprevalence Survey of Women Attending Public Antenatal Clinics in South Africa 2002,* Department of Health, www.doh.ac.za.

4. "Shock AIDS Figures for Nurses Prompts Probe," *The Star,* 5 September 2000; "AIDS Taking a Massive Toll on Mining Industry," *Pretoria News,* 23 February 2004; "What Future Awaits HIV-Positive Soldiers," *The Star,* 18 August 2004.

5. Rob Dorrington, "The Demographic Impact of HIV/AIDS in South Africa by Province, Race and Class," paper presented at AIDS in Context Conference, April 2001; "AIDS to Cut Life Expectancy by 15 Years," *Cape Times,* 3 March 2003; Rob Dorrington, "New AIDS Models Reflects Significant Impact of Interventions," press release, ASSA 2002, July 2004. Original documents available at rdorring@commerce.uct.ac.za.

6. Olive Shisana and Leickness Simbayi, *Nelson Mandela/HSRC Study of HIV/AIDS* (Pretoria: HSRC, 2002). Of the 13,518 persons initially drawn by lots (rate of acceptance 62.3 percent), the survey covered 8,428 persons.

7. "Statistics Row Inflames New AIDS Debate," *Reuters,* 19 January 2004; "Stats Row over Stranglehold on Africa," *Reuters,* 27 February 2004. As Reuters news correspondent Helen Nyambura notes interrogatively, "AIDS has Africa in its claws, but how strongly?"

8. Where, according to a survey done in four provinces by the Human Science Research Council, the rate of seroprevalence reached 15.7 percent among personnel, while it was 28 percent for patients. It is indeed an exceptional situation when an illness affects almost equally those who do the caring and those who are cared for. See "16% of Health Workers Are HIV-Positive," *Pretoria News,* 11 December 2003.

9. L. Calabrese, M. Albrecht, J. Young et al., "Successful Cardiac Transplantation in an HIV-1 Infected Patient with Advanced Disease," *New England Journal of Medicine* 348, no. 23 (2003): 2323–2328; R. Steinbrok, "HIV Infection—A New Drug and New Costs," *New England Journal of Medicine* 348, no. 22 (2003): 2171–2172.

10. A survey of the living conditions of 771 families affected by AIDS in South Africa shows that 55 percent of the households in the rural areas declare they have reduced their food intake and are suffering from hunger. The loss of revenue due to the illness, observed in two-thirds of the cases, affects particularly those 44 percent of households living on less than 1,000 rands a month. As in the case reported here, the loss is mainly due, on the one hand, to the fact that the persons helping the patient or replacing him or her to care for the children are obliged to give up their employment and, on the other, to the fact that the sick person is unable to contribute to the financial efforts of the family. If medical expenses represent one-third of the household budget on average, the greatest expense is represented by the cost of a funeral, the average price of which is over 5,000 rands. See Malcolm Steinberg, Saul Johnson, Gill Schierhout, and David Ndegwa (2002), "Hitting Home: How Households Cope with the Impact of the HIV/AIDS Epidemic," Abt Associates, Inc., Kaiser Family Foundation, 42 pp., mimeo.

11. This is hardly new. A few years ago, when the problem of maternal mortality was "discovered"—incidentally, long after infantile mortality, which is an ancient preoccupation—its seriousness was mainly justified by the consequences of a mother's death on the children's lives, as if the benefits expected for the women were insufficient to make public action in their direction legitimate. On this point, see my study on reproductive health (Fassin 2000b).

12. For example, Nicoli Nattrass, in "AIDS and Human Security in Southern Africa," CSSR Working Paper no. 18, University of Cape Town, 2002, and Rachel Bray, in "Predicting the Social Consequences of Orphanhood in South Africa," CSSR Working Paper no. 29, University of Cape Town, 2003, warn against this tendency, which in the end turns against the orphans themselves: from threatened, they become threatening.

13. See Olive Shisana and Leickness Simbayi, *Nelson Mandela/HSRC Study of HIV/AIDS* (Pretoria: HSRC, 2002); and Helen Meitjes, Debbie Budlender, Sonja Giese, and Leigh Johnson, *Children in Need of Care or in Need of Cash?* (Cape Town: CARE, 2003).

14. The policy of providing foster care grants also induces inequalities among families affected by AIDS since the grants are three times higher for tutors raising children alone than the child support grant received by poor parents. What is more, the need to obtain a decision from the children's court in order to be eligible for the foster care allowance creates great differences according to whether families have access to the judicial system or not, which translates to a ratio of 1 to 5 between the number of beneficiaries of that grant and the estimated number of orphans potentially concerned.

15. She gives an example: "Peace, Fathers and Mothers in Zion! / I am oppressed. / My heart is sore. / My child is sick. / His stomach runs like water. / One already died while I was working in Randfontein. / It is correct, Lord!

Amen! / There I had no kin, no help. / Here I am at home. / It is correct, Lord! Amen!" Jean Comaroff (1985: 209) speaks of "ritual verbalizations."

16. At this time the two men were close and shared the same views on the African Renaissance. Two years earlier Mbeki had even written the preface to Makgoba's book on the affair that had opposed the latter to academic circles at the University of Witwatersrand. It is the AIDS controversy that divided them a year later.

17. See in particular the speech on the African way of volunteering given by Minister of Social Development Zola Skweyiya on 5 December 2002 and analyzed by Katinka De Wet (2004).

18. The South African Initiative for a Vaccine counts among the ten or so ongoing African experiments, as Jon Cohen points out in "Africa Boosts AIDS Vaccine R&D," *Science* 288 (2000): 2165–2167. It is probably the most "national" of all the experiments.

19. For a global view of the diversity of these Afrocentric trends, see Fauvelle-Aymar, Chrétien, and Perrot 2000.

20. The speech has been reproduced many times, notably in Hadland and Rantao 1999 and on the ANC web site, www.anc.co.za. Contrary to what is claimed about the racialization of the president's rhetoric, European migrants and Afrikaner farmers as well as slaves and Asian workers are included in his definition of African identity.

21. These discourses are translated into the politics of "Black empowerment" that particularly aim to promote the access of "non-Whites" to capital. They started out practically from zero. After progressing rapidly until 1997 (reaching 9.3 percent of the volume of stocks), capitalization of the private sector on the Johannesburg Stock Exchange then fell back sharply (with a growing participation of Afrikaners at the same time). In the public sector, where voluntarism is obviously more efficient, contracts granted to companies included in the preferential politics amounted to 40 percent of the total on the national and provincial levels. See *South Africa Survey 2000/2001* (Johannesburg: South African Institute of Race Relations, 2001). Operations associating "Black empowerment" capital are always well publicized, such as the takeover by the Association of Veterans in the Fight against Apartheid (MKVA), which acquired the majority in SNO, the second most important South African telecommunications company: "Struggle Vets in Telecoms Bid," *Business Report*, 17 April 2003. In this news coverage, everyone gets their due.

22. To my knowledge, the only person to have participated in both was Mahmood Mamdani, then director of the Centre for African Studies at the University of Cape Town: a theoretician of the African Renaissance, he criticized the theoretical orientations of the Symposium on Globalization in Africa. Bernard Makhosezwe Magabane had not been invited to participate in the latter but intervened in the discussion: the historian of the African Renaissance rejected the

analyses made in the field of African social sciences. Too postcolonial for the former, the event seemed too neocolonial to the latter.

23. That both arguments appear in the same discourse puts us in the middle of the tensions of the African Renaissance as political movement or identity project. "Is Mbeki an Africanist or a Globalist?" wonder Peter Valeand and Sipho Maseko (2002). It is probably best to answer this question not by saying he is both, which would be too vague, but by saying that he is playing the African card on the global stage—for better and for worse, say foreign observers. For this project can be found in the support given the regime of Robert Mugabe and in the sympathy shown to Jean-Bertrand Aristide just as much as in the growing diplomatic role that South Africa plays in the wars in the Great Lakes or in the political place occupied in the economic negotiations in the World Organization of Commerce. In fact, the logic is the same, even down to its ambiguities and contradictions.

24. According to the 1996 census, the Zion Christian Church is in first place among South African churches, with 11 percent of the faithful, followed by the Dutch Reformed Church, the Apostolic Church, and the Catholic Church, each with a little under 9 percent. See Statistics South Africa, *The People of South Africa: Population Census 1996*. This type of statistics is, however, moderately dependable because several simultaneous affiliations are possible and because of the versatility of membership rolls.

25. On the history and uses of trauma as a category of psychiatric nosography but also of public action, read Allan Young's book on North America (1995) and the article I wrote with Estelle d'Halluin, Stéphane Latté, and Richard Rechtman (2004) on the French case and its humanitarian ramifications throughout the world.

26. Address by Deputy President Zuma to the Moral Regeneration Movement national consultative meeting, 23 November 2001; address by Deputy President Zuma to the Moral Regeneration Movement campaign rally, 12 May 2002; opening address by President Nelson Mandela to the Fiftieth National Conference of the ANC, Mafeking, 16 December 1997. A series of financial and sexual scandals in 2005 and 2006 profoundly altered Jacob Zuma's legitimacy in representing the moral regeneration combat.

27. "Jacques Derrida: 'Je suis en guerre contre moi-même (I'm at war with myself),' " *Le Monde*, 19 August 2004. The interview is entirely centered on the question of what it means to be alive. It begins with a question by Jean Birnbaum in the form of a retrospective of the philosopher's work: "At the threshold of this interview, let us return to *Spectres de Marx*. A crucial work, totally dedicated to the question of the justice to come, which begins with the enigmatic exordium, 'Someone, you or I, comes forward and says, I would like to learn to live at last.'"

28. The quote is from *Nicomachean Ethics* I.6.1096a, where physical existence is also called the "simple fact of living," an expression picked up by Walter Ben-

jamin in particular. The passage from Aristotle's *Politics* III.6.1278b relates "man by nature a political animal" to what would therefore be its opposite, man as a biological animal, an opposition further analyzed by Agamben.

29. See "Probe Manto and Mbeki for Genocide," *Sapa,* 23 February 2003; interview of Malegapuru William Makgoba, *Weekly Mail and Guardian,* 6 October 2000; "AIDS Denial and Holocaust Denial—AIDS, Justice and the Courts in SA," Justice Edwin Cameron, Edward Smith Annual Lecture, Harvard Law School, 8 April 2003; intervention by Zachie Achmat at the AIDS in Context Conference, April 2001.

30. A long version of this difficult reflection on what is at stake in the AIDS controversy exists in a mimeographed document: Ulrike Kirstner, "Sovereign Power and Bare Life with HIV/AIDS: Biopolitics South African Style," no date, 23 pp. A short version was published under a slightly different title (2002).

31. Nazism, which Foucault discussed but did not elaborate on (and it is known that Agamben criticized him for that), is both the paradigm and the borderline case of such practices. It is noteworthy that certain South African commentators do not hesitate to refer to it when discussing the South African government: "Has Mbeki Heard of Nuremberg?" *Weekly Mail and Guardian,* 7 December 2001.

32. Though Posel (2001) has convincingly shown that behind the rhetoric and ideology of biological racialism the practical stakes of the definition, hierarchization, and uses of these groups were in fact social, economic, and cultural—not biological.

33. See my text on life politics and the politics of the living (2000a). This category joins Arendt's idea (1963) of "life as a supreme good."

34. As I analyzed in an earlier article (2003b). This acceptance of sovereignty defines the "foundation of modern power" since Bodin, as Gérard Mairet (1997) demonstrates.

35. For Zachie Achmat's story, read the article by Samantha Power (2003); and for Edwin Cameron's gesture, the text by Tim Trengrove-Jones (2001).

BRIEF CHRONOLOGY OF
SOUTH AFRICAN HISTORY

From Thompson 2000; Beinart 2001; Saunders and Southey 2001

1 million–3 million years B.P.	*Australopithecus africanus* in southern Africa.
90,000–1 million years B.P.	*Homo erectus* in southern Africa.
30,000–90,000 years B.P.	*Homo sapiens* in southern Africa.
26,000 years B.P.	Earliest dated rock art in southern Africa.
15,000 years B.P.	San hunter-gatherers in southern Africa.
2,200 years B.P.	Migration to the south of the San, later known as Khoikhoi.
3d century A.D.	Establishment of cultivators, ancestors of Bantu-speaking in modern South Africa, south of the Limpopo River.
14th–15th centuries	Settlements of Sotho-Tswana groups in the High Veld, of Nguni groups on the southeastern coast and around the Drakensberg, and of Khoisan groups in the southern and southwestern Cape.
1487	Portuguese expedition led by Bartolomeu Dias reaches Mossel Bay and rounds the Cape, opening the sea route to the East.

1590	Dutch and British ships start to put in regularly at Table Bay and develop trade with the Khoikhoi.
1652	Foundation by Jan van Riebeeck of a supply station for the Dutch East India Company at the Cape of Good Hope.
1658	First slaves brought to the Cape. They will be progressively imported from Indonesia, Malaysia, India, and Mozambique.
1659–1677	First and second wars of white Dutch farmers, the Boers, against the Khoikhoi, who are vanquished.
1690–1702	Progression of Trekboers, migrant farmers, toward the Cape interior and first encounters with Bantu-speaking populations.
1779–1793	First and second frontier wars, east of the Cape region, against the Xhosa populations, the result of which remains uncertain.
1795–1806	First occupation of the Cape Colony by the British. The Dutch, under the Batavian Republic, regain it, then lose it again.
1808–1812	Abolition of slave trade by the British. War against the Xhosa, who are expelled from the Zuurveld.
1816–1828	Creation of the Zulu kingdom by Shaka, followed by several years of war among African groups, known as Mfecane.
1835–1840	Beginning of the Great Trek. Five thousand Afrikaners leave the Cape Colony with their Coloured clients. They defeat the Zulu at Blood River.
1843–1854	Annexation of Natal by the British, who, however, recognize Transvaal and Orange Free State as independent Afrikaner republics.
1856–1857	Xhosa mass slaughter of their cattle after a prophecy. In the following months, forty thousand people die of famine.
1867–1886	Discovery of diamonds near Bloomfontein, mainly in Kimberley, and of gold in the Witwatersrand, leading to the foundation of Johannesburg.
1899–1902	War between the British and the Afrikaners, who are defeated and lose their republics.
1910	Creation of the Union of South Africa, composed of Cape Colony, Natal, the Transvaal, and Orange Free State.

1912	Foundation of the South African Native National Congress, which eleven years later will become the African National Congress (ANC).
1913	Natives Land Act, which limits Africans' properties to "reserves," representing 7 percent of the territory, and makes racial segregation official.
1916	Opening of the South African Native College, the first academic institution exclusively for Africans.
1919	Beginning of the mandate given to the Union of South Africa for South West Africa, later to become Namibia.
1923	Natives Urban Areas Act, which expands racial segregation to towns by instituting native locations for African populations.
1924	National elections won by an alliance of the National Party and the white Labour Party.
1927	Immorality Act, which prohibits sexual relations between Whites and other racially defined groups.
1934	Joining of J. B. M. Hertzog's National Party and Jan Smuts's South African Party and the creation of D. F. Malan's Purified National Party.
1940	Alliance between J. B. M. Hertzog and D. F. Malan, who form the Herenigde Nasionale Party in favor of Afrikaner nationalism.
1948	Electoral victory of the Herenigde Nasionale Party with a program of apartheid and with D. F. Malan as prime minister.
1949	Prohibition of Mixed Marriage Act, which makes illegal all interracial marriages.
1950	Population Registration Act, which imposes the official classification of all South Africans according to their supposed racial group.
1951	Bantu Authorities Act, which institutes the homelands, ethnically defined territories placed under African administration.
1952	Abolition of Passes Act, which provides that all Africans must carry passes. Defiance campaign leading to mass arrests and mass protests.
1953	Bantu Education Act, which provides for a separate and inferior school system for Africans. Declaration of the state of emergency.

1955	Destruction of Sophiatown, a Johannesburg African neighborhood where an intellectual and cultural life had been preserved.
1959	Foundation of Robert Sobukwe's Pan Africanist Congress, resulting from a schism of the ANC by a fraction opposed to multiracialism.
1960	Sharpeville massacre, south of Johannesburg, when the police open fire on anti–pass law demonstrators, killing sixty-nine. Banning of African parties.
1961	Proclamation of the independence of the Republic of South Africa, which leaves the Commonwealth. Adoption of armed struggle by the ANC.
1963	Arrest of the ANC's armed branch, Umkhonto weSizwe, High Command, at a Rivonia farm.
1964	Life sentence for the eight leaders of the ANC and the Pan Africanist Congress arrested in Rivonia, among them Nelson Mandela.
1975	Independence of former Portuguese colonies of Angola and Mozambique. Reestablishment of the Inkatha by Mangosuthu Buthelezi.
1976	Soweto uprising beginning with the death of an adolescent, Hector Petersen, shot by the police. Over seven hundred people killed.
1977	Steve Biko beaten to death in jail. Independence of Bophuthatswana. UN embargo against South Africa.
1980	Independence of Rhodesia, which becomes Zimbabwe with an African government.
1983	New constitution instituting a tricameral parliament with separate representation for Whites, Coloured, and Indians and none for Africans.
1986	Repeal of laws on passes, marriages, and sexual relations. Urban riots in the townships and proclamation of a state of emergency.
1990	Lifting of ban on African parties, in particular the ANC. Liberation of Nelson Mandela. Beginning of political transition. Independence of Namibia.
1994	Violence between Inkatha and the ANC. First democratic elections, won by the ANC. Nelson Mandela forms a government of National Unity.

1996	First hearings of the Truth and Reconciliation Commission. The new constitution is signed. The National Party leaves the government.
1999	General elections won by the ANC. The Democratic Party becomes the principal opposition party. Thabo Mbeki becomes president.
2000	Convening of the Presidential Panel, including AIDS dissidents. Thirteenth International AIDS Conference in Durban.
2001	Nonsuit in the Pretoria High Court case brought by thirty-seven international drug companies against the South African government.
2002	Condemnation of the government by the Pretoria High Court for delayed implementation of prevention of mother-to-child transmission of HIV.
2004	General elections that give the ANC its widest victory since 1994. Thabo Mbeki is confirmed as president. The National Party announces its dissolution and its leaders join the ANC. South Africa is elected to be the first African country to organize the Football World Cup in 2010. The tenth anniversary of the new South Africa is celebrated.

MAPS

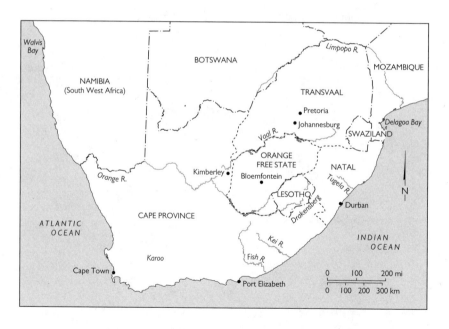

Map 1. South Africa between 1910 and 1940. From Saunders and Southey 2001.

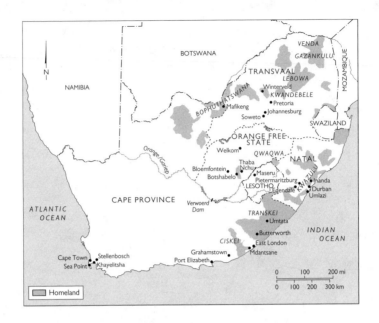

Map 2. South Africa under apartheid. From Beinart 2001.

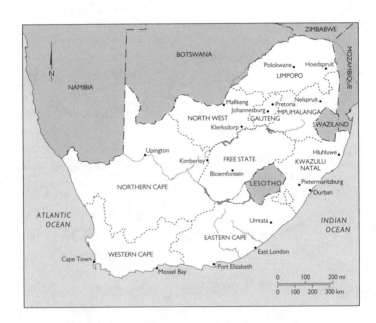

Map 3. South Africa today. From www.places.co.za 2005.

BIBLIOGRAPHY

Only social sciences texts and general literature appear here. Medical papers, newspaper and magazine articles, and unpublished documents are cited in the notes.

Abu-Lughod, Lila
   2002   "Do Muslim Women Really Need Saving? Anthropological Reflections on Cultural Relativism and Its Others." *American Anthropologist* 104 (3): 783–790.
Achebe, Chinua
   1995   "Colonialist Criticism." In *The Postcolonial Studies Reader,* ed. Bill Ashcroft, Gareth Griffith, and Helen Tiffin, 57–61. London: Routledge.
Agamben, Giorgio
   1997   *Homo sacer: Le pouvoir souverain et la vie nue.* Paris: Seuil. (1st ed. 1995.)
Aldrin, Philippe
   2003   "Penser la rumeur: Une question discutée des sciences sociales." *Genèses* 50: 126–141.
Aliber, Michael, and Reuben Mokoena
   2003   "The Land Question in Contemporary South Africa." In *State of the Nation: South Africa, 2003–2004,* ed. John Daniel, Adam Habib, and Roger Southall, 330–346. Cape Town: Human Science Research Council.

Althabe, Gérard
    1969   *Oppression et libération dans l'imaginaire.* Paris: Maspéro.

Anderson, Benedict
    1983   *Imagined Communities: Reflections on the Origin and Spread of Nationalism.* London: Verso.

Arendt, Hannah
    1951   *The Origins of Totalitarianism: Imperialism.* New York: Harcourt.
    1963   *On Revolution.* New York: Viking Press.
    1959   *The Human Condition.* Garden City, NY: Doubleday. (1st ed. 1958.)
    1995   *Qu'est-ce que la politique?* Paris: Seuil. (1st ed. 1993.)

Aristotle
    1995   *La politique.* Paris: Librairie Philosophique J. Vrin.
    1997   *Ethique à nicomaque.* Paris: Librairie Philosophique J. Vrin.

Arnold, David
    1993   *Colonizing the Body: State Medicine and Epidemic Disease in Nineteenth-Century India.* Berkeley: University of California Press.

Ashforth, Adam
    2000   *Madumo: A Man Bewitched.* Chicago: University of Chicago Press.
    2002   "An Epidemic of Witchcraft? The Implications of AIDS for the Post-Apartheid State." *African Studies,* special issue "AIDS in Context," 61 (1): 121–143.

Atkinson, Paul, and David Silverman
    1997   "Kundera's Immortality: The Interview Society and the Invention of the Self." *Qualitative Inquiry* 3 (3): 304–325.

Auden, W. H.
    1991   "The Age of Anxiety." In *Collected Poems,* 447–536. New York: Vintage International.

Austin, J. L.
    1970   *Quand dire c'est faire.* Paris: Seuil. (1st ed. 1962.)

Balandier, Georges
    1974   *Anthropologiques.* Paris: Presses Universitaires de France.

Bauman, Zygmunt
    1998   *Globalization: The Human Consequences.* Cambridge: Polity Press.
    2004   *Wasted Lives: Modernity and Its Outcasts.* Cambridge: Polity Press.

Beck, Ulrich
    1992   *Risk Society: Towards a New Modernity.* London: Sage.

Becker, Gay
    1997   *Disrupted Lives: How People Create Meaning in a Chaotic World.* Berkeley: University of California Press.

Becker, Howard
    1963   *Outsiders: Studies in the Sociology of Deviance.* New York: Free
                Press of Glencoe.
Beinart, William
    2001   *Twentieth-Century South Africa.* Oxford: Oxford University Press.
                (1st ed. 1994.)
Benjamin, Walter
    1968   "Theses on the Philosophy of History." In *Illuminations,* 255–266.
                New York: Harcourt, Brace & World. (1st ed. 1942.)
Berridge, Virginia
    1992   "The Early Years of AIDS in the United Kingdom, 1981–1986:
                Historical Perspectives." In *Epidemics and Ideas: Essays on the His-
                torical Perception of Pestilence,* ed. Terence Ranger and Paul Slack,
                303–328. Cambridge: Cambridge University Press.
Bhabha, Homi
    1994   *The Location of Culture.* London: Routledge.
Bibeau, Gilles
    1991   "L'Afrique, terre imaginaire du sida: La subversion du discours
                scientifique par le jeu des fantasmes." *Anthropologie et Sociétés* 15
                (2–3): 125–147.
Biehl, João
    2005   *Vita: Life in a Zone of Abandonment.* Berkeley: University of Cal-
                ifornia Press.
Blaauw, Duane
    2004   "Transformations de l'Etat et réforme de la santé: Le cadre his-
                torique et institutionnel de la mise en œuvre des actions de lutte
                contre le sida." In *Afflictions: L'Afrique du sud, de l'apartheid au
                sida,* ed. Didier Fassin, 111–138. Paris: Karthala.
Bloch, Marc
    1993   *Apologie pour l'histoire ou Métier d'historien.* Paris: Armand Colin.
                (1st ed. 1949.)
    1999   *Réflexions d'un historien sur les fausses nouvelles de la guerre.* Paris:
                Allia. (1st ed. 1921.)
Boltanski, Luc
    1993   *La souffrance à distance: Morale humanitaire, médias et politique.*
                Paris: Métailié.
Boltanski, Luc, and Eve Chiapello
    1999   *Le nouvel esprit du capitalisme.* Paris: Gallimard.
Bonner, Philip, and Lauren Segal
    1998   *Soweto: A History.* Cape Town: Maskew Miller Longman.
Boris, Staci
    2001   "The Process of Change: Landscape, Memory, Animation and

Felix in Exile." In *William Kentridge,* 28–37. Chicago: Museum of Contemporary Art; New York: New Museum of Contemporary Art.

Bourdieu, Pierre

1971   "Genèse et structure du champ religieux." *Revue Française de Sociologie* 12: 295–334.

1979   *La distinction: Critique sociale du jugement.* Paris: Editions de Minuit.

1980   *Le sens pratique.* Paris: Editions de Minuit.

1986   "L'illusion biographique." *Actes de la Recherche en Sciences Sociales* 62–63: 69–72.

Bourgois, Philippe

1995   *In Search of Respect: Selling Crack in El Barrio.* New York: Cambridge University Press.

Bouveresse, Jacques

1976   *Le mythe de l'intériorité: Expérience, signification et langage privé chez Wittgenstein.* Paris: Edition de Minuit.

Bozzoli, Belinda, with the assistance of Mmantho Nkotsoe

1991   *Women of Phokeng: Consciousness, Life Strategy and Migrancy in South Africa, 1900–1983.* Portsmouth: Heinemann; London: James Currey.

Brandt, Allan

1985   *No Magic Bullet: A Social History of Venereal Disease in the United States since 1880.* Oxford: Oxford University Press.

Briggs, Charles, and Clara Mantini-Briggs

2003   *Stories in the Time of Cholera: Racial Profiling during a Medical Nightmare.* Berkeley: University of California Press.

Brink, André

1998   "Stories of History: Reimagining the Past in Post-Apartheid Narrative." In *Negotiating the Past: The Making of Memory in South Africa,* ed. Sarah Nuttall and Carli Coatzee, 29–56. Oxford: Oxford University Press.

Burger, Marlene, and Chandré Gould

2002   *Secrets and Lies: Wouter Basson and South Africa's Chemical and Biological Warfare Programme.* Cape Town: Zebra Press.

Bury, Michael

1982   "Chronic Illness as Biographical Disruption." *Sociology of Health and Illness* 4 (2): 167–182.

Butchart, Alexander

1998   *The Anatomy of Power: European Constructions of the African Body.* London: Zed Books.

Butt, Leslie

2002   "The Suffering Stranger: Medical Anthropology and International Morality." *Medical Anthropology* 21: 1–24.

Caldwell, John C., and Pat Caldwell

1996   "The African AIDS Epidemic." *Scientific American* 274: 40–46.

Callon, Michel

1999   "Ni intellectuel engagé, ni intellectuel dégagé: La double stratégie de l'attachement et du détachement." *Sociologie du Travail* 41: 65–78.

Campbell, Catherine

1997   "Migrancy, Masculine Identities and AIDS: The Psychosocial Context of HIV Transmission in the South African Gold Mines." *Social Science and Medicine* 45 (2): 273–281.

2000   "Selling Sex in the Time of AIDS: The Psychosocial Context of Condom Use by Sex Workers in a Southern African Mine." *Social Science and Medicine* 50: 479–494.

2003   *Letting Them Die: Why HIV/AIDS Interventions Fail.* Oxford: James Currey.

Campbell, Catherine, and Brian Williams

1999   "Beyond the Biomedical and the Behavioural: Towards an Integrated Approach to HIV Prevention in the Southern African Mining Industry." *Social Science and Medicine* 48: 1625–1639.

Cassin, Barbara, Olivier Cayla, and Joseph Philippe Salazar

2004   *Vérité, réconciliation, réparation.* Le genre humain. Paris: Seuil.

Castells, Manuel

1996   *The Rise of the Network Society.* Oxford: Blackwell.

Cavell, Stanley

1997   "Comments on Veena Das' Essay: 'Language and Body: Transactions in the Construction of Pain.'" In *Social Suffering*, ed. Arthur Kleinman, Veena Das, and Margaret Lock, 207–244. Berkeley: University of California Press.

Certeau, Michel de

1987   *Histoire et psychanalyse entre science et fiction.* Paris: Gallimard.

Chalmers, Alan

1987   *Qu'est-ce que la science?* Paris: La Découverte. (1st ed. 1976.)

Cipolla, Carlo

1976   *Public Health and the Medical Profession in the Renaissance.* Cambridge: Cambridge University Press.

Clifford, James

1988   *The Predicament of Culture: Twentieth-Century Ethnography, Literature, and Art.* Cambridge, Mass: Harvard University Press.

Clifford, James, and George Marcus

    1986   *Writing Culture: The Poetics and Politics of Ethnography.* Berkeley: University of California Press.

Cohen, Stanley

    2001   *States of Denial. Knowing about Atrocities and Suffering.* Cambridge: Polity Press.

Comaroff, Jean

    1985   *Body of Power, Spirit of Resistance: The Culture and History of a South African People.* Chicago: University of Chicago Press.

Comaroff, John, and Jean Comaroff

    1991   *Of Revelation and Revolution.* Vol. 1: *Christianity, Colonialism, and Consciousness in South Africa.* Chicago: University of Chicago Press.

    1992   "Le fou et le migrant: Travail et peine dans la conscience historique d'un peuple sud-africain." *Actes de la Recherche en Sciences Sociales* 94: 41–58.

    1997   *Of Revelation and Revolution.* Vol. 2: *The Dialectics of Modernity on a South African Frontier.* Chicago: University of Chicago Press.

Connerton, Paul

    1989   *How Societies Remember.* Cambridge: Cambridge University Press.

Coplan, David

    2001   *In the Times of Cannibals: The Word Music of South Africa's Basotho Migrants.* Johannesburg: Witwatersrand University Press. (1st ed. 1994.)

Cottereau, Alain

    1999   "Dénis de justice, dénis de réalité: remarques sur la réalité sociale et sa dénégation." In *L'expérience du déni,* ed. Pascale Gruson and Renaud Dulong, 159–178. Paris: Editions de la Maison des Sciences de l'Homme.

Crais, Clifton

    2002   *The Politics of Evil: Magic, State Power and the Political Imagination in South Africa.* Cambridge: Cambridge University Press.

Csordas, Thomas

    2002   *Body/Meaning/Healing.* Houndmills: Palgrave-Macmillan.

    2004   "Asymptote of the Ineffable: Embodiment, Alterity and the Theory of Religion." *Current Anthropology* 45 (2): 163–185.

Curtin, Philip

    1992   "Medical Knowledge and Urban Planning in Colonial Tropical Africa." In *The Social Basis of Health and Healing in Africa,* ed. Steven Feierman and John Janzen, 235–255. Berkeley: University of California Press.

D'Andrade, Roy
    1995   "Moral Models in Anthropology." *Current Anthropology* 36 (3): 399–408.

Daniel, Valentine
    2000   "Mood, Moment, and Mind." In *Violence and Subjectivity*, ed. Veena Das, Arthur Kleinman, Mamphela Ramphele, and Pamela Reynolds, 333–66. Berkeley: University of California Press. (1st ed. 1996.)

Das, Veena
    1997   "Language and Body: Transactions in the Construction of Pain." In *Social Suffering*, ed. Arthur Kleinman, Veena Das, and Margaret Lock, 67–91. Berkeley: University of California Press.

Dean, Jodi
    1998   *Aliens in America: Conspiracy Cultures from Outerspace to Cyberspace.* Ithaca: Cornell University Press.

De Beer, Cedric
    1984   *The South African Disease: Apartheid Health and Health Services.* Johannesburg: South African Research Service.

Dejours, Christophe
    1993   *Travail, usure mentale: De la psychopathologie à la psychodynamique du travail.* Paris: Bayard.

Deleuze, Gilles
    1962   *Nietzsche et la philosophie.* Paris: Presses Universitaires de France.

Delius, Peter
    1996   *A Lion amongst the Cattle: Reconstruction and Resistance in the Northern Transvaal.* Johannesburg: Ravan Press; Portsmouth: Heinemann; Oxford: James Currey.

Delius, Peter, and Clive Glaser
    2002   "Sexual Socialization in South Africa: A Historical Perspective." *African Studies,* special issue "AIDS in Context," 61 (1): 27–54.

Denis, Philippe
    2001   "La croisade du président Mbeki contre l'orthodoxie du sida." *Esprit* (January): 81–97.

De Wet, Katinka
    2004   "Un militantisme social: Le volontariat associatif dans les soins à domicile pour les malades du sida." In *Afflictions: L'Afrique du sud, de l'apartheid au sida,* ed. Didier Fassin, 159–201. Paris: Karthala.

Dilthey, Wilhelm
    1976   *Selected Writings.* Ed. H. P. Rickman. Cambridge: Cambridge University Press. (1st ed. 1914.)

Dodier, Nicolas

2001　"La bataille des universalismes: Les traitements du sida et la construction d'une médecine transnationale." *Ruptures: Revue Transdisciplinaire en Santé* 8 (2): 6–20.

Douglas, Mary

1992　*Risk and Blame: Essays in Cultural Theory.* London: Routledge.

Dozon, Jean-Pierre, and Didier Fassin

1989　"Raison épidémiologique et raisons d'Etat: Les enjeux sociopolitiques du sida en Afrique." *Sciences Sociales et Santé* 7 (1): 21–36.

Du Bois, W. E. B.

1994　*The Souls of Black Folk.* New York: Dover Publications. (1st ed. 1903.)

Dubow, Saul

1989　*Racial Segregation and the Origins of Apartheid in South Africa, 1919–1936.* Houndmills: Macmillan.

Eaton, Liberty, Alan Flisher, and Leif Aaro

2003　"Unsafe Sexual Behaviour in South African Youth." *Social Science and Medicine* 56: 149–165.

Elbourne, Elisabeth

2002　*Blood Ground: Colonialism, Missions and the Contest for Christianity in the Cape Colony and Britain, 1799–1853.* Montreal: McGill-Queen's University Press.

Elias, Norbert

1956　"Problems of Involvement and Detachment." *British Journal of Sociology* 7 (3): 226–252.

1982　*The Civilizing Process: State Formation and Civilization.* Oxford: Blackwell.

2002　*Ecrits sur l'art africain.* Paris: Kimé.

Elster, Jon

1990　*Psychologie politique.* Paris: Editions de Minuit.

Epstein, Helen

2000　"The Mystery of AIDS in South Africa." *New York Review of Books,* 20 July.

Epstein, Steven

1996　*Impure Science: AIDS, Activism, and the Politics of Knowledge.* Berkeley: University of California Press.

Fabian, Johannes

1983　*Time and the Other: How Anthropology Makes Its Object.* New York: Columbia University Press.

1995　"Ethnographic Misunderstanding and the Perils of Context." *American Anthropologist* 97 (1): 41–50.

Farmer, Paul

1997   "On Suffering and Structural Violence: A View from Below." In *Social Suffering,* ed. Arthur Kleinman, Veena Das, and Margaret Lock, 261–283. Berkeley: University of California Press.

1999   *Infections and Inequalities: The Modern Plagues.* Berkeley: University of California Press.

2003   *Pathologies of Power.* Berkeley: University of California Press.

Fassin, Didier

1994   "Le domaine privé de la santé publique: Pouvoir, politique et sida au Congo." *Annales. Histoire, Sciences Sociales* 49 (4): 745–775.

1998   "Politique des corps et gouvernement des villes." In *Les figures urbaines de la santé publique: Enquête sur des expériences locales,* ed. Didier Fassin, 7–46. Paris: La Découverte.

1999a   "L'anthropologie, entre engagement et distanciation: Essai de sociologie des recherches en sciences sociales sur le sida en Afrique." In *Sciences sociales et sida en Afrique: Bilan et perspectives,* ed. Charles Becker, Jean-Pierre Dozon, Christine Obbo, and Moriba Touré, 41–66. Paris: Karthala.

1999b   "L'indicible et l'impensé: La 'question immigrée' dans les politiques du sida." *Sciences Sociales et Santé* 19 (4): 5–36.

2000a   "Entre politiques du vivant et politiques de la vie: Pour une anthropologie de la santé." *Anthropologie et Société,* special issue "Terrains d'avenir," 24 (1): 195–215.

2000b   "La production de la santé reproductive." In *Les enjeux politiques de la santé: Etudes sénégalaises, équatoriennes et françaises,* ed. Didier Fassin, 161–174. Paris: Karthala.

2001a   "Au cœur de la cité salubre: La santé entre les mots et les choses." In *Critique de la santé publique: Une approche anthropologique,* ed. Jean-Pierre Dozon and Didier Fassin, 47–73. Paris: Balland.

2001b   "Culturalism as Ideology." In *Cultural Perspectives on Reproductive Health,* ed. Carla Makhlouf Obermeyer, 300–317. Oxford: Oxford University Press.

2002a   "Le sida comme cause politique." *Les temps modernes,* special issue "Afriques du monde," 57 (620–621): 312–331.

2002b   "Embodied History: Uniqueness and Exemplarity of South African AIDS." *African Journal of AIDS Research* 1 (1): 63–68.

2003a   "Anatomie politique d'une controverse: La démocratie sud-africaine à l'épreuve du sida." *Critique Internationale* 20: 93–112.

2003b   "Sovereignty vs. Biolegitimacy: The Contradictory Foundations of the Politics of AIDS." *Debate: Voices from the South African Left* 9 (August): 23–26.

2004a   "Et la souffrance devient sociale." *Critique,* special issue "Frontières de l'anthropologie," nos. 680–681: 16–29.

2004b   "L'incorporation de l'inégalité: Condition sociale et expérience historique dans le post-apartheid." In *Afflictions: L'Afrique du sud, de l'apartheid au sida,* ed. Didier Fassin, 19–44. Paris: Karthala.

2005   "L'ordre moral du monde: Essai d'anthropologie de l'intolérable." In *Les constructions de l'intolérable,* ed. Didier Fassin and Patrice Bourdelais, 17–50. Paris: La Découverte.

Fauvelle-Aymar, François-Xavier, Jean-Pierre Chrétien, and Claude-Hélène Perrot

2000   *Afrocentrismes: L'histoire des Africains entre Egypte et Amérique.* Paris: Karthala.

Fee, Elisabeth, and Daniel Fox

1988   *AIDS: The Burdens of History.* Berkeley: University of California Press.

Feldman, Allen

1994   "On Cultural Anesthesia: From Desert Storm to Rodney King." *American Ethnologist* 21 (2): 404–418.

Foucault, Michel

1976   *Histoire de la sexualité. 1. La volonté de savoir.* Paris: Gallimard.

1994   *Dits et écrits.* Vol. 4. Paris: Gallimard.

1997   *"Il faut défendre la société": Cours au Collège de France, 1976.* Paris: Hautes Études, Gallimard-Seuil.

2001   *L'herméneutique du sujet: Cours au Collège de France, 1981–1982.* Paris: Hautes Études, Gallimard-Seuil.

Freidson, Eliot

1970   *The Profession of Medicine.* New York: Harper & Row.

Fujimora, Joan, and Danny Chou

1994   "Dissent in Science: Styles of Scientific Practice and the Controversy over the Cause of AIDS." *Social Science and Medicine* 38 (8): 1017–1036.

Geschiere, Peter

1997   *The Modernity of Witchcraft: Politics and the Occult in Postcolonial Africa.* Charlottesville: University Press of Virginia.

Giddens, Anthony

1984   *The Constitution of Society: Outline of a Theory of Structuration.* Berkeley: University of California Press.

Gilman, Sander

1985   *Differences and Pathology: Stereotypes of Sexuality, Race and Madness.* Ithaca: Cornell University Press.

Gisselquist, David
  2003   "Emergence of the HIV Type 1 Epidemic in the Twentieth Cen-
              tury." *AIDS Research and Human Retroviruses* 19 (12): 1071–1078.
Glaser, Clive
  2000   *Bo-Tsotsi: The Youth Gangs of Soweto, 1935–1976*. Portsmouth:
              Heinemann; Oxford: James Currey; Cape Town: David Phillips.
Good, Byron
  1994   *Medicine, Rationality and Experience: An Anthropological Perspec-
              tive*. Cambridge: Cambridge University Press.
Grmek, Mirko
  1989   *Histoire du sida*. Paris: Payot.
Gusterson, Hugh
  2003   "Anthropology and the Military—1968, 2003, and Beyond?" *An-
              thropology Today* 19 (3): 25–26.
Hacking, Ian
  1990   *The Taming of Chance*. Cambridge: Cambridge University Press.
Hadland, Adrian, and Jovial Rantao
  1999   *The Life and Times of Thabo Mbeki*. Rivonia: Zebra Press.
Hahn, Aloïs
  1986   "Contribution à la sociologie de la confession et autres formes in-
              stitutionnalisées d'aveu: Autothématisation et processus de civil-
              isation." *Actes de la Recherche en Sciences Sociales,* nos. 62–63:
              54–68.
Hahn, Aloïs, Willy Eirmbter, and Jacob Rüdiger
  1994   "Le sida: savoir ordinaire et insécurité." *Actes de la Recherche en
              Sciences Sociales* 104: 81–89.
Hall, Stuart
  1996   "New Ethnicities." In *Stuart Hall: Critical Dialogues in Cultural
              Studies,* ed. David Norvey and Kuan-Hsing Chen, 441–449. Lon-
              don: Routledge.
Hammersley, Martyn
  1993   "The Rhetorical Turn in Ethnography." *Social Science Information*
              32 (1): 23–37.
Hammond-Tooke, David
  1970   "Urbanization and the Interpretation of Misfortune." *Africa* 40:
              25–39.
Hartog, François
  2003   *Les régimes d'historicité: Présentisme et temps de l'histoire*. Paris: Seuil.
Hartog, François, and Jacques Revel, eds.
  2001   *Les usages politiques du passé*. Paris: Editions de l'Ecole des Hautes
              Études en Sciences Sociales.

Heller, Agnes
    1996   "Has Biopolitics Changed the Concept of the Political? Some Further Thoughts about Biopolitics." In *Biopolitics: The Politics of the Body, Race and Nature,* ed. Agnes Heller and Sonja Puntscher Riekmann, 3–15. Aldershot: Avebury–European Center Vienna.

Herzfeld, Michael
    1991   *A Place in History: Social and Monumental Time in a Cretan Town.* Princeton: Princeton University Press.

Herzlich, Claudine, and Janine Pierret
    1988   "Une maladie dans l'espace public: Le sida dans six quotidiens français." *Annales ESC* (5): 1109–1134.

Hilgartner, Stephen, and Charles Bosk
    1988   "The Rise and Fall of Social Problems: A Public Arenas Model." *American Journal of Sociology* 94 (1): 53–78.

Hofstadter, Richard
    1964   "The Paranoid Style in American Politics." *Harper's Magazine* 11: 77–86.

Horton, Richard
    1996   "Truth and Heresy about AIDS." *New York Review of Books* 43 (9).

Howe, Stephen
    1998   *Afrocentrism: Mythical Pasts and Imagined Homes.* London: Verso.

Hrdy, Daniel
    1987   "Cultural Practices Contributing to the Transmission of Human Immunodeficiency Virus in Africa." *Reviews of Infectious Diseases* 9 (6): 1109–1119.

Hughes, Everett
    1945   "Dilemmas and Contradictions of Status." *American Journal of Sociology* 50: 353–359.

Hunter, Mark
    2002   "The Materiality of Everyday Sex: Thinking beyond 'Prostitution.'" *African Studies,* special issue "AIDS in Context," 61 (1): 99–120.

Jacobs, Sean, and Richard Calland
    2002   "Thabo Mbeki : Myth and Context. An Introduction." In *Thabo Mbeki's World: The Politics and Ideology of the South African President,* ed. Sean Jacobs and Richard Calland, 1–24. Pietermaritzburg: University of Natal Press.

Jeeves, Alan, and Jonathan Crush
    1995   "The Failure of the Stabilisation Experiments on South African Gold Mines." In *Crossing Boundaries: Mine Migrancy in Democratic South Africa,* ed. Jonathan Crush and James Wilmot, 2–13. Cape Town: Idasa.

Jewkes, Rachel, and Naeema Abrahams

2002   "The Epidemiology of Rape and Sexual Coercion in South Africa: An Overview." *Social Science and Medicine* 55: 1231–1244.

Jewsiewicki, Bogumil

2002   "De la vérité de la mémoire à la réconciliation: Comment travaille le souvenir." *Le Débat* 122 (November–December): 63.

Jochelson, Karen

2001   *The Colour of Disease: Syphilis and Racism in South Africa, 1880–1950.* Basingstoke: Palgrave.

Jones, James

1981   *Bad Blood: The Tuskegee Syphilis Experiment.* New York: Free Press.

Katz, Elaine

1994   *The White Death: Silicosis in the Witwatersrand Gold Mines.* Johannesburg: University of Witwatersrand Press.

Kelly, Michael, and David Field

1996   "Medical Sociology, Chronic Illness, and the Body." *Sociology of Health and Illness* 18 (2): 241–257.

Kleinman, Arthur

1988   *The Illness Narratives: Suffering, Healing and the Human Condition.* New York: Basic Books.

Kleinman, Arthur, and Joan Kleinman

1994   "How Bodies Remember: Social Memory and Bodily Experience of Criticism, Resistance, and Delegitimation following China's Cultural Revolution." *New Literary History* 25: 707–723.

Koselleck, Reinhardt

1990   *Le futur passé: Contribution à la sémantique des temps historiques.* Paris: Editions de l'Ecole des Hautes Études en Sciences Sociales. (1st ed. 1979.)

1997   *L'expérience de l'histoire.* Paris: Hautes études, Gallimard-Seuil. (1st ed. 1975.)

Kuhn, Thomas

1962   *The Structure of Scientific Revolutions.* Chicago: University of Chicago Press.

Lahire, Bernard

1998   *L'homme pluriel: Les ressorts de l'action.* Paris: Nathan.

Latour, Bruno

1988   "Le Grand Partage." *Revue du MAUSS,* n.s., 1: 27–64.

Leclerc-Madlala, Suzanne

2002   "On the Virgin-Cleansing Myth: Gendered Bodies, AIDS and Ethnomedicine." *African Journal of AIDS Research* 1 (2): 87–95.

Le Marcis, Frédéric
2004   "L'empire de la violence: Un récit de vie aux marges d'un township." In *Afflictions: L'Afrique du sud, de l'apartheid au sida,* ed. Didier Fassin, 237–273. Paris: Karthala.

Lloyd, Geoffrey
1990   *Demystifying Mentalities.* Cambridge: Cambridge University Press.

Lock, Margaret
1997   "Displacing Suffering: The Reconstruction of Death in North America and Japan." In *Social Suffering,* ed. Arthur Kleinman, Veena Das, and Margaret Lock, 207–244. Berkeley: University of California Press.

Lodge, Tom
1983   *Black Politics in South Africa since 1945.* London: Longman.
1999   *South African Politics since 1994.* Cape Town: David Phillips.
2002   *Politics in South Africa: From Mandela to Mbeki.* Cape Town and Oxford: David Philip–James Currey.

London, Leslie
1999   "The 'Dop' System, Alcohol Abuse and Social Control amongst Farm Workers in South Africa: A Public Health Challenge." *Social Science and Medicine* 48: 1407–1414.

Magubane, Bernard Makhosezwe
1999   "The African Renaissance in Historical Perspective." In *African Renaissance: The New Struggle,* ed. Malegapuru William Makgoba, 10–36. Sandton: Mafube; Cape Town: Tafelberg.

Mairet, Gérard
1997   *Le principe de souveraineté: Histoires et fondements du pouvoir moderne.* Paris: Gallimard.

Malkki, Liisa
1995   *Purity and Exile: Violence, Memory and National Cosmology among Hutu Refugees.* Chicago: University of Chicago Press.

Mannoni, Octave
1969   "Je sais bien, mais quand même . . . " In *Clefs pour l'imaginaire ou L'autre scène,* 9–33. Paris: Seuil.

Marais, Hein
2000   *To the Edge: AIDS Review 2000.* Pretoria: Centre for the Study of AIDS.

Marcus, George
1999   "Introduction: The Paranoid Style Now." In *Paranoia within Reason: A Casebook on Conspiracy as Explanation,* ed. George Marcus, 1–11. Chicago: University of Chicago Press.

Marks, Harry

1997   *The Progress of Experiment: Science and Therapeutic Reform in the United States, 1900–1990.* Cambridge: Cambridge University Press.

Marks, Shula

2002   "An Epidemic Waiting to Happen? The Spread of HIV/AIDS in South Africa in Social and Historical Perspective." *African Studies,* special issue "AIDS in Context," 61 (1): 13–26.

Marks, Shula, and Neil Andersson

1992   "Industrialization, Rural Health, and the 1944 National Health Services Commission in South Africa." In *The Social Basis of Health and Healing in Africa,* ed. Steven Feierman and John Janzen, 131–161. Berkeley: University of California Press.

Marmot, Michael, and Richard Wilkinson, eds.

1999   *Social Determinants of Health.* Oxford: Oxford University Press.

Marwick, Max, ed.

1987   *Witchcraft and Sorcery: Selected readings.* Harmondsworth: Penguin Books. (1st ed. 1970.)

Mauss, Marcel

1980   "Les techniques du corps." In *Sociologie et anthropologie,* 363–386. Paris: Presses Universitaires de France. (1st ed. 1934.)

Mbembe, Achille

2001   *On the Postcolony.* Berkeley: University of California Press.

2002   "African Modes of Self-Writing." *Public Culture* 14 (1): 239–273.

2003   "Necropolitics." *Public Culture* 15 (1): 11–40.

M'Bokolo, Elikia

1984   "Histoire des maladies, histoire et maladies: L'Afrique." In *Le sens du mal: Anthropologie, histoire et sociologie de la maladie,* ed. Marc Augé and Claudine Herzlich, 155–186. Paris: Editions des Archives Contemporaines.

McCulloch, Jock

1995   *Colonial Psychiatry and "the African Mind."* Cambridge: Cambridge University Press.

Merton, Robert K.

1968   *Social Theory and Social Structure.* New York: Free Press.

Mitchell, J. Clyde

1987   "The Meaning of Misfortune among Urban Africans." In *Witchcraft and Sorcery,* ed. Max Marwick, 381–390. Harmondsworth: Penguin Books. (1st ed. 1965.)

Mignolo, Walter

2000   *Local Histories, Global Designs: Coloniality, Subaltern Knowledges and Border Thinking.* Princeton: Princeton University Press.

Minaar, Anthony

1995   "Violent Conflicts in Mine Hostels: Post 1990." In *Crossing Boundaries: Mine Migrancy in Democratic South Africa,* ed. Jonathan Crush and James Wilmot, 43–55. Cape Town: Idasa.

Molapo, Matsheliso Palesa

1995   "Job Stress, Health and Perceptions of Migrant Mineworkers." In *Crossing Boundaries: Mine Migrancy in Democratic South Africa,* ed. Jonathan Crush and James Wilmot, 88–100. Cape Town: Idasa.

Moodie, Dunbar

2001   "Black Migrant Mine Labourers and the Vicissitudes of Male Desire." In *Changing Men in Southern Africa,* ed. Robert Morrell, 297–315. Pietermaritzburg: University of Natal Press.

Morrell, Robert

2001   "The Times of Change: Men and Masculinity in South Africa." In *Changing Men in Southern Africa,* ed. Robert Morrell, 3–37. Pietermaritzburg: University of Natal Press.

Naepels, Michel

1998   "Une étrange étrangeté: Remarques sur la situation ethnographique." *L'Homme* 148: 185–200.

Nattrass, Nicoli

2004   *The Moral Economy of AIDS in South Africa.* Cambridge: Cambridge University Press.

Nattrass, Nicoli, and Jeremy Seekings

2001   "Democracy and Distribution in Highly Unequal Economies: The Case of South Africa." *Journal of Modern African Studies* 39 (3): 471–498.

Niehaus, Isak

2001   "Witchcraft in the New South Africa: From Colonial Superstition to Postcolonial Reality." In *Magical Interpretations, Material Realities,* ed. Henrietta Moore and Todd Sanders, 184–205. London: Routledge.

Nora, Pierre

1997   "Entre mémoire et histoire: La problématique des lieux." In *Les lieux de mémoire,* vol. 1, 23–43. Paris: Gallimard. (1st ed. 1984.)

Nuttall, Sarah

1998   "Telling 'Free' Stories? Memory and Democracy in South Africa since 1994." In *Negotiating the Past: The Making of Memory in South Africa,* ed. Sarah Nuttall and Carli Coetzee, 75–88. Oxford: Oxford University Press.

Oppenheimer, Gerald
    1988   "In the Eye of the Storm: The Epidemiological Construction of AIDS." In *AIDS: The Burdens of History,* ed. Elisabeth Fee and Daniel Fox, 267–300. Berkeley: University of California Press.

Oppong, Joseph, and Ezekiel Kalipeni
    2004   "Perceptions and Misperceptions of AIDS in Africa." In *HIV and AIDS in Africa: Beyond Epidemiology,* ed. Ezekiel Kalipeni, Susan Craddock, Joseph Oppong, and Jayati Ghosh, 47–57. Malden: Blackwell.

Orubuloye, I. O., John Caldwell, Pat Caldwell, and Gigi Santow
    1994   *Sexual Networking and AIDS in Sub-Saharan Africa: Behavioural Research and the Social Context.* Canberra: Australian National University.

Ory, Pascal, and Jean-François Sirinelli
    1986   *Les intellectuels en France, de l'Affaire Dreyfus à nos jours.* Paris: Armand Colin.

Packard, Randall
    1989   *White Plague, Black Labor: Tuberculosis and the Political Economy of Health and Disease in South Africa.* Berkeley: University of California Press.

Packard, Randall, and Paul Epstein
    1992   "Medical Research on AIDS in Africa: A Historical Perpective." In *AIDS: The Making of a Chronic Disease,* ed. Elisabeth Fee and Daniel Fox, 346–376. Berkeley: University of California Press.

Pandolfo, Stefania
    1997   *Impasse of the Angels: Scenes from a Moroccan Space of Memory.* Chicago: University of Chicago Press.

Parish, Jane
    2001   "The Age of Anxiety." In *The Age of Anxiety: Conspiracy Theory and the Human Sciences,* ed. Jane Parish and Martin Parker, 17–30. Cambridge: Blackwell.

Pels, Peter
    1999   "Professions of Duplexity: A Prehistory of Ethical Codes in Anthropology." *Current Anthropology* 40 (2): 101–36.

Penn-Kekana, Loveday
    2004   "Chronique hospitalière: Les professions de santé à l'épreuve du sida." In *Afflictions: L'Afrique du sud, de l'apartheid au sida,* ed. Didier Fassin, 139–159. Paris: Karthala.

Petryna, Adriana
    2002   *Life Exposed: Biological Citizens after Chernobyl.* Princeton: Princeton University Press.

Pettit, Philip

1996   "Conséquentialisme." In *Dictionnaire d'éthique et de philosophie morale,* ed. Monique Canto-Sperber, 313–320. Paris: Presses Universitaires de France.

Phillips, Harry

1993   "The 1945 Gluckman Report and the Establishment of South Africa's Health Centers." *American Journal of Public Health* 83 (7): 1937–1056.

Pickering, Andrew

1992   "From Science as Knowledge to Science as Practice." In *Science as Practice and Culture,* ed. Andrew Pickering, 1–26. Chicago: University of Chicago Press.

Pollak, Michaël

1992   "Attitudes, Beliefs and Opinions." In *AIDS: A Problem for Sociological Research,* ed. Michaël Pollak, with Genneviève Paicheler and Janine Pierret, 24–35. London: Sage.

Polliak, Claude

2002   "Manières profanes de 'parler de soi.'" *Genèses: Sciences Sociales et Histoire* 47: 4–20.

Popper, Karl

1959   *The Logic of Scientific Discovery.* London: Hutchinson & Co. (1st ed. 1934.)

Portilla, Miguel León

1989   *Visión de los vencidos: Relaciones indígenas de la Conquista.* Mexico, D.F.: Universidad Nacional Autónoma de México. (1st ed. 1958.)

Posel, Deborah

1991   *The Making of Apartheid, 1948–1961: Conflict and Compromise.* Oxford: Oxford University Press.

2001   "What's in a Name? Racial Categorizations under Apartheid and the Afterlife." *Transformation* 47: 50–74.

2002   "The TRC Report: What Kind of History? What Kind of Truth?" In *Commissioning the Truth: Understanding South Africa's Truth and Reconciliation Commission,* ed. Deborah Posel and Graeme Simpson, 147–172. Johannesburg: Witwatersrand University Press.

2004   "Politiques de la vie et politisation de la sexualité: Lectures de la controverse sur le sida." In *Afflictions: L'Afrique du sud, de l'apartheid au sida,* ed. Didier Fassin, 45–73. Paris: Karthala.

Power, Samantha

2003   "The AIDS Rebel." *New Yorker,* 19 May, 54–67.

Rabinow, Paul
    1977   *Reflections on Fieldwork in Morocco.* Berkeley: University of California Press.
    1996   *Making PCR: A Study in Biotechnology.* Chicago: University of Chicago Press.
    1999   *French DNA: Trouble in Purgatory.* Chicago: University of Chicago Press.

Ramphele, Mamphela
    1993   *A Bed Called Home: Life in the Migrant Labour Hostels of Cape Town.* Claremont, South Africa: David Philip.

Rancière, Jacques
    1998   *Aux bords du politique.* Paris: La Fabrique.

Renan, Ernest
    1947   "Qu'est-ce qu'une nation?" In *Œuvres,* vol. 1, 887–906. Paris: Calmann-Lévy.

Reynolds, Pamela
    2000   "The Ground of All Making: State Violence, the Family and Political Activists." In *Violence and Subjectivity,* ed. Veena Das, Arthur Kleinman, Mamphela Ramphele, and Pamela Reynolds, 141–170. Berkeley: University of California Press.

Ricoeur, Paul
    1990   *Soi-même comme un autre.* Paris: Seuil.
    2000   *La mémoire, l'histoire, l'oubli.* Paris: Seuil.

Rosenberg, Charles
    1988   "Diseases and Social Order in America: Perceptions and Expectations." In *AIDS: The Burdens of History,* ed. Elisabeth Fee and Daniel Fox, 12–32. Berkeley: University of California Press.

Rushton, Philippe, and Anthony Bogaert
    1989   "Population Differences in Susceptibility to AIDS: An Evolutionary Analysis." *Social Science and Medicine* 28 (12): 1211–1220.

Said, Edward
    1978   *Orientalism.* London: Routledge & Kegan Paul.

Samarbakhsh-Liberge, Lydia
    2000   "L'African Renaissance en Afrique du sud: De l'utilité ou de l'utilisation de l'histoire." In *Afrocentrismes: L'histoire des Africains entre Egypte et Amérique,* ed. François-Xavier Fauvelle-Aymar, Jean-Pierre Chrétien, and Claude-Hélène Perrot, 381–400. Paris: Karthala.

Saunders, Christopher, and Nicholas Southey
    2001   *A Dictionary of South African History.* 2d ed. Cape Town: David Philip.

Scheper-Hughes, Nancy

    1992   *Death without Weeping: The Violence of Everyday Life in Brazil.* Berkeley: University of California Press.

    1995   "The Primacy of the Ethical: Propositions for a Militant Anthropology." *Current Anthropology* 36 (3): 409–420.

Schneider, Helen

    2002   "On the Fault-Line: The Politics of AIDS Policy in Contemporary South Africa." *African Studies,* special issue "AIDS in Context," 61 (1): 145–167.

    2004   "Le passé dans le présent: Epidémiologie de l'inégalité face au sida et politiques de justice sociale." In *Afflictions: L'Afrique du sud, de l'apartheid au sida,* ed. Didier Fassin, 75–110. Paris: Karthala.

Schneider, Helen, and Didier Fassin

    2002   "Denial and Defiance: A Socio-political Analysis of AIDS in South Africa." *AIDS,* special issue "2002: A Year in Review," 16 (suppl. 4): S45–S51.

Schneider, Helen, and Joanne Stein

    2001   "Implementing AIDS Policy in Post-Apartheid South Africa." *Social Science and Medicine* 52: 723–731.

Schoepf, Brooke Grundfest

    1992   "Women at Risk." In *The Time of AIDS: Social Analysis, Theory and Method,* ed. Gilbert Herdt and Shirley Lindenbaum, 259–286. Newbury Park, Calif.: Sage.

Schutz, Alfred

    1962   *Collected Papers, Vol. 1: The Problem of Social Reality,* ed. Maurice Natanson. The Hague: Martinus Nijhoff.

Sennett, Richard

    1974   *The Fall of Public Man.* New York: Knopf.

Seremetakis, Nadia

    1994   "Intersection: Benjamin, Bloch, Braudel, Beyond." In *The Senses Still: Perception and Memory as Material Culture in Modernity,* ed. Nadia Seremetakis, 19–22. Chicago: University of Chicago Press.

Showalter, Elaine

    1997   *Hystories: Hysterical Epidemics and Modern Culture.* New York: Columbia University Press.

Smith, Adam

    1976   *The Theory of Moral Sentiments.* Oxford: Oxford University Press. (1st ed. 1753.)

Soyinka, Wole

    1999   *The Burden of Memory, the Muse of Forgiveness.* Oxford: Oxford University Press.

Sperber, Dan

1985   "Anthropology and Psychology: Towards an Epidemiology of Representations." *Man* 20: 73–89.

Starn, Orin

1992   "Missing the Revolution: Anthropologists and the War in Peru." In *Re-reading Cultural Anthropology,* ed. George Marcus, 99–112. Durham: Duke University Press.

Stillwaggon, Eileen

2003   "Racial Metaphors: Interpreting Sex and AIDS in Africa." *Development and Change* 34 (5): 809–832.

Stoczkowski, Wiktor

2001   "Rires d'ethnologues." *L'Homme* 160: 91–114.

Strathern, Marilyn

2000   "New Accountabilities: Anthropological Studies in Audit, Ethics and the Academy." In *Audit Cultures,* ed. Marilyn Strathern, 1–18. London: Routledge.

Swanson, Maynard

1977   "The Sanitation Syndrome: Bubonic Plague and Urban Native Policy in the Cape Colony, 1900–1909." *Journal of African History* 18: 387–410.

Thompson, Leonard

1985   *The Political Mythology of Apartheid.* New Haven: Yale University Press.

2000   *A History of South Africa.* New Haven: Yale University Press.

Tilly, Charles

1978   *From Mobilization to Revolution.* Reading, Mass.: Addison-Wesley.

Treichler, Paula

1999   *How to Have Theory in an Epidemic: Cultural Chronicles of AIDS.* Durham: Duke University Press.

Trengrove Jones, Tim

2001   *Who Cares? AIDS Review 2001.* Pretoria: University of Pretoria.

Turner, Victor

1986   "Dewey, Dilthey and Drama: An Essay in the Anthropology of Experience." In *The Anthropology of Experience,* ed. Victor Turner and Edward Bruner, 33–44. Urbana: University of Illinois Press.

Tutu, Desmond

2004   *Amnistier l'apartheid: Travaux de la Commission Vérité et réconciliation.* Ed. Philippe-Joseph Salazar. Paris: Seuil.

Vale, Peter, and Sipho Maseko

2002   "Thabo Mbeki, South Africa and the Idea of an African Renaissance." In *Thabo Mbeki's World: The Politics and Ideology of the*

South African President, ed. Sean Jacobs and Richard Calland, 121–142. Scottsville: University of Natal Press.

Vaughan, Megan

1991   *Curing Their Ills: Colonial Power and African Illness.* Stanford: Stanford University Press.

1992   "Syphilis in Colonial East and Central Africa: The Social Construction of an Epidemic." In *Epidemics and Ideas: Essays on the Historical Perception of Pestilence,* ed. Terence Ranger and Paul Slack, 269–302. Cambridge: Cambridge University Press.

van der Vliet, Virginia

2001   "AIDS: Losing 'The New Struggle'?" *Daedalus,* special issue, "Why South Africa Matters," 130 (1): 151–184.

Vernant, Jean-Pierre

1989   *L'individu, la mort, l'amour: Soi-même et l'autre en Grèce ancienne.* Paris: Gallimard.

Veyne, Paul

1971   *Comment on écrit l'histoire.* Paris: Seuil.

Vidal, Laurent

1996   *Le silence et le sens: Essai d'anthropologie du sida en Afrique.* Paris: Anthropes-Economice.

Walker, Liz, and Leah Gilbert

2002   "HIV/AIDS: South African Women at Risk." *African Journal of AIDS Research* 1 (1): 75–85.

Walzer, Michael

1983   *Spheres of Justice: A Defense of Pluralism and Equality.* New York: Basic Books.

Wax, Murray

2003   "Wartime Dilemmas of an Ethical Anthropology." *Anthropology Today* 19 (3): 23–24.

Weber, Max

1959   *Le savant et le politique.* Paris: Plon. (1st ed. 1919.)

Whiteside, Alan, and Clem Sunter

2000   *AIDS: The Challenge for South Africa.* Cape Town: Human & Rousseau-Tafelberg.

Williams, Brian, Catherine Campbell, et al.

2000   *The Natural History of HIV/AIDS in South Africa: A Biomedical and Social Survey in Carletonville.* Johannesburg: Council for Scientific and Industrial Research.

Wilson, Francis

2001   "Minerals and Migrants: How the Mining Industry Has Shaped South Africa." *Daedalus,* special issue, "Why South Africa Matters," 130 (1): 99–121.

Wittgenstein, Ludwig
  2004   *Recherches philosophiques.* Paris: Gallimard. (1st English ed.
            1953.)
Wojcicki, Janet Maia
  2002   " 'She Drank His Money': Survival, Sex and the Problem of Vio-
            lence in Taverns in Gauteng Province, South Africa." *Medical An-
            thropology Quarterly* 16 (3): 267–293.
Wolpe, Harold
  1995   "Capitalism and Cheap Labour Power in South Africa: From Seg-
            regation to Apartheid." In *Segregation and Apartheid in Twentieth-
            Century South Africa,* ed. William Beinart and Saul Dubow,
            60–90. London: Routledge.
Wood, Kate, and Rachel Jewkes
  2001   "Dangerous Love: Reflections on Violence among Xhosa Town-
            ship Youth." In *Changing Men in Southern Africa,* ed. Robert
            Morrell, 317–340. Pietermaritzburg: University of Natal Press.
Young, Allan
  1995   *The Harmony of Illusions: Inventing Post-traumatic Stress Disorder.*
            Princeton: Princeton University Press.
Zemon Davis, Natalie
  1987   *Fiction in the Archives: Pardon Tales and Their Tellers in Sixteenth-
            Century France.* Stanford: Stanford University Press.
Zempléni, András
  1975   "De la persécution à la culpabilité." In *Prophétisme et thérapeu-
            tique,* ed. Marc Augé, René Bureau, Colette Piault et al., 153–218.
            Paris: Hermann.
Zwi, Anthony, and Antonio Jorge Cabral
  1991   "Identifying 'High Risk Situations' for Preventing AIDS." *British
            Medical Journal* 303: 1527–1529.
Zwi, Anthony, and Deborah Bachmayer
  1990   "HIV and AIDS in South Africa: What Is an Appropriate Public
            Health Response?" *Health Policy and Planning* 5 (4): 316–326.

INDEX

Abdool-Karim, Quarraisha, 108
Abdool-Karim, Salim, 8
Abrahams, Naeema, 198
Abu-Lughod, Lila, 12
Achebe, Chinua, 296n20
Achmat, Zachie, 68, 106, 109, 110, 112, 114,
   115, 265, 269, 284n17, 294n6, 299n48
Ackerman, Anton, 164
Activism, anti-AIDS, 105–7, 109, 111–15,
   173–74, 268–70
Act Up organization, 53, 68
Adler, Gary, 40
Adorno, Theodor W., xii
African National Congress (ANC), 1, 46,
   54, 83, 102, 104, 105, 107, 108, 109, 155,
   159–60, 189, 211, 214, 258, 265, 271,
   286n9, 300nn50,54, 323–25
African Renaissance, xx, 249–54, 258, 259,
   317–18nn22–23, 317n16
African Union, 291n35
Afrocentrism, 251–52
Agamben, Giorgio, 263, 319nn28,31
Agriculture, 128, 137, 138, 186, 193, 218–23
AIDS: apartheid as factor in, xvii, 16, 61,
   62; apartheid compared to, 3–4, 14,
   266; Black Death compared to, 250;

cholera compared to, 33; dissident scientists' views on, 8, 34, 54, 55–62, 70,
81; government ministers' views on,
75–76, 80, 98, 99, 102; iatrogenic factors in, 61, 153, 304n25; malnutrition
as factor in, 15, 31, 56, 58, 61, 78, 116,
304n24; Mbeki's views on, 5–17, xvii,
5–17, 29, 30–31, 34–35, 56–59, 62, 67,
80, 97–104, 116, 121–22, 189; multiple
infections as factor in, 15, 31, 61, 78;
orthodox scientists' views on, 36, 59–
62, 70, 81, 107–8; political aspects of,
xvii–xviii, 4, 34–35, 53–54, 102, 108–9,
268–69, 274–76; poverty as factor in,
xvii, 15, 16, 31, 58, 59, 61, 62, 100, 116,
118, 153, 189, 190, 194; sexual promiscuity as factor in, 147–49, 153–54, 157–
58, 170, 284n20; social factors in, 5, 16,
61, 116, 273, 304n25; viral etiology of,
xvii, 7, 30–31, 34, 54, 56–62, 70, 75–76,
78, 97, 99, 100, 116, 118, 122; witchcraft
as cause of, 93–95. See also HIV entries
AIDS Consortium, 43, 173–74, 282n7
AIDS Foundation, 40
AIDS in Context conference, 10, 109,
   282n7, 284n18

Dubos, René, 304n21
Dubow, Saul, 138
Duesberg, Peter, 8, 34, 55, 56, 60, 77, 100, 285n5, 289n24, 290nn29–30, 293n1
Dufoix, Georgina, 48, 287n13
Du Plessis, Dirk, 42, 43–44
Durban: HIV infection rates in, 2; international AIDS conference in, xvi, 3, 6, 13, 36, 60, 63, 66, 72, 73, 99, 325
Durban Declaration, 36, 121
Durkheim, Emile, xxiii, 203

Economic relations: and Black empowerment, 317n21; and HIV infection rates, 191–92; and New Partnership for Africa's Development (NEPAD), 251, 291n35; and racial inequality, 190–91
Education: and AIDS prevention, 36–37, 59, 116, 134, 157–58, 205; and HIV infection rates, 191
Egypt, 48
Eirmbter, Willy, 208
Elbourne, Elizabeth, 130
Elections, 1, 27, 33, 53–54, 83, 108–9, 180, 271, 286n9, 305n28, 309n57; chronology of, 323–25
Elias, Norbert, 10, 265
Ellis, Mike, 38, 39, 46
Elster, Jon, 118
Employment of HIV-infected persons, 193, 217, 221, 242–45
Employment statistics: and HIV infection rates, 191–92; and racial inequality, 190
Epidemiology, 32–33, 65, 88, 127, 130, 134, 136, 140, 153, 208
Epstein, Helen, 67, 275–76
Epstein, Paul, 25, 149, 304n25
Epstein, Steven, 78, 106–7, 285n5
Erwin, Alexander, 113
Ethics, 16, 42, 47, 87–92, 241, 262–63, 295n15
Ethiopia, 90
Ethnic divisions: colonial imposition of, 302n11; and hospital treatment, 128–29, 145; and violence, 129
Ethnography, xiv, xv, xxi, 21, 93, 124, 150, 179, 190, 192, 195, 201–2, 208, 230, 274, 301n7. *See also* Anthropological research; Social science
European Union, 47, 271–72, 277, 291n35
Evans-Pritchard, Edward, 166, 296n22
Even, Philippe, 48

Fabian, Johannes, xiii, 124
Family relations, xx, 149, 157, 187, 188; and case studies of HIV-infected persons, 193–94, 197–98, 212–14, 216, 220–21, 241–47; and sexual violence, 197–98, 212–14, 216
Farmer, Paul, 16, 25, 100, 200
Feldman, Allen, xii
Felix in Exile (film), 180
Fiala, Christian, 8
Field, David, 238
Folb, Peter, 42, 45, 46
Food and Drug Administration, U.S., 87
Forrest, Drew, 122
Fort Hare University, 122
Foucault, Michel, xxi, 22, 144, 209, 263, 265, 266, 319n31
France, 32, 48, 82, 103, 208, 271, 272, 282n8, 287n13, 292n37, 306n34, 309n2
Freidson, Eliot, 84
Freud, Sigmund, 125, 230, 314n1
Fujimura, Joan, 61
Fuller, Bernard, 129

Gallo, Robert, 7, 285n5
Gandhi, Mahatma, 299n50
Gauteng Province, 2, 104, 168, 218, 304n24
Gayle, Helen, 7
Gazankulu homeland, 128, 129, 145
Gazi, Costa, 53, 108, 282n7
Gellman, Barton, 7
Geneva, international AIDS conference in, 52
Genocide, xiii, xix, 13, 52, 83, 115–16, 231, 252, 265, 278
Geschekter, Charles, 8, 57, 61, 100
Geschiere, Peter, 94
Gevisser, Mark, 285n8
Ghana, 159
Gibb, Diane, 51
Giddens, Anthony, 223–24

Home Affairs department, South African, 64, 66
Homelands under apartheid, 64, 128, 129, 304n22, 313n34
Homosexual transmission of AIDS, 1, 9, 155–56, 157, 208
Horton, Richard, 55
Hospitals: AIDS treatment in, 2, 52, 69, 82; and ethnic divisions, 128–29, 145; and racial divisions, 143, 144
Howe, Stephen, 251
Hrdy, Daniel, 148, 284n20
Hughes, Everett, 176
Human Rights Commission, 104, 108, 113
Hunter, Mark, 199
Huys, Pieter-Dierk, 265

Iatrogenic factors in AIDS, 61, 153, 304n25
Immigration, 158–59. *See also* Migrant workers
Industrialization, 136, 142, 302n10
Inequalities, social and racial, 189–92; as factor in AIDS epidemic, 5, 16, 61, 116, 180; increase in, 28, 92, 116, 118, 268, 277, 278, 316n14; legacy of, 61, 104, 144, 169, 177, 211, 253, 267; reduction of, 91, 102, 107, 269; and violence, 25, 224, 225, 270, 272, 274
Infant mortality, 62, 133, 191
Innes, James Rose, 131
Interferon, 48
Internet, 56, 57, 61, 70, 71, 95–96, 109, 114, 293n1
Interviews with HIV-infected persons, xvii, 17–20, 193–94, 204–8, 210–25, 228–30, 254–57, 259–60, 262
Iraq, 217, 218, 271
Isaacson, Maureen, 162
Ivory Coast, 48, 90, 159

Jacobs, Sean, 33
Jara, Mazibuko, 174
Jeeves, Alan, 137, 185–86
Jewkes, Rachel, 96, 108, 198
Jochelson, Karen, 134, 142, 143
Johannesburg: African Renaissance conference in, 249–54; AIDS conferences in,
10, 173; HIV infection rates in, 2; mortality rates in, 191, 231–32; sexual violence in, 198; stock exchange in, 317n21; wealthiest neighborhood in, 178
Johannesburg General Hospital, 133, 144
Johns Hopkins University, 87, 88
Johnson, Leigh, 191
Johnson, Nkosi, 284n17
Jones, James, 91
Joubert, Elsa, 221, 314n37

Kaiser Foundation, 99
Kalipeni, Ezekiel, 122
Kangwane homeland, 133
Kani, John, 1, 281n4
Kark, Sidney and Emily, 143
Katz, Elaine, 135
Kazatchkine, Michel, 283n11
Kelly, Michael, 238
Kemron (presented as anti-AIDS drug), 48, 49
Kentridge, William, 179–80
Kenya, 48, 90, 119, 235
Khumalo, Nonkosi, 113
Khuzwayo, Zazah, 215, 313n31
Kirstner, Ulrike, 265
Kleinman, Arthur, xvi, 238, 283n15
Köhlnlein, Claus, 70
Koselleck, Reinhardt, 27, 168–69, 301n4
Krog, Antjie, 201
Kuhn, Thomas, 55, 60, 289n24
Kunene, Mazizi, 80
KwaZulu Natal Province, 2, 36, 96, 112, 199, 234, 284n18

Labor: agricultural, 218–23; in mines, 135–37, 181, 185–88
Lahire, Bernard, 178–79
Lamont, Gary, 38, 52
Lancet (medical journal), 7, 55, 142
Landauer, Kallie, 42
Lane, Clifford, 7
Latour, Bruno, 33–34
Lebowa homeland, 128, 129, 145
Leclerc-Madlala, Suzanne, 96
Legal proceedings. *See* Litigation

Sierra Leone, xiii, 311n18
Silverman, David, 22
Simelela, Nono, 103, 109–11, 299n46
Simmons, Leo, 230
Sisulu, Walter, 300n50
Sitas, Ari, 55–56
Slabber, Coan, 156
Smallpox, 130–31
Smart, Rose, 44, 52
Smith, Adam, 4
Smith, Charlene, 195, 196, 312n24
Social science: and biographical narrative, 22–23, 238; and bodily inscription, 175, 177–78; and dissident views on AIDS, 15–17, 76–80; and epidemiology, 32–33; and habitus theory, 178, 179; and hermeneutic interpretation, 124, 179, 226; and Mbeki's views on AIDS, 15–17; objectivity of, xxii, 264; phenomenological approach to, 177, 178, 226; and political activism, xxiii, 112–14; and public health policy, 31–35; and social suffering, 264, 283n15; and witchcraft, 94
Social workers, 129, 198, 221
South African Medical Journal, 64, 142, 232
South African Medical Record, 141
Soweto, 2, 4, 259, 266, 296n19, 324
Soyinka, Wole, 127
Sperber, Dan, 57
Starn, Orin, 273
Statistics. *See* Employment statistics; HIV infection rates; Life expectancy; Mortality rates
Stillwaggon, Eileen, 153
Stoczkowski, Wiktor, 167
Strathern, Marilyn, 16
Subjectivity, 26, 261–62, 263
Suffering, sociology of, 264, 283n15
Survival, meaning of, 260–65
Swanson, Maynard, 129, 131
Syphilis, xviii, 31, 91, 134, 142, 143, 149, 151, 303n19

Talayesva, Don, 230
Tanzania, 90, 288n17
Terrorism, 12, 164, 274–75
Tess, Beatriz, 51

Thailand, 51
Therastim (presented as anti-AIDS drug), 48
Thompson, Leonard, 96, 302n11
Thoreau, Henry David, 299n50
Tickyline, 94, 217–18, 242
Tilly, Charles, 112–13
Time magazine, 30–31, 67
Toms, Ivan, 161
Toxicity of anti-AIDS drugs, 54–55, 58, 69, 72, 82, 83, 118
Trade unions, 3, 106, 173–74, 184, 186
Transkei homeland, 64
Transvaal Medical Journal, 132
Treatment Action Campaign (TAC), 3, 40, 53–54, 66–68, 70, 104–7, 109, 111–15, 173–74, 217, 233, 236, 266, 269, 300nn51–53
Treichler, Paula, 32
Trengrove-Jones, Timothy, 75, 86, 300n52
Trials. *See* Clinical trials; Litigation
Truth and Reconciliation Commission (TRC), 4–5, 28, 126, 127, 161–66, 172, 226, 308nn51–52, 325
Tshabalala-Msimang, Manto, 13, 38, 54, 59, 63, 75–76, 80, 83, 98, 102, 104, 111–12, 292n41
Tuberculosis, xviii, 15, 58, 62, 135–40, 149, 158, 181, 188, 243, 304nn23–24
Turner, Victor, 226
Tuskegee experiment, 90–91
Tutu Desmond, 184, 266

Uganda, 86, 87, 88, 90, 158
Umkhonto weSizwe, 1
UNAIDS, 2, 7, 53, 236
United Nations Population Fund, 149
United States: AIDS cases in, 155; discrimination against immigrants in, 159; Gini index of, 311n18; HIV testing in, 208; invasion of Iraq by, 217, 271
Urbanization, 16, 136, 142, 150, 302n10
USAID, 37, 95
Uys, Pieter-Dirk, 296n16

Vancouver, AIDS conference in, 38
Van Herden, Brood, 166
Van Niekerk, Willie, 157

Text:	Garamond 11.25/13.5
Display:	Garamond
Compositor:	Binghamton Valley Composition
Indexer:	Andrew Joron
Cartographer	Bill Nelson
Printer and Binder:	Thomson-Shore, Inc.